T0234373

Handbook of Old Age Liaison Psychiatry

Handbook of Old Age Liaison Psychiatry

Edited by

George Tadros
Aston University, Birmingham, UK

George Crowther
Leeds and York Partnership NHS Foundation Trust, Leeds, UK

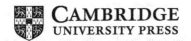

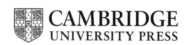

Shaftesbury Road, Cambridge CB2 8EA, United Kingdom

One Liberty Plaza, 20th Floor, New York, NY 10006, USA

477 Williamstown Road, Port Melbourne, VIC 3207, Australia

314–321, 3rd Floor, Plot 3, Splendor Forum, Jasola District Centre,
New Delhi – 110025, India

103 Penang Road, #05-06/07, Visioncrest Commercial, Singapore 238467

Cambridge University Press is part of Cambridge University Press &
Assessment, a department of the University of Cambridge.

We share the University's mission to contribute to society through the
pursuit of education, learning and research at the highest international
levels of excellence.

www.cambridge.org
Information on this title: www.cambridge.org/9781108408516

DOI: 10.1017/9781108292252

© Cambridge University Press & Assessment 2024

First published 2024

A catalogue record for this publication is available from the British Library.

Library of Congress Cataloging-in-Publication Data
Names: Tadros, George, 1962- editor. | Crowther, George, editor.
Title: Handbook of old age liaison psychiatry / edited by George Tadros,
  George Crowther.
Description: Cambridge, United Kingdom ; New York, NY : Cambridge
  University Press, 2023. | Includes bibliographical references and index.
Identifiers: LCCN 2023027441 (print) | LCCN 2023027442 (ebook) |
  ISBN 9781108408516 (paperback) | ISBN 9781108292252 (epub)
Subjects: MESH: Mental Disorders–therapy | Psychosocial Functioning |
  Hospitalization | Aged
Classification: LCC RC480.5 (print) | LCC RC480.5 (ebook) | NLM WT 161
  | DDC 616.89/1–dc23/eng/20230727
LC record available at https://lccn.loc.gov/2023027441
LC ebook record available at https://lccn.loc.gov/2023027442

ISBN 978-1-108-40851-6 Paperback

Contents

Contributors

Khalid Ali, MBBS, FRCP, MD
Senior lecturer in geriatrics at the Brighton
and Sussex Medical School, Brighton

Cate Bailey
Royal London Hospital and East London
Foundation NHS Trust

Ayesha Bangash, MBBS, MRCPsych
Consultant and old age psychiatrist at the
South West Yorkshire Partnership NHS
Foundation Trust

Susan Benbow
Old age psychiatrist, director of Older
Mind Matters Ltd, Manchester, and
professor of mental health at the Centre
for Ageing Studies, University of
Chester

Sarmishtha Bhattacharyya
Consultant psychiatrist at the Wrexham
Maelor Hospital, Betsi Cadwaladr
University Health Board, and professor at
the Centre for Ageing Studies, University of
Chester

Eve Braithwaite
Clinical and digital change leader at the
Leeds Teaching Hospitals NHS Trust

Wendy Burn, CBE
Professor and consultant in old age
psychiatry, Leeds and York Partnership
NHS Foundation Trust

Peter Byrne
Consultant liaison psychiatrist at the Royal
London Hospital and the East London
Foundation NHS Trust

George Crowther
Consultant in old age liaison psychiatry at
the Leeds and York Partnership NHS
Foundation Trust and visiting senior
lecturer at the University of Leeds

Eimear Devlin MBChB BA MRCPsych
ST5 Old Age Psychiatry, Mental Health
Assessment and Liaison Team,
Tees Esk and Wear Valleys NHS
Foundation Trust

Christiana Elisha-Aboh
Consultant Psychiatrist, York Outreach
Recovery Team, Tees, Esk and Wear
Valley NHS Foundation Trust, York

Ravinder Kaur Hayer
Consultant in old age psychiatry,
Midlands Partnership NHS
Foundation Trust

**Josie Jenkinson, MBBS BSc MSc PhD
MRCPsych**
Consultant psychiatrist for older people
at the Surrey and Borders Partnership
NHS Foundation Trust, Psychiatric
Liaison Service Ashford and St Peters

David Jolley, MSc FRCPsych
Honorary reader in old age psychiatry
at Social Care and Society, Manchester

Sally A. Jones
Consultant physician and geriatrician
with specialist interest in Parkinson's
disease, Ysbyty Gwynedd,
Betsi Cadwaladr University
Health Board

**Farooq Khan, MBBS MD MRCPsych
FIPS MSc Med Ed**
Clinical director and consultant
psychiatrist for Birmingham and
Solihull Mental Health NHS Foundation
Trust, senior lecturer at the Centre for
Ageing and Mental Health, University

of Chester, and senior clinical lecturer at
Aston Medical School, Aston University

Mani Santhana Krishnan, FRCPsych
Chair, Faculty of Old Age Psychiatry,
Royal College of Psychiatrists, consultant
in old age psychiatry and liaison
psychiatry, senior clinical director at
MHSOP Trust-wide, and dean and
regional delirium lead for health education
in England

**Atef Michael, MD MSc MSc MB BCh
FRCP**
Medical service head, the Dudley Group
NHS Foundation Trust

Sarah Murphy
Senior strategic safeguarding adult lead at
Tower Hamlets Local Authority, London

**Rashi Negi, MBBSMD FRCPsych MSc.Med
PGCME**
Consultant psychiatrist for older adults,
associate medical director for quality
improvement and MHA, honorary senior
clinical fellow Keele University, specialty lead
CRN DENDRON West Midlands,
and foundation training programme director,
Midlands Partnership Foundation Trust

Sean Ninan
Consultant in geriatric medicine at the
Leeds Teaching Hospitals NHS Trust

Nonyelum Obiechina
Consultant physician and geriatrician in
the Department of Medicine/Geriatrics,
University Hospitals of Derby and Burton
NHS Foundation Trust

**Andrew Papadopoulos, BSc, MSc, PhD,
AFBPsS**
Consultant clinical psychologist at the
Spire Parkway Hospital, Solihull

**Sabeena Pheerunggee, MUDR, MRCGP,
DCH**
Clinical lead for mental health and
learning disabilities at Waltham Forest,
London, and GP for safeguarding adults
at Newham, Tower Hamlets, and
Waltham Forest, London

**Tareq Qassem, MBBCh MSc MD
FRCPsych**
Consultant in old age psychiatry and
lead for the Older Adult Clinical
Academic Group, Maudsley Health,
Al-Amal Hospital, Dubai, UAE

Tony Rao
Consultant psychiatrist in old age at the
South London and Maudsley NHS
Foundation Trust and visiting clinical
fellow at King's College, London

Osama Refaat, MD
Professor of psychiatry in the Faculty of
Medicine, Cairo University

Brenda Roe, PhD, RN, RHV, FRSP
Professor of health research, Faculty of
Health & Social Care, Edge Hill
University, Lancashire

Hugh Series
Consultant old age psychiatrist at the
Oxford Health NHS Foundation Trust
and member of the Faculty of Law at
the University of Oxford

Emad Sidhom
Clinical research associate in the
Department of Clinical Neurosciences,
University of Cambridge,
and in the Windsor Research Unit,
Gnodde Goldman Sachs Translational
Neuroscience, Fulbourn Hospital,
Cambridge

Caroline Sutcliffe, MSc
Research associate at Social Care and
Society, Manchester

**Cathy Symonds, PhD, MRCP,
MRCPsych**
Consultant in old age liaison psychiatry at
the Royal Bolton Hospital,
Greater Manchester

George Tadros
Consultant psychiatrist, professor of
psychiatry and dementia at Aston Medical
School, Aston University, and adjunct
professor of psychiatry at Cairo Medical
School, Cairo University

Rosalind Tandy
GP and mental health clinical lead, West

Suffolk CCG, Clements and Christmas
Maltings Practice, Haverhill

Simon Thaker
Consultant in old age psychiatry,
Derbyshire Healthcare Foundation NHS
Trust, Radbourne

Benjamin R. Underwood
Assistant professor at the University of
Cambridge and honorary consultant old
age psychiatrist, Cambridgeshire and
Peterborough NHS Foundation Trust,
Windsor Research Unit, Gnodde
Goldman Sachs Translational
Neuroscience, Fulbourn
Hospital, Cambridge

Katie Ward
Consultant physician,
Imperial College NHS Trust and
Nightingale Hospital

**Rob Wears, MB ChB MSc FRCP FRCP
(Glasg)**
Consultant geriatrician physician, South
Warwick NHS Foundation Trust

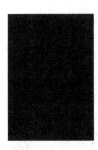

Introduction
Geriatric Medicine and Old Age Psychiatry

Rob Wears

The Evolution of Specialties

Geriatric medicine has been defined as 'a branch of general internal medicine that is concerned with the clinical, preventative, remedial and social aspects of illness in old age. The challenges of frailty, complex comorbidity, different patterns of disease presentation, slower response to treatment and requirements for rehabilitation or social support require special medical skills' (1). Geriatric medicine is one of the largest specialties in the United Kingdom (2). The original pioneers of geriatric medicine in the 1940s demonstrated the value of specialised assessment of older adults and defined the problems most often faced by this group of patients. The 'geriatric giants' of instability, immobility, incontinence, intellectual impairment and memory loss, and impaired independence (3) form the basis of the required specialty's skill.

Old age psychiatry developed as a specialty designed to deliver the specialist knowledge and skills needed to provide effective care for older people with mental illness. It recognises the increased prevalence of dementia in this age group, as well as the prevalence of social, psychological, and medical problems in this population (4).

Liaison psychiatry is a subspecialty of psychiatry that acknowledges the importance of recognising and treating mental illness in a general hospital population. It aims to integrate the assessment and treatment of mental disorders into routine care (5). Improvements in providing for mental health problems, including mental health liaison in acute hospitals and dementia care, were placed among the nine 'must dos' for the NHS in the two-year planning guidance of 2017–19 (6). Almost all UK hospitals have access to a liaison psychiatry service (7). This is also the cornerstone of the National Confidential Enquiry into Patient Outcome and Death's 'Treat as One' report (8).

Within the past thirty years many, but not all, liaison psychiatry teams in the United Kingdom have developed services to specifically assess and treat older people (9, 10). Traditionally in UK psychiatry the age of 65 is used as a cut-off point in determining when a person is 'older'; yet some services are delivered according to patient need, for example frailty. The perceived advantage of mental health services for older people is that they have specialist experience in meeting the care needs of a population that often has complex communication, social, medical, and mental health problems (11).

Geriatric medicine and liaison psychiatry teams vary in size and remit from hospital to hospital, but are generally made up of multidisciplinary professionals who, in addition to the geriatrician or psychiatrist, can include specialist nursing staff, healthcare support workers, psychologists, physiotherapists, and occupational therapists.

1

Both geriatric medicine and old age psychiatry will tend to attract doctors who have an interest in general medical and psychiatric illness, have good communication skills, and work well in teams. Although these specialties retain a strong hospital focus, both recognise the need to provide expert opinion in the community setting and to work effectively across the traditional divide between primary and secondary care. Clinicians working in these specialties will have the skills required to address the challenges of providing safe and effective health care for an ageing population. In recent years there has been an increasing emphasis on the need to supply all possible 'organ specialists' on in-patient specialty wards, as well as acute physicians with sufficient skills in geriatric medicine to care for older adults with predominantly specialty-defining illnesses complicated by frailty, dementia, and complex comorbidities.

Our Aging Population

There is considerable evidence to support the contention that the UK population is ageing. The Office for National Statistics provides detailed figures that clearly show tremendous changes in the UK population over the past century, and notes that changes in lifestyle, health care, and technology have allowed us to live longer on average than we had done previously. English life tables show that, for a male child born in 1901, the expectation of life was just over 48 years. When the NHS was founded in 1948, around 48 per cent of people died before the age of 65. Now that figure is around 12 per cent, as men and women at 65 are expected to live respectively 18 and 20 more years on average. In 1997, around one in every six people (15.9 per cent) were aged 65 years and over; the proportion increased to one in every five people (18.2 per cent) in 2017 and is projected to reach around one in every four people (24 per cent) by 2037. The Office for National Statistics estimates that by mid-2039 the number of people aged 75 and over would rise by 89.3 per cent, to 9.9 million. The number of people aged 85 and over is projected to more than double, namely to reach 3.6 million by mid-2039; and the number of centenarians is projected to rise nearly six times, from 14,000 in mid-2014 to 83,000 in mid-2039. The situation is further complicated by falling fertility rates in the United Kingdom: these rates have declined from 1.87 children per woman in 2007 to 1.79 in 2016. Thus, at the same time as we are living longer, our declining birth rate tips the overall age structure of the United Kingdom further towards the later-life age groups. The UN demographic yearbook defines the United Kingdom as an ageing society since 1930, when those aged over 65 years reached 7 per cent of the total population. By 2041, the 1960s baby boomers will have aged into their 70s and 80s and by 2069 an additional 7.5 million people aged 65 years and over are projected, by comparison with 2019 figures. This would take the United Kingdom's 65+ age group to 19.8 million people, accounting for 26.2 per cent of the projection population, which would define the United Kingdom as having reached 'super-aged' status (12–15).

This demographic change has significantly impacted the case mix of acute hospitals. Medical specialties in the early years of the NHS tended to focus on short-lived illness usually limited to single-organ pathology, and generally in patients of working age. Recent studies have suggested that now 65 per cent of the people admitted to hospital are over 65 years old and that this population accounts for approximately 70 per cent of hospital bed days (16). Hospital-admitted patient care activity for 2017–18 showed that the age group with the highest number of episodes was the 70–74-year group (1.8 million), which accounted for 7.9 per cent of all episodes for that year (17).

It is important to note, however, that the ageing population itself does not cause problems for health and social services. Simply put, the problem is not that we are living longer, but rather that we are not getting healthier. People are living longer with a growing number of long-term chronic conditions such diabetes, heart disease, and dementia. It is estimated that by the age of 75 an older adult living in the United Kingdom will have, on average, two long-term conditions. There is often no cure for such conditions, and managing them is more about care than about cure. In addition to surviving longer with a long-term condition, more people nowadays have multiple long-term conditions. The number of people in England with four or more medical conditions is predicted to double between 2015 and 2035, from 9.8 per cent to 17.6 per cent (18). It should be stressed that not all people with multimorbidity are old. Studies have shown a strong link between socioeconomic status and multimorbidity. Patients from disadvantaged areas were more likely to develop multimorbidity ten to fifteen years earlier than those from more advantaged areas (19).

The Scale of the Problem

In 2012, the Royal College of Physicians produced a report entitled 'Hospitals on the edge? The time for action' (20). In the introduction, the report noted: 'All hospital inpatients deserve to receive safe, high quality, sustainable care centred around their needs and delivered in an appropriate setting be respectful, compassionate, expert health professionals. Yet it is increasingly clear that our hospitals are struggling to cope with the challenge of an ageing population and increasing hospital admissions.' This report was followed by a wide-ranging examination of service provision and training within the health service. This culminated in the General Medical Council producing the Shape of Training review in 2013 (21). The review noted that the needs of patients in the United Kingdom were changing and that doctors would be expected to care for patients with chronic illness and multiple comorbidities. There was a recognised need to achieve 'a better balance between doctors who are trained to provide care across a general specialty area and those prepared to deliver more specialised care'. The consensus view was that doctors needed to be better prepared for working in multiprofessional teams and that the service needed more generalists. Since the 1940s, in the United Kingdom this role of 'expert generalist' in medicine has been filled by geriatricians and general physicians. Along with acute physicians and emergency department consultants, these doctors are defined more by a group of patients than by a system or organ disease. These physicians are now seen as having a crucial role in making the acute hospitals work more effectively.

The burgeoning population of older people in hospitals is not spared of mental disorder; in fact the rate of prevalence of most mental disorders in hospitals is higher than community prevalence figures (for details, see chapter 2, on epidemiology) (5). This is relevant because mental illness and its consequences can complicate a person's hospital journey, causing significant distress for the patients, worry for their carers and families, and anxiety among the hospital staff. Perhaps most importantly, hospital outcomes are often worse for people with mental illness in hospital with longer in-patient stays; increased hospital-acquired infections, increased mortality, and increased dependence on care on discharge are frequently cited consequences of admission (5).

It is the role of the liaison psychiatrist to navigate the patient and the hospital teams through this journey, trying both to reduce the impact of mental disorder on the hospital admission and the impact of the hospital admission on the mental disorder.

Both the geriatrician and the liaison psychiatrist will have a role in signposting on discharge and linking patients with appropriate community services after discharge. In some areas, these clinicians may also be actively involved in the ongoing treatment of these patients in the community.

Frailty and Assessment

In addition to ageing and having multiple medical conditions, we need to recognise the concept of frailty as an entity that has a major role in ill health. Frailty is a distinctive health state related to the ageing process in which multiple body systems gradually lose their in-built reserves. This state results in a loss of function, a loss of physiological reserve, and an increased vulnerability to disease and death. Around 10 per cent of people aged over 65 years have frailty, and in those aged over 85 the proportion raises to something between a quarter and a half. People with multimorbidity may not be frail, and people with frailty may have only a single long-term condition. Multiple instruments have been developed in recent years to try to provide a standardised definition of frailty so as to render it objectively measurable (22). Currently there are two broad models of frailty most commonly used. The first, known as the frailty phenotype, is based on a predefined set of patient characteristics (unintentional weight loss, reduced muscle strength, reduced gait speed, self-reported exhaustion, and sedentary behaviour) that, if present, can predict poorer outcomes (23). This model can be applied at the first contact with the person. Generally individuals with three or more of the characteristics listed here are said to have frailty. The second model is known as the frailty index or the cumulative deficit model and assumes an accumulation of deficits from a long checklist of clinical conditions and diseases (24). The original version of the frailty index had seventy items, but shorter versions with as few as twenty conditions have been described. This system requires a detailed clinical assessment of the patient before it can be completed. The two models should be seen as complementary rather than interchangeable. The frailty phenotype model can be applied at the first contact with the patient whereas the frailty index requires a comprehensive geriatric assessment of the patient and can be used for continuous follow-up.

Whichever model is used, the key feature of frailty is the person's loss of physiological reserve, which results in significant illness and prolonged disability from relatively minor triggers. A common method of depicting this scenario is shown in Figure 0.1.

Frailty syndromes usually present in crisis. Frailty is strongly associated with increased use of health and community services (25). In the acute hospital setting, frailty is associated with high readmission and high mortality rates (26). One of the most important skills of the geriatrician is to be able to recognise the underlying problems hidden behind the presenting 'minor' illness. A key component in the geriatrician's ability to identify underlying problems is comprehensive geriatric assessment (CGA). Comprehensive geriatric assessment can be defined as the process of carrying out a multidimensional assessment of an older person's health and well-being, formulating a planned intervention to address areas of concern both to the older person and to his or her family and carers (where applicable), reviewing the older person's progress, and reconsidering the interventions accordingly. It has been shown that a CGA can reduce hospital admissions and readmissions, and also the impact of frailty on the older adult (27).

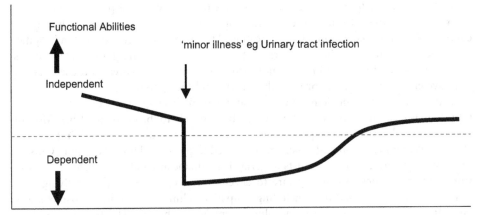

Figure 0.1 The impact of minor triggers on functional ability in frail older people

Comprehensive geriatric assessment also increases the older person's likelihood of survival and of living in his or her own home after an emergency admission to hospital (28). The British Geriatrics Society (BGS) has developed a CGA toolkit for use in primary care (29). Further details can be found in chapter 19.

Embedding comprehensive geriatric assessment in any interaction with a frail older adult is an important strategy; it helps the health service to manage the problems associated with an ageing population. Developing a skilled workforce able to deliver this assessment in the community, in care homes, and in the emergency departments as well as on more traditional geriatric medicine units should be regarded as essential to securing good, patient-centred care in the future.

A similar emphasis should be placed on removing the perceived barriers between physical and mental health services. This is particularly relevant in the management of frail older adults because of the prevalence of significant mental health issues among this population. For example, 29 per cent of older people in hospital will have diagnosable depression (30). It is currently estimated that approximated 850,000 people in the United Kingdom have dementia and that that this figure will rise to 1.6 million by 2040 (31). It is therefore likely that older adults with existing dementia will be admitted to an acute hospital setting even if the dementia is not the primary reason for hospital admission. Forty-two per cent of over 75-year-olds in hospitals are likely to have dementia (32). Once inside the hospital system, the patient with dementia can face a variety of challenges and risk serious adverse outcomes unless the need to provide appropriate care for his or her cognitive issues is recognised as being just as important as the need to provide care for his or her physical illness (33). Sixty-six per cent of patients with dementia admitted to an acute hospital will develop delirium during their hospital stay (34). Even experts can sometimes struggle to differentiate accurately between dementia and delirium, and the two conditions can coexist. Delirium is often poorly recognised and poorly managed in the acute hospital setting. In the United Kingdom, a nationwide audit of forty-five hospitals was carried out in 2018. This audit showed that the regular care team screened only 27 per cent of patients for delirium before the audit assessment.

Among those found to have it, delirium was recognised only in 34.9 per cent (35). Some older patients present to the acute hospital with delirium, others develop it during the course of their hospitalisation. Delirium can lead to increased lengths of stay in hospital, increased mortality, and increased risk of institutional placement (36). Delirium is preventable in up to a third of cases and early attention to the acutely confused patient can have enormous benefits for both the patient and the hospital.

Although geriatric medicine is a hospital-based medical specialty, one of its attractions to many geriatricians is that it is not confined purely to the hospital setting. Most of the acutely ill older patients require skilled rehabilitation and discharge planning, and are at risk of decompensation and disability if exposed to prolonged hospitalisation. Outside the hospital environment, specialists in geriatric medicine and old age psychiatry seek to work with colleagues in primary care to develop services for older people living with frailty in a variety of settings, including outpatient clinics, community hospitals and other intermediate care settings, and older people's own homes. The British Geriatrics Society has published recommendations for the recognition and management of frailty in community and outpatient settings (37) and advice and guidance on the development, commissioning, and management of services for people living with frailty in community settings (38). For many geriatricians and psychiatrists, the requirement to provide good medical care across a range of settings, together with being granted the privilege of seeing the patient in their own home, is a strong incentive to work within the specialties.

All these facts clearly indicate the need for a workforce fit for the future; and consultant geriatricians and old age psychiatrists are a key part of it.

References

1. Mulley, G. *Geriatric Medicine Defined.* London: British Geriatrics Society, 2010.

2. Joint Royal Colleges of Physicians Training Board (JRCPTB). Geriatric medicine, 2014. www.jrcptb.org.uk/specialties/geriatric-medicine.

3. Isaacs, B. *An Introduction to Geriatrics.* London: Balliere, Tindall and Cassell, 1965.

4. Wattis, J. Caring for older people: What an old age psychiatrist does. *BMJ* 1996, 313: 101–4.

5. British Geriatrics Society. Who cares wins, 2021. www.bgs.org.uk/resources/who-cares-wins.

6. NHS Operational Planning and Contracting Guidance 2017–19. www.england.nhs.uk/wp-content/uploads/2016/09/NHS-operational-planning-guidance-201617-201819.pdf.

7. Joint Commissioning Panel for Mental Health. *Guidance for Commissioners of Liaison Mental Health Services to Acute Hospitals*, 2012. https://mentalhealthpartnerships.com/wp-content/uploads/sites/3/jcpmh-liaison-guide.pdf.

8. The National Confidential Enquiry into Patient Outcome and Death. *Mental Health in General Hospitals: Treat as One*, 2017. www.ncepod.org.uk/2017mhgh.html#:~:text=This%20NCEPOD%20report%20highlights%20the,patients%20might%20have%20been%20improved.

9. Barrett, J., Aitken, P.L.W., and Lee, W. *Report of the 3rd Annual Survey of Liaison Psychiatry in England*, 2016. www.hee.nhs.uk/sites/default/files/documents/Report%20of%20the%203rd%20Annual%20Survey%20of%20Liaison%20Psychiatry%20in%20England%20FINAL.pdf.

10. Palmer, L., Hodge, S., Ryley, A., and Bolton, J.W.C. *Psychiatric Liaison Accreditation Network (PLAN) National Report, 2012–2015.* 2016. www.rcpsych.ac.uk/docs/default-source/improving-care/

ccqi/quality-networks/psychiatric-liaison-services-plan/plan-publications-and-links-national-report-2012-15.pdf?sfvrsn=3814f12_2.

11. Crowther, G., Chinnasamy, M., Bradbury, S., Shaw, L., Ormerod, S., Wilkinson, A. et al. (2021). Trends in referrals to liaison psychiatry teams from UK emergency departments for patients over 65. *International Journal of Geriatric Psychiatry*, 36(9): 1415–22. doi: 10.1002/gps.5547.

12. Office for National Statistics. *Overview of the UK population*. 2021. www.ons.gov.uk/peoplepopulationandcommunity/populationandmigration/populationestimates/articles/overviewoftheukpopulation/january2021.

13. Office for National Statistics. *Interim Life Tables*. 2019. www.ons.gov.uk/peoplepopulationandcommunity/birthsdeathsandmarriages/lifeexpectancies/bulletins/interimlifetables/englandandwales20102012.

14. Office for National Statistics. *Release Edition Reference Tables*. 2019. https://webarchive.nationalarchives.gov.uk/20160108060625/http://www.ons.gov.uk/ons/publications/re-reference-tables.html?edition=tcm%3A77-224936.

15. United Nations. *Demographic Yearbook*. New York: United Nations, 2005.

16. Cornwell, J. et al. *Continuity of Care for Older Hospital Patients: A Call for Action*. London: King's Fund, 2012.

17. Hospital Admitted Patient Care and Adult Critical Care Activity, 2017–18. 2019. https://files.digital.nhs.uk/B3/DCC543/hosp-epis-stat-admi-summ-rep-2017-18-rep.pdf.

18. Kingston, A., Robinson, L., Booth, H., Knapp, M., and Jagger, C. Projections of multi-morbidity in the older population in England to 2035: Estimates from the Population Ageing and Care Simulation (PACSim) model. *Age Ageing* 2018, 47: 374–80.

19. Stafford, M. et al. Briefing: Understanding the health care needs of people with multiple health conditions. 2018. www.health.org.uk/sites/default/files/upload/publications/2018/Understanding%20the%20health%20care%20needs%20of%20people%20with%20multiple%20health%20conditions.pdf.

20. Royal College of Physicians. Hospitals on the edge? The time for action. 2015. www.rcplondon.ac.uk/guidelines-policy/hospitals-edge-time-action.

21. General Medical Council. Shape of training review. 2021. www.gmc-uk.org/education/standards-guidance-and-curricula/guidance/shape-of-training-review.

22. Cesari, M., Gambassi, G., Van Kan, G.A., and Vellas, B. The frailty phenotype and the frailty index: Different instruments for different purposes. *Age & Ageing* 2014, 43(1): 10–12.

23. Fried, L.P., Tangen, C.M., Walston, J., et al. Frailty in older adults: Evidence for a phenotype. *J Gerontol A Biol Sci Med Sci* 2001, 56: M146–56.

24. Rockwood, K., Song, X., MacKnight, C., et al. A global clinical measure of fitness and frailty in elderly people. *CMAJ* 2005, 173: 489–95.

25. Rochat, S., Cumming, R.G., Blyth, F., Creasey, H., Handelsman, D., Le Couteur, D.G., Naganathan, V., Sambrook, P.N., Seibel, M.J., andWaite, L. Frailty and use of health and community services by community-dwelling older men: The Concord Health and Ageing in Men Project. *Age & Ageing* 2010, 39(2): 228–33.

26. Conroy, S.P., Stevens, T., Parker, S.G., and Gladman, J.R. A systematic review of comprehensive geriatric assessment to improve outcomes for frail older people being rapidly discharged from acute hospital: 'Interface geriatrics'. *Age & Ageing* 2011, 40(4): 436–43.

27. Stuck, A.E., Siu, A.L., Wieland, G.D., et al. Comprehensive geriatric assessment: A meta-analysis of controlled trials. *Lancet* 1993, 342: 1032.

28. Ellis, G. et al. Comprehensive geriatric assessment for older adults admitted to

hospital: Meta-analysis of randomised controlled trials. *BMJ* 2011, 343: d6553.

29. British Geriatric Society. *Comprehensive Geriatric Medicine Assessment Toolkit for Primary Care Practitioners.* 2021. www .bgs.org.uk/sites/default/files/content/ resources/files/2019-02-08/BGS% 20Toolkit%20-%20FINAL%20FOR% 20WEB_0.pdf.

30. Depression Survey Team at Royal College of Psychiatrists Centre for Quality Improvement. *Survey of Depression Reporting in Older Adults Admitted to Acute Hospitals.* 2021. www.rcpsych.ac .uk/docs/default-source/improving-care/ ccqi/ccqi-research-and-evaluation/capss/ studies/depression-survey-report-older-adults-2018.pdf?sfvrsn=3ed9de11_4.

31. Wittenburg, R., Hu, B., Barraza-Araiza, L., and Rehill, A. Projections of older people with dementia and costs of dementia care in the United Kingdom, 2019–2040. CPEC Working Paper 5, Care Policy and evaluation Centre, London School of Economics and Political Sciences, November 2019.

32. Sampson, E., Blanchard, M., Jones, L., Tookman, A., and King, M. 2009. Dementia in the acute hospital: Prospective cohort study of prevalence and mortality. *British Journal of Psychiatry* 1009, 195(1): 61–6.

33. Leung, D., and Todd, J. Dementia care in the acute district general hospital. *Clinical Medicine* 2010, 10(3): 220–2.

34. Inouye, S. 1999. Predisposing and precipitating factors for delirium in hospitalized older patients. *Dementia and Geriatric Cognitive Disorders* 1999, 10(5): 393–400.

35. Geriatric Medicine Research Collaborative (GeMRC). *Delirium Audit: Round 2: Guidance.* 2019. www .gemresearchuk.com/copy-of-world-delirium-day-guidance.

36. Potter, J. et al. The prevention, diagnosis and management of delirium in older people: Concise guidelines. *Clinical Medicine* 2006, 6(3).

37. British Geriatrics Society. *Fit for Frailty.* 2021. https://www.bgs.org.uk/resources/ resource-series/fit-for-frailty.

38. British Geriatrics Society. Commissioning services for frailty. 2014. https://www.bgs.org.uk/resources/ commissioning-services-for-frailty.

Psychological Well-Being in Later Life

Andrew Papadopoulos

Introduction

Ageing can be considered in three fundamental ways:

First, as a process of physical and cognitive change where such factors as genetics, occupation, lifestyle, environment, diet, mental health, illness, disability, and life events can all have a considerable influence upon how our bodies function and respond to challenges in later life.

Research on biological ageing has identified several factors that influence the aging process. These include: accumulation in the body, over the lifespan, of pathological substances that trigger cell senescence (e.g. atherosclerotic plaques and amyloid proteins); disruption of regulatory pathways (e.g. as a result of frequent inflammatory diseases); mutations in mitochondrial DNA leading to poor energy metabolism; age corruption of the DNA telomeres that affect cell copying processes; and the pre-programmed cessation of stem cell renewal in late life.

Research into cognitive ageing suggests that, while there are wide individual differences in cognitive functioning in later life, people are likely to benefit from established wisdom and pre-existing skills and abilities. However, our speed of information processing, immediate recall, and word-finding ability are all likely to suffer reduced functioning as we age, particularly in those over eighty years of age. Accordingly, people affected with multimorbidities are likely to experience a greater range of adverse life events and outcomes, including lengthy hospital stays, frequent care transfers, poor quality of life, and increased mortality. Physical multimorbidity is strongly correlated with unplanned admission to hospital, particularly when also associated with existing mental health conditions and socioeconomic deprivation (1).

Second, as a time of particular social and material change and transition in our lives, triggered for example by retirement, loss of loved ones, rehousing, and a satisfactory level of available financial and social resources. Thus, while older adults are often more experienced than younger adults in coping with major life events, they also face some of life's hardest challenges, such as chronic illness, disability, and bereavement. These factors, in addition to social context, cohort differences, and idiosyncratic coping styles, have a significant relevance to the presentation of older people in care settings and to working with them therapeutically (2).

Third, from an existential perspective, in terms of whether we experience our lives as being meaningful or meaningless in relation to our values, activities, interests, level of social inclusion, status, and value within the community, and in terms of our view of our lives as having been accomplished. According to Erikson (3), people are faced with a number of psychological tasks throughout their lives, from birth to senescence, that support our personal and social development. These reflect trust, independence, accomplishment, identity, relationship formation and maintenance, contribution to society, and, finally, reflection from the age of 65 years on. This latter task reflects a need to retain one's sense of self-integrity or wholeness by considering one's life as having worth and by being able to accept the regrets in one's life rather than experiencing the sense of despair induced by the thought that one's life has been fruitless, insignificant, or morally deficient.

Within this perspective, how a given society views and responds to its older people plays a major role in the experience of being older and in the meaning we draw from our lives. The lack of meaning and purpose to one's life is a strong predictor of mental health problems, specifically in relation to depression (4), suicidal behaviour (5), and poor recovery from illness in older adults (6).

Drawing upon these perspectives, the term 'successful ageing' has been applied to reflect a field of study that explores predictive processes and mechanisms in late life that promote well-being and an adaptive ability. Rowe and Kahn (7, 8) have developed one of several models of successful ageing and define this as the ability to maintain a low risk of disease and disease-related disability by adopting a healthy lifestyle, high mental and physical functioning, and active engagement in life. Alternatively, Baltes and Baltes (9) suggest that successful ageing reflects our effectiveness at adapting to life's challenges regardless of health status and involves our ability to select and apply what we are good at while compensating for what we are least good at. They call this 'selective optimisation' and 'compensation'. Nevertheless, both the experience of growing older and the factors that influence it in positive and negative ways are complex and multifaceted and show a great deal of variation across individuals. Accordingly, the clinical problems and needs of older people admitted to acute care are often more complex and substantially different from those of younger people. Older people are more likely to experience a combination of multimorbidities as well as general frailty, polypharmacy, financial, social, and mental health problems (10).

In addition to the medical and psychiatric factors that trigger admission to hospital, many problems that affect an older person's well-being and quality of life may have been evident and building in intensity over time. These are often financial, social, or environmental problems, such as social isolation and loneliness, inadequate income or support, caring for other dependent people, struggling to maintain their home, and managing other demands in relation to their interests and activities (11). Accordingly, in assessing and responding to the needs of older people in hospital settings, significant challenges arise for clinicians and other professionals.

Understanding Psychological Well-Being in Older People

The psychology of ageing reflects a complex and often complicated interplay of biological, cognitive, emotional, behavioural, social, cultural, environmental, and economic factors that determine the experience of being older. Hence no single factor can be predictive of well-being and longevity in later life.

In later life, well-being is as much to do with *living a meaningful life* (an existential definition that reflects one's way of being in the world) as it is about *being well* in oneself (a biomedical definition that indicates being free from illness and disability) (12).

In addition, *quality of life* concerns those culturally and personally valued life domains through which well-being is experienced (13).

Accordingly, contemporary research on well-being and quality of life in later life suggests that well-being comprises of a number of principal properties or needs that enable people to experience their lives as contented and meaningful (12). These include:

1. **Integrity of self:** The range of intrapersonal characteristics (cognitive, emotional, and behavioural) that inform and influence the extent to which one can face and overcome major challenges and transgressions to oneself.
2. **Integrity of other:** Being concerned with and contributing to the welfare and quality of life of valued others.
3. **Belonging:** Attachment or connection to one's material, social, or spiritual environments and relationships that engenders commitment, closeness, inclusion, and involvement.
4. **Agency:** Both being able and having the opportunity to exert influence over one's life (and those of others) in accordance with one's personal choices and spiritual beliefs.
5. **Enrichment:** Engagement in activities and conventions that hold personal interest and serve to motivate, stimulate, and enrich one's life and give it moral worth.
6. **Security:** Adequacy of one's physical, mental, financial, spiritual, social, and material resources in securing welfare.

Quality of life domains that support well-being and psychological resilience in later life include: having good social relationships, which foster a sense of positive affirmation, respect, and value; having help and support when needed, both practical and financial; living in a home and in a neighbourhood that are perceived to give pleasure, security, meaning, and access to local facilities and services; engaging in hobbies, interests, and leisure activities; having a social role and maintaining social activities, including by contributing to the lives and well-being of others; having a positive psychological outlook and being able to accept circumstances that cannot be changed; having good health and mobility supported by a Mediterranean diet, exercise, and ongoing education; enjoying financial security and sufficiency to meet basic needs and enjoy life; retaining one's independence and control over one's life (14, 15).

Conversely, *ill-being* can be considered to reflect a life that is experienced as *meaningless* (16), where the following characteristics are salient:

➢ **A difficult life** (experiencing daily struggles with health, frailty, social isolation and loneliness, poverty, pain, and loss of independence);
➢ **A sense of purposelessness** (feeling that life lacks any purpose or meaning or that it is pointless);
➢ **Bitterness** (directed mainly at conditions and circumstances outside the self);
➢ **Negative self** (characterised by low self-worth, low self-confidence, and an abundance of self-criticism);
➢ **Negative world** (characterised by negative attitudes towards society and politics).

Meaninglessness is a strong predictor of mental health problems in later life, particularly depression (4) and suicidal behaviour (5, 17), and is also a predictor of poor recovery from illness (6). Conditions that give rise to the experience of meaninglessness in many older people often involve social exclusion or isolation, poverty, abuse and exploitation, loss of personhood, loss of independence and functionality, persistent and severe pain, multiple transitions, cognitive impairment, and loss of purpose in life (14). This is particularly the case for those who are much older or who experience frailty and age-related decline in physical ability, multiple pathologies, and dementia and where admission to an acute medical ward is often the consequence of a minor stressor or illness that leads to a breakdown in the person's ability to care for him- or herself or to be cared for by others.

The Psychological sequelae of Illness and Acute Admission

The psychological sequelae of illness and acute admission to hospital in older people reflects a complex and dynamic interplay between *illness-specific factors* or *symptoms* and various *idiosyncratic* and *contextual variables* that influence an individual's response to illness and that would affect that individual's well-being, recovery, and readjustment, these are described in Table 1.1.

While illness-specific effects reflect key influences upon a person's presentation and ability to recover, there is a great degree of fluctuation that can be accounted for by *idiosyncratic variables*. These include:

- *Compounding physical and mental health difficulties or frailty, for example drug interactions.*

Around 25 per cent of adverse drug interactions are experienced by older people, particularly those with advanced frailty. Those who experience chronic anxiety, depression, and self-neglect are also likely to have poor immunity, while people who have suffered frequent infections are likely to show chronic fatigue and persistent pain (18).

- *Level of awareness.*

Many older people coming into acute care are, by their very nature, likely to be experiencing limited awareness as a result of distress, delirium, dementia, or other physical health problems that may affect their cognition.

Table 1.1 Illness-specific factors and their causes

Illness-specific conditions	Common causes
acute organic reactions/confusional states/delirium	*toxicity, anoxia, dehydration, shock, psychological trauma*
neuropsychological impairment	*stroke, dementia, cardiovascular insufficiency, respiratory diseases, raised intracranial pressure, space-occupying lesions*
situational anxiety/phobic reactions	*falls, general frailty, abuse/psychological trauma*
depression	*cerebrovascular disease/stroke secondary to long-term disability/treatment regimens, chronic pain after viral diseases, loss/bereavement*
behavioural disturbance	*acute organic reactions, CVA middle cerebral and anterior cerebral artery occlusions, frontal lobe dementias, brain cancer, substance misuse/addiction*

- *Ability to communicate effectively.*

Even in those who remain cognitively able, communication may be an issue by virtue of impaired motor functioning (dysarthria or dyspraxia after stroke, Parkinson's disease, etc.), depression, anxiety, fear, or even inability to speak English.

- *Compliance with treatment regimes.*

A person's ability to comply with treatment regimens, particularly where there are multiple and complex treatments of long duration, is likely to be limited. Compounding factors may also be present, for example motivation to live, existing frailty, responsiveness to treatment, nature and level of support from family and friends, and ability to engage with the treatment process.

- *Severity of handicap imposed.*

The impact that illness or disability has upon a person's life will be reflected in that person's identity, valued activities and lifestyle, and overall quality of life; in addition, it will be reflected in how it impacts upon that person's family and friends. For example, the loss of mobility will affect differently a person who values running and a person whose quality of life is grounded in writing.

- *Coping styles.*

There is now wealth of literature that evidences the significance of coping strategies or coping styles in influencing both a patient's response to illness and a patient's recovery from illness or adaptation to it. However, most patients in acute care settings are likely to face many challenges, which may require very different coping styles across a range of different domains – physical, functional, social, financial, and environmental.

Adapting to Hospitalisation, Illness, and Disability

Weiten et al. (19) have identified four main types of adaptive coping strategies that may be used generically across different illness scenarios.

Appraisal-Focused Strategies

These involve modifying the ways in which we may think or make sense of an experience. Often termed 'reframing', appraisal focused strategies often involve *challenging* people's views, beliefs, or understanding of their difficulties, orienting them towards a more positive attitude via education, demystifying beliefs, testing reality, or providing positive case examples. Such methods are a core component of cognitive behavioural therapy.

For example, a patient may believe that having a diagnosis of cancer means that one will inevitably die of it, thus developing anxiety or a sense of hopelessness and despair. Providing relevant information and education about treatment options and outcomes, lifestyle changes, and access to patients who have themselves recovered from cancer can all help to change the patient's negative appraisal of his or her illness and prognosis. Sometimes humour can be a very powerful way of reframing a situation or an experience. Psychologically, humour has the function of converting what could be viewed as violating or abhorrent events into benign or normalised events, thus rendering them more acceptable and providing an opportunity for sharing values (20).

Solution-Focused Strategies

Whereas appraisal-focused approaches aim to change the way a person makes sense of or thinks about his or her difficulties, solution- or problem-focused strategies are aimed at dealing directly with the triggers – the conditions that give rise to, or appear to be maintaining, the person's difficulties. Paradoxically, what people may identify as the problem can in fact be the *solution* to it. This idea is a central component of systemic or family therapy. For example, a patient may be frightened at the prospect of being discharged back home, even though he or she is medically fit. The reason may be fear of abuse perpetrated by the patient's spouse. However, for various reasons, the patient is reluctant to report this fear. Instead, the patient may locate the problem with going home in lack of confidence about being able to use his or her new assisted bath. In spite of various attempts by the occupational therapist to help the patient build reasonable ability and confidence to use the bath during home visits, the patient still maintains that he or she lack sufficient confidence to return home. Here the *problem* is that, by returning home, the patient is likely to experience abuse. Once abuse is recognised and thus identified as the problem, discharge planning can be more accurately and meaningfully developed with the patient.

Having identified the problem, a range of relevant and meaningful solutions are generated, then evaluated – either directly (in vivo) or by thinking it through (simulation) – on the basis of how effective, safe, and practical they are likely to be. The best solution is then accordingly attempted, ensuring that it is adequately resourced and supported; this will give it the best chance of success. The process may involve a degree of skill learning, accessing aids and adaptations, gaining the support of others, and so on (21). Taking control and being proactive is central to a problem-solving approach, and may also entail strategies that assist in anticipating and preventing future difficulties.

Emotion-Focused Strategies

Experiencing any range of emotions in the face of adverse conditions is a natural and essential aspect of being human. Emotions serve to communicate our status and needs to others, help us to express pent-up tension, grief, or anger, and can be important drivers to our becoming able to make necessary changes to our circumstances. However, emotions can also become overwhelming, disabling, and at times destructive. Some psychotherapists would argue that reactive depression involves the internalisation of anger (22).

In responding to and managing emotions, a number of non-destructive strategies or interventions can be helpful in addition to appraisal and problem-focussed strategies. These include *expressing emotions* (talking or confronting, crying, writing, sculpting, drawing, acting, playing music, running, etc.), *distraction* (reading, counting backwards, cooking, exercising, playing a computer game, cleaning, etc.), *distancing oneself* (non-engagement with the source or trigger of the emotion), *resolution* (conflict, hostility, guilt, blame, distance, hurt, abuse may require professional counselling, psychotherapy, or support), and *managing one's feelings* (relaxation, mindfulness exercises or meditation, physical exercise, compassionate acceptance, seeking comfort and affection from others; gaining sufficient sleep and having appropriate nutrition are also essential). On occasion, emotional distress may require professional help and support from practitioners such as mental health nurses, the liaison psychiatry team, clinical and counselling psychologists, counsellors, and psychotherapists.

Occupation- or Activity-Focused Strategies

Occupation-focused strategies embrace a range of psychological components and processes that aim to address the impact of a person's illness or disability upon their functionality and physical and psychological well-being. Often directed by occupational therapists, the underlying philosophy that underpins the importance and benefit of occupation is the MOHOST (Model of Human Occupation Screening Tool) (23). The MOHOST assesses patients' motivation for activity, their occupational patterns, their communication and relational style, their motor skills, and the environment as reflecting the degree of congruency or fit between their functioning, their needs, and the environmental capability to support these needs. Strategies may involve discrete activities such as preparing a meal as well as more programmed approaches to assisting mobility, self-esteem, relational competence, activities of daily living, self-expression, cultural meaning, and so on (24).

While adaptive coping strategies are associated with recovery and improved quality of life, *negative* coping strategies are more likely to maintain, or even cause further disruption to, a person's existing status or situation. They often occur because of a number of reasons such as observing others – for instance parents, friends, or relatives who may have used similar methods at some point in their lives; paired association learning, where an action has led to a short-term benefit, then has become the norm; self-blame, self-hatred, or self-reproach; suppressed anger towards others or towards their illness or the impact it has had on one's life; pessimistic outlook or loss of hope that things could get better; other mental health issues (depression, psychosis, paraphrenia, dementia).

Examples of negative strategies are (25):

Overcompensation

- *Aggression/hostility*: Person counterattacks by defying, abusing, blaming, attacking, or criticizing others.
- *Dominance/excessive self-assertion*: Person controls others through direct means of accomplishing goals.
- *Recognition-seeking/status-seeking*: Person overcompensates by impressing, through high achievement, status, attention-seeking, and so on.
- *Manipulation/exploitation*: Person meets own needs through covert manipulation, seduction, dishonesty, or conning.
- *Passive-aggressiveness/rebellion*: Person appears overtly compliant while punishing others or rebelling covertly through procrastination, pouting, 'backstabbing', lateness, complaining, rebellion, non-performance, and so on.
- *Excessive orderliness/obsessionality*: Person maintains strict order, tight self-control, or high level of predictability through order and planning, excessive adherence to routine or ritual, or undue caution. They may devote inordinate amounts of time to finding the best way to accomplish tasks or avoid negative outcomes.

Surrender

- *Compliance/dependence*: Person relies on others, gives in, seeks affiliation, is passive, dependent, submissive, or clinging, avoids conflict, is people-pleasing.

Avoidance

- *Social withdrawal/excessive autonomy*: Person copes through social isolation, disconnection, and withdrawal. They may demonstrate an exaggerated focus on independence and self-reliance rather than involvement with others. Sometimes they may retreat through private activities such as excessive television watching, reading, recreational computing, or solitary work.
- *Compulsive stimulation-seeking*: Person seeks excitement or distraction through compulsive socialising, shopping, sex, gambling, risk-taking, physical activity, drug use, and so on.
- *Addictive self-soothing*: Person avoids discomfort through addictions involving the body, such as to alcohol, drugs, overeating, excessive masturbation, self-cutting, and so on.
- *Psychological withdrawal*: Person copes through dissociation, numbness, denial, fantasy, or other internal forms of psychological escape.

Well-Being in Relation to Culture, Faith, and Ethnicity

People from ethnic minority groups, particularly Pakistani, Bangladeshi, and Black African Caribbean people, tend consistently to report the poorest health, older people showing the greatest diversity in inequality across age groups (26).

But the relationship between ethnicity and well-being is complex in terms of the range of factors associated with the latter and the way in which they interact to affect health. Factors that have been identified across ethnic groups as having a significant influence on both physical and mental health and well-being include:

Socioeconomic Status

There is a wealth of literature on older people that clearly shows consistently poor socioeconomic status among Black minority ethnic groups in Britain (27). In older people, low socioeconomic status appears to have both a direct effect on well-being, via lower functional ability, depression, and disorders related to inadequate nutrition, and a secondary effect, through poor living conditions and social isolation.

Racial Discrimination

Burke (28) argues that racism maintains social and economic deprivation, limited access to care, and subordination to and social control by the majority culture. Littlewood and Lipsedge (29) go on to suggest that dominant cultures actively alienate people who do not belong to them. Such cultures lack an adequate frame of reference for understanding the experience, opinions, values, and needs of individuals from other cultures and hence are more likely to marginalise and socially exclude such individuals.

Social Support

Social support has been shown to have an important role in reducing the risk of depression after loss and in facilitating recovery from physical illness and disability

(30). There is also evidence to suggest that the nature and level of social support vary across ethnic minority groups (31, 32) and that, in addition, such variation accounts in part for differences in the levels of subjective well-being and suicide rates among ethnic minority groups (17).

Faith

Set in the context of spirituality and ageing, there exists a wide body of research identifying the role and importance of spirituality as a mediator of well-being in older people (33–35). Here spirituality is considered both as reflecting one's faith in a higher transcendent and as reflecting the ultimate meaning in life that derives from a person's sense of self-worth and relationship with others (36, 37).

Well-Being and the Hospital Environment

Over recent years there has been a growing body of research that has explored environmental effects upon recovery and prognosis. This has been influenced in part by a growing emphasis on patient perspective and engagement – as the experience of patients and their families is a key factor in service design and strategic planning – and in part by academic research, which has identified key aspects of care environments that can facilitate recovery and reduce the cost of inpatient care.

For the majority of older people, research suggests that the experience of hospital care, particularly acute care, reflects mainly high levels of satisfaction. Where negative experiences are reported, they tend to relate to staff attitudes, behaviour, and poor communication (38). Key themes include occurrences that involve deterioration in health or perceived poor care; unmet and unexplored expectations; difficult relationships with staff that pertain to poor communication and conflict over care. Older patients in the hospital may feel worthless, fearful, or not in control of what happens, especially if they have impaired cognition or communication difficulties.

Jurgens et al. (39) propose 'a cycle of discontent' in which events or crises are associated with expectations unmet by patients or their carers. When this cycle occurs, people become uncertain or suspicious, which leads to a period of 'hyper vigilant monitoring' in which people will seek out evidence of poor care, culminating in challenge, conflict with staff, or withdrawal. This scenario can itself become a crisis.

Concerning specifically the experience of hospital care by people living with dementia, a review of the literature suggests that there are mainly negative consequences and outcomes associated with these people's admission to general hospitals (40). Such consequences and outcomes relate to factors such as the hospital's physical environment – which can present significant challenges in terms of spatial location, lack of privacy, lack of familiarity and normative cues; co-morbidity in relation to both physical and mental health conditions; the type of interventions required; enduring multiple treatments; poor detection and diagnosis of illnesses and chronic pain; the failure of care staff to interpret behavioural communication and presentation as an expression of unmet need, distress, pain, or fear; and a culture of care that devalues people or that emphasises task focus and not person centeredness. All these factors increase the risk of long hospital stay, poor quality of life, falls, dehydration and malnutrition, functional decline, and death.

Developing a Positive Culture of Care

According to Bridges et al. (41), what these findings highlight is the importance of including the perspectives of older people themselves and their relatives in the planning and delivery of care in medical settings. They also lend support to the notion of creating a culture of care that is both personalised and relationship-centered. Factors reflecting such a culture of care would normally have the following components:

First, *a value base* informed from a person-centred perspective (42) that

- asserts the absolute value of all people, regardless of age, gender, ethnicity, physical or cognitive disability and places the individuals and their social relationships at the centre of services and interventions;
- recognises that people have a right to a dignified and meaningful life defined by themselves, regardless of illness or disability;
- recognises the unique nature of individuals, reflected in their identity, ethnicity, preferences, personal narratives, and life story.

Second, an individualised approach to assessment, treatment, and personalised care that

- ➤ is informed by an understanding of the perspective and experience of each individual, their story, and their lifestyle;
- ➤ focuses upon empowering the patient, their family members, and their friends, to have influence over their care and quality of life on the ward;
- ➤ creates personalised care plans that are co-produced and frequently monitored by both patients and their relatives;
- ➤ enables and supports positive and trusting relationships with care staff and other professionals;
- ➤ provides a well-managed treatment regime that considers and responds to the impact of the treatment upon the ability of the patient to tolerate and comply with it;
- ➤ minimises the need for excessive care transitions;
- ➤ seeks to maximise the patient's strengths and abilities regardless of the stage of their illness, or their capabilities;
- ➤ protects vulnerable patients from abuse and exploitation;
- ➤ enables and supports patients to take managed and normative risks (risk enablement);
- ➤ offers expertise, activities, and resources in partnership with patients and their families to achieve their goals and aspirations;
- ➤ works towards breaking down the barriers to discharge and re-homing;
- ➤ emphasises, considers, and addresses a range of factors that have an impact on a patient's well-being and personhood, including physical and mental health needs, functional ability, history, self-esteem and self-confidence, living environment, education and employment where relevant, and family and social relationships (43–45).

As applied specifically to professional person-centred practice, these principles can be usefully articulated under the acronym *CAREING*.

- C= *care* (with warmth, empathy, compassion, curiosity, and respect: care for and with patients, their families, one's colleagues, and the local community, thereby engendering a sense of value, belonging, containment, and continuity throughout).
- A= *accept* (people for who they are, and that they have the right to take risks; embrace risk as a necessary and meaningful condition of living; enable people to experience

meaningful and appropriate levels of risk regardless of illness, disability, or capacity: this is *risk enablement*).

- R= *restore* (and maintain self-esteem, self-confidence, personhood, and optimal functioning through the experience of valuing, affirming, supportive, and non-stigmatising relationships).

- E= *empower* (patients to remain in control of their lives and to make meaningful and relevant choices regardless of illness, disability, or capacity).

- I= *include* (patients and their families in decision-making, planning, and provision at all levels; ensure that their perspectives, opinions, and choices are embedded in everything we do).

- N= *nurture* (engagement in activities that provide a sense of meaning, purpose, and enrichment to life).

- G= *get to know* (patients from their perspectives, their culture, their life histories, and from those who know them well; renew your understanding of them each and every day, and through each and every challenge they face).

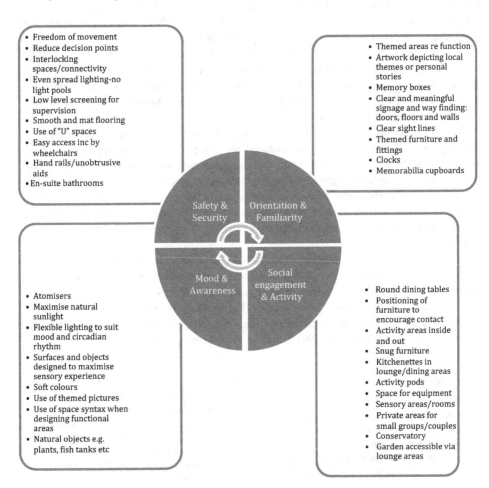

Figure 1.1 Environmental factors promoting recovery and quality of life on in-patient wards

Third, the provision of a *ward environment* that enables patients, their families, and their friends to feel safe and to have sufficient privacy and that offers sufficient opportunities for normative activities and experiences (46).

While there is now a wealth of research that identifies those models of care, interventions, services and ways of engaging vulnerable people, particularly those experiencing dementia, that make a positive difference to their lives and those of their families (47, 48), the physical environment has a large part to play in the well-being of those people and in the experience of their care (49). Environmental design characteristics that are known to play a crucial role in facilitating positive well-being and experience can be summarised in Figure 1.1.

Conclusions

Well-being in later life reflects two principal themes: first, that of *being well* in relation to illness and disability and, second, that of *being well* in relation to a *way of being* where life is considered to have meaning, purpose, agency, a sense of belonging, sufficient resources to meet one's needs (material, social, and financial), the resilience, personal integrity, and self-confidence for people to respond positively to its challenges, and the knowledge that those who we love are happy and healthy.

As we age, difficulties encountered in any of these areas can give rise to significant mental and physical health problems that may require hospitalisation. Both the difficulties a person may be experiencing before admission and those experienced within the hospital environment can further compound that person's health status and lead to poor recovery and, possibly, high dependency.

Factors predictive of a good recovery within hospital settings include positive relationships with family, friends, and hospital staff, a person-centred approach to care planning and delivery, meaningful and culturally relevant ward-based activities, regular monitoring of treatment regimens, a pro-recovery-designed hospital environment, continuity of care in the person's natural environment after discharge, and a staff team whose members are themselves physically and mentally well, are well supported and resourced, receive regular supervision and training, and are suitably protected from adverse ward conditions.

Understanding and responding to the needs and experiences of older people in acute hospital settings should never reflect an 'us and them' paradigm but should be driven by an 'us and us' paradigm. In this context, care provision is about delivering robust, evidence-based interventions, combined with empathic awareness, a commitment to working in partnership with patients and their families, and ring-fencing time for self-reflection. It's about being and caring *with*, not just caring *for*.

References

1. Payne, R.A., Abel, G.A., Guthrie, B., and Mercer, S.W. The effect of physical multimorbidity, mental health conditions and socioeconomic deprivation on unplanned admissions to hospital: a retrospective cohort study. *CMAJ* 2013, 185(5): 221–8.

2. Knight, B.G., and Lee, L.O. Contextual adult lifespan theory for adapting psychotherapy. In Laidlaw, K., and Knight, B. (eds), *Handbook of Emotional Disorders in Later Life: Assessment and Treatment*. Oxford: Oxford University Press, 2008, pp. 59–88.

3. Erickson, E.H. *Identity and the Life Cycle.* New York: Norton, 1980.

4. Harlow, L.L., Newcomb, M.D., and Bentler, P.M. Depression, self-derogation, substance use, and suicide ideation: lack of purpose in life as a mediational factor. *Journal of Clinical Psychology* 1986, 42(1): 5–21.

5. Stillion, J.M., and McDowell, E.E. *Suicide across the Lifespan.* Bristol: Taylor Francis, 1996.

6. King, K.B., Porter, L.A., Norsen, L.H., and Reis, H.T. Patient perceptions of quality of life after coronary heart surgery: Was it worth it? *Research in Nursing and Health* 1992, 15(5): 327–34.

7. Rowe, J.W., and Kahn, R.L. Human aging: Usual and successful. *Science* 1987, 237: 143–9.

8. Rowe, J.W., and Kahn, R.L. Successful aging. *Gerontologist* 1997, 37: 433–40.

9. Baltes, P.B., and Baltes, M.M. *Successful Aging: Perspectives from the Behavioral Sciences.* Cambridge: Cambridge University Press, 1993.

10. Summary report: The state of ageing in 2020. Centre for Ageing Better, 19n November 2020. https://ageing-better.org.uk/publications/state-of-ageing-2020.

11. Living well in older years. National Mental Health Intelligence Network, Gov. UK. www.gov.uk/government/publications/better-mental-health-jsna-toolkit/7-living-well-in-older-years.

12. Papadopoulos, A., Biggs, S., and Tinker, A. Well-being in later life: A proposed eco-systemic framework. *British Journal of Well-Being* 2011, 2(6): 22–31.

13. Bond, J., and Corner, L. The future of well-being: Quality of life of older people in the twenty-first century. In Vincent, J.A., Phillipson, C.R., and Downs, M. (eds), *The Futures of Old Age.* London: Sage, 2006, pp. 147–53.

14. Gabriel, Z., and Bowling, A. Quality of life in old age from the perspectives of older people. In Walker, A., and Hennessy, C.A. (eds), *Growing Older: Quality of Life in Old Age.* Maidenhead: Open University Press, 2004, pp. 14–34.

15. Green, M., Iparraguirre, J., Davidson, S., Rossall, P., and Zaidi, A. Index of wellbeing in later life. Age UK, 2017. www.ageuk.org.uk/our-impact/policy-research/wellbeing-research/index-of-wellbeing.

16. Dittman-Kohli, F.D., and Westerhof, G.J. The SELE Sentence Completion Questionnaire: A new instrument for the assessment of personal meaning in research on aging. *Anuario de Psicologia* 1997, 73: 7–18.

17. Baker, F.M. Suicide among ethnic elders. In Kennedy, G.J. (ed.), *Suicide and Depression in Late Life: Critical Issues in Treatment, Research, and Public Policy.* New York: John Wiley & Sons, 1996, pp. 51–79.

18. Berko, P. Make do and mend: An evaluation of an intervention for pain management within limited resources. *Clinical Psychology Forum* 2017, 296: 28–33

19. Weiten, W., Dunn, D.S., and Hammer, E.Y. *Psychology Applied to Modern Life: Adjustment in the 21st Century* (11th ed.). Belmont, CA: Wadsworth Publishing, 2014.

20. McGraw, A.P., and Warren, C. Benign violation theory. In Attardo, S. (ed.), *Encyclopedia of Humor Studies*, vol. 1. Thousand Oaks, CA: Sage, 2014, pp. 75–7.

21. Papadopoulos, A., and La Fontaine, J.H. *Elder Abuse: Therapeutic Perspectives in Practise.* Chipping Norton: Winslow Press, 2000.

22. Sahu, S., Gupta, P., and Chatterjee, B. Depression is more than just sadness: A case of excessive anger and its management in depression. *Indian J Psychol Med.* 2014, 36(1): 77–9.

23 Parkinson, S., Chester, A., Cratchley, S., and Rowbottom, J. Application of the Model of Human Occupation Screening Tool (MOHOST Assessment) in an acute psychiatric setting. *Occup Ther Health Care* 2009; 22(2–3): 63–75.

24. Clarke, C., Stack, C., and Martin, M. Lack of meaningful activity on acute physical hospital wards: Older people's experiences. *British Journal of Occupational Therapy* 2017, 81(1): 15–23.

25. Young, J.E., Klosko, J.S., and Weishaar, M.E. *Schema Therapy: A Practitioner's Guide*. New York: Guilford Press, 2003.

26. Ethnicity and health. POSTnote 276. British Parliamentary Office of Science and Technology, 2007. https:// researchbriefings.files.parliament.uk/ documents/POST-PN-276/POST-PN-276 .pdf.

27. Nazroo, J., Bajekal, M., Blane, D., and Grewal, I. Ethnic inequalities. In:Walker, A., and Hennessy, C.H. (eds), *Growing Older: Quality of Life in Old Age*. Maidenhead: Open University Press, 2004, pp. 35–59.

28. Burke, A. Racism, prejudice and mental illness. In Cox, J. (ed.), *Transcultural Psychiatry*. London: Croom Helm, 1986, 139–57.

29. Littlewood, R., and Lipsedge, M. *Aliens and Alienists: Ethnic Minorities and Psychiatry* (3rd ed.). London: Unwin Hyman, 1997.

30. Drew, L.M., and Silverstein, M. Intergenerational role investments of great grandparents: Consequences for psychological wellbeing. *Ageing and Society* 2004, 24(1): 95–111.

31. Butt, J., and Moriarty, J. Social support and ethnicity in old age. In Walker, A., and Hennessy, C.H. (eds), *Growing Older: Quality of life in Old Age*. Maidenhead: Open University Press, 2004, pp. 167–88.

32. Katz, R. Intergenerational family relations and subjective well-being in old age: A cross-national study. *European Journal of Ageing* 2009, 6(2): 79–90.

33. Kraus, N. Religious meaning and subjective wellbeing in late life. *Journal of Gerontology, Social Sciences, 58B* 2003, 3: 160–70.

34. Kirby, S.E., Coleman, P.G., and Daley, D. Spirituality and well-being in frail and non-frail older adults. *Journal of Gerontology, Series B: Psychological Sciences and Social Sciences* 2004, 59(3): 123–9.

35. Keyes, C.L., and Reitzez, D.C. The role of religious identity in the mental health of older working and retired adults. *Aging and Mental Health* 2007, 11(4): 434–43.

36. MacKinlay, E. *The Spiritual Dimension of Ageing*. London: Jessica Kingsley Publishers Ltd, 2001.

37. Marcoen, A. Spirituality and personal well-being in old age. *Ageing and Society* 1987, 14: 537–73.

38. Day, J., and Higgins, I. Existential absence: The lived experience of family members during their older loved one's delirium. *Qual Health Res* 2015, 25(12): 1700–18.

39. Jurgens, F.J., Clissett, P., Gladman, J.R.F., and Harwood, R.H. Why are family carers of people with dementia dissatisfied with general hospital care? A qualitative study. *BMC Geriatrics* 2012, 12(57): 1–10.

40. Dewing, J., and Dijk, S. What is the current state of care for older people with dementia in general hospitals? A literature review. *Dementia* 2016, 15(1): 106–24.

41. Bridges, J., Flatley, M., and Meyer, J. Older people's and relatives' experiences in acute care settings: Systematic review and synthesis of qualitative studies. *International Journal of Nursing Studies* 2010, 47(1): 89–107.

42. Kitwood, T. *Dementia Reconsidered: The Person Comes First*. Buckingham: Open University Press, 2010.

43. Majeed, N., and Williams, E. Improving mental and physical health care for older adults: An inpatient service development project by frontline staff. *FPOP Bulletin* 2016, 133: 72–77.

44. Baillie, L., Gallini, A., Corser, R., Elworthy, G., Scotcher, A., and Barrand, A. Care transitions for frail, older people from acute hospital wards within an integrated healthcare system in England: A qualitative case study. *International*

Journal of Integrated Care 2014, 14(1). DOI: http://doi.org/10.5334/ijic.1175.

45. Brooker, D., and Latham, I. *Person Centred Dementia Care: Making Services Better with the VIPS Framework* (2nd ed.). London: Jessica Kingsley, 2016.

46. Røsvik, J., and Rokstad, A.M.M. What are the needs of people with dementia in acute hospital settings, and what interventions are made to meet these needs? A systematic integrative review of the literature. *BMC Health Services Research* 2020, 20(1), 723. doi: 10.1186/s12913-020-05618-3.

47. Fossey, J., and James, I. (eds). *Evidence-Based Approaches for Improving Dementia Care in Care Homes*. London: Alzheimer Society, 2007.

48. Carpenter, C., Banerjee, J., and Conroy, S. Silver book II: Quality care for older people with urgent care needs. British Geriatrics Society, 2021. www.bgs.org.uk/resources/resource-series/silver-book-ii.

49. Waller, S., Masterson, A., and Finn, H. Improving the patient experience: Developing supportive design for people with dementia: The King's Fund's enhancing the healing environment programme, 2009–12. The King's Fund, London, 2013. www.kingsfund.org.uk/sites/default/files/field/field_publication_file/developing-supportive-design-for-people-with-dementia-kingsfund-jan13_0.pdf.

The Epidemiology of Mental Illness in Older People in Acute Hospitals

A Growing Challenge for the Liaison Psychiatrist

Christiana Elisha-Aboh and George Crowther

Introduction and Background

Epidemiology is the study of how regularly diseases occur in different groups of people and why. As the backbone of public health, the information gathered from this process is used to plan and evaluate strategies tested to prevent illness. It also guides the management and rational planning of resources for patients in whom disease has already developed (1, 2). Older people in psychiatry in the United Kingdom are traditionally described as persons of 65 years or above that age, although, as biologically people age at different rates, it is sometimes argued that the cut-off should be based on needs, frailty, comorbid conditions, and presentation (3). It is important that ageing be seen as a normal biological and social process rather than as a problematic disease process to which a figurative cut-off point can be applied.

The cost of mental disorders in older people is considerable and far-reaching, the impacts being borne by the patients, their families, and the wider society, including the taxpayer. It is estimated that the social and economic impacts of mental health disorders cost the United Kingdom economy £70 to £100 billion each year, or 4.5 per cent of GDP (4, 5), and that older people take up approximately 40 per cent of healthcare resources in England and Wales (6). An estimated 13.5 billion pounds per annum in extra financial costs is borne by physical health trusts for people with comorbid physical and mental health illnesses, including medically unexplained symptoms (7). Mental health services are frequently underfunded and understaffed, despite the government's attempts to close the gap between physical and mental illness. Unsurprisingly, patients with dual pathologies end up with more adverse outcomes (8). Projections suggest that an additional investment of up to £1 billion per year would be necessary to plug the gaps in mental health service provision, while more proactive steps are taken towards preventive strategies and early interventions (5).

Generally the presence of mental illness predicts worse physical healthcare outcomes.

- Having a long-term physical illness is associated with a higher rate of complications if superimposed mental health problems arise, raising the cost of care by an average of 45 per cent (5).
- People with severe mental health problems die 15–20 years earlier than age-matched controls (9).

- In the United Kingdom, older people occupy two thirds of NHS beds and 60 per cent of older people admitted to general hospital will have, or go on to develop, a mental disorder (6).
- 30 per cent of people with a long-term physical health problem also have a history of mental illness, and 46 per cent of people with a mental health problem also have a chronic physical health problem (10).
- It can be extrapolated that on acute wards there are four times as many older people with a mental disorder as there are on in-patient mental health wards for older people (6).

These statistics further illustrate the intricate connection between physical and mental health; if ignored, this connection can have far reaching consequences.

Ultimately, the preferred end goal in liaison psychiatry is to improve various health-care outcomes while incurring the lowest possible costs and generating savings where possible (7, 11, 12). This is a mammoth task, which requires a challenge of current practice for all those involved in health service design and delivery, if these goals are to be realised. It is therefore essential that health commissioners, acute hospital trusts, and mental health services carefully consider their individual and collective roles in address-ing the shortfalls in elderly care (4, 6, 7, 11, 13).

When epidemiological parameters are correctly applied to a population, they can help to inspire change in that community and among the health professionals who serve it. It is also important to be aware of the cultural views upheld in any community, as they can influence the uptake and acceptance of epidemiological principles, potentially affecting engagement (2). Caring for an older patient not only involves physical care but delves much deeper, requiring careful consideration of what emotional, psycho-logical, and social factors may underlie illness. It demands the adoption of holistic models of care that meet the patients' needs in a meaningful way.

As the number of people who access mental health services increases, this has had a direct impact on the number of older people who need access to liaison psychiatry services after their admission to general hospitals (14–16).

These figures further buttress the importance of liaison psychiatry in acute hospitals, whose role it is to unpick the often multifactorial aetiologies of diseases in older persons. They also draw attention to a conspicuous gap, both in understanding and research, calling for a more thoughtful exploration and reconciliation of confounding factors to improve general health outcomes. The evidence for demonstrating the impact of liaison psychiatry in these settings is limited and sometimes variable; however, most data suggest that this specialty can shorten hospital stay and is broadly welcomed by staff, patients, and their relatives alike (17).

Liaison psychiatry for older people is a relatively young specialty and is, arguably, less established than the services available for adults of working age. Some United Kingdom hospitals provide an ageless service, but in areas where these systems are separate it is important that services be adaptable to patient care needs when the perception is that these needs would better be met by another service and not rely on age as the main criterion for referrals.

Several different models exist within liaison services, but the general consensus is to opt for one that uses proactive and collaborative strategies to assess and treat patients in acute settings (18). Liaison psychiatrists are often the driving force behind coordinated service developments, which aim to give careful thought and resolution to problems, ultimately ensuring a smooth transition to the appropriate community service (7).

Access to appropriate treatment in acute hospital settings is often not straightforward, because mental disorders are sometimes minimised and may not always be identified by staff on general wards or emergency departments (EDs) to begin with. Other times they can be blurred by other medical conditions that present in a similar manner, which delays contact with mental health services (8). Generally, people in acute hospitals have a higher prevalence for mental health-related problems because of physical health complexities, chronic comorbidities, presentations that mimic physical and somatoform illnesses – to name only a few factors (14). Sadly, it is reported that only 50 per cent of patients predicted to require input from liaison psychiatry are referred from the ED. This makes it a national priority to improve access to high quality care (8, 19). Mental health disorders exist comorbidly with other medical conditions, and this makes them difficult to disentangle. A high index of suspicion, patience, and expertise is required in order to manage this complex and intricate relationship.

Important Epidemiological Terms

It is essential to consider the basic epidemiological terms which are fundamental in defining and understanding the mental health disorders that occur in the older population seen in acute hospitals. Generally, studies on incidence are more laborious and expensive, thus there are a greater number of prevalence studies (20–22). Table 2.1 outlines the common epidemiological terms to be aware of.

Life Expectancy

Life expectancy in the United Kingdom is lengthening, albeit at a slower rate by comparison with pre-2011 figures (6, 23). The population aged 80 years and over is growing in number at a faster rate that its younger counterparts (11). This is reflected in the number of people with secondary care episodes; there is also a 65 per cent increase in over-75s, compared to a 31 per cent increase in those aged 15–59 (24). There are more than 2 million unplanned annual admissions for over-65s, and there has been a 37 per cent increase in emergency admissions over the past decade (24, 25). When one bears in mind that the number of acute and general hospital beds has decreased by a third during the past 25 years (as a result of the emphasis placed on moving from the traditional hospital-based practice to care in the community), it has become even more important than ever to manage the limited resources available with greater effectiveness (25). Systems need to cater for the expanding needs of the older person, pre-emptively taking collaborative steps to forestall a crisis where services become overwhelmed and unable to safely meet their care demands (24).

Prevalence of Mental Health Disorders in Older People in Emergency Departments

Year after year, increasing numbers of older people continue to present to emergency services in a crisis. Emergency departments (EDs) constitute one of the most frequently used settings for assessing acute mental health problems in patients with known or newly presenting mental health disorders (26). After a recent review of crisis care in the United

Table 2.1 Common epidemiological terminologies (20–22)

Terminology	Definition
Prevalence	The prevalence of a condition in a population is the total number of cases over the number of individuals in that population at a given time. It is determined by the disease duration and the number of new cases, and it tells us how common a condition is in a particular place at a particular time.
Incidence	The incidence is the extent to which something happens. It looks at the risk of developing a new condition within a specified period and relates it to new cases.
Lifetime risk	The lifetime risk factor looks at the risk for a disease over a long period (not just a year). It considers the probability that a person who is currently disease-free will develop the condition at some point during the remainder of their expected lifespan.
Disability-adjusted life years (DALYs)	The disability-adjusted life years measure considers the overall disease burden and is designed to measure the global burden. It pays specific attention to the years lost due to mortality and the years lost due to disability (morbidity) in a single tool.
Morbidity	Morbidity refers to any departure from a state of physiological or psychological well-being, whether it be based on subjective or on objective reports.
Mortality rate	The mortality rate considers a specified time interval and tries to measure the frequency of occurrence of death in a defined population.
Trends	Trends are upward or downward movements that describe changes in frequency.

Kingdom, the Care Quality Commission found a low level of satisfaction (14 per cent) with the care received by the adults surveyed. The report also highlighted that only a minority of EDs had 24/7 cover from a liaison psychiatry or a mental health team. This situation sometimes resulted in long waiting times, especially over the weekends, which further delayed access to what should be basic health care (5).

There are currently very few data around the prevalence of mental health disorders in working-age adults in EDs, and there is an even greater scarcity of data for older people. This paucity raises questions about a possible underestimation of the magnitude of the problem and its consequent impact on strategic health service planning.

The number of people attending EDs who require mental health care or are in crisis is likely to be influenced by local community mental health provision or by wider external drivers (2). After the outbreak of the Covid-19 pandemic, EDs have reported record low figures in terms of general presentations to acute departments. It is suggested that some older persons have delayed seeking help for fear of possibly contacting the virus, and this contributed to a late presentation that sometimes occurs in crisis, although more research and information are needed on this issue (27). At the time of writing, it remains to be seen whether a predicted surge in mental health crises materialises after the pandemic.

A study by NHS England that described attendance to EDs in people over the age of 60 showed a two-third increase in attendance between 2007/8 and 2013/4 – a much higher increase than was expected on the basis of demographic change alone (28). The same report highlights an increase in the number of patients who presented to EDs with psychiatric conditions: this number rose by 56 per cent between 2016/17 and 2019/20. It is also important to bring to the fore that over the same time period there was an even higher percentage increase (84 per cent) in the number of people who presented with 'poisoning', which includes overdoses. An increase (albeit a less severe one) is seen in presentations with social problems, including chronic alcoholism and homelessness (29).

A study by Casser et al. (26) described the prevalence of mental disorders in working-age adults who attended the emergency department in St Thomas Hospital, London. In descending order, these were self-harm (31 per cent), substance misuse (mostly alcohol) (20 per cent), psychosis (17 per cent), and mood disturbance (15 per cent).

The largest study to date reporting ED presentations for mental health needs in over-65-year-olds in the United Kingdom was published in 2021. A retrospective service evaluation study across 28 EDs analysed more than 18,000 patient records in England and Scotland (30). Over a six-year period, it reported a year-on-year rise in the number of people referred to liaison psychiatry after attending the ED and in the rate of these referrals (in 2018, the rate was 20 patients per 1,000 ED over 65-year-old attenders). Perhaps more significant than the upward trend in referral rates was the observed and reported interdepartmental variation: liaison referral rates ranged between 0.1 and 25 referrals per 1,000 ED attenders. This would suggest that local community mental health provision has a profound effect on how ED is used by people in mental health crisis. In the same study the most common documented reasons for referral (and therefore presentation at ED) were low mood, self-harm, and suicidal ideation. These three categories accounted for one third of all referrals to liaison psychiatry. Presentations associated with cognition (dementia and confusion) formed the second most common reason, followed by psychosis and substance misuse. People across the

Table 2.2 Prevalence rates of psychiatric disorders in 7207 patients who attended EDs in the United Kingdom (30)

ICD-10 classification	Rate per referral to LP % (95% confidence interval)
Mood disorders F30–F39	20.3 (19.4–21.2)
Organic mental disorders F00–F09	15.7 (14.9–16.6)
Neurotic, stress-related, and somatoform disorders F40–48	8.0 (7.4–8.7)
No identifiable mental disorder	7.6 (7.0–8.2)
Schizophrenia F20–F29	7.4 (6.8–8.0)
Mental disorders due to substance misuse F10–F19	4.0 (3.5–4.4)
Disorders of adult personality F60–F69	1.62 (1.3–1.9)
Disorders of mental retardation F70–F79	0.25 (0.13–0.36)
Behavioural syndromes associated with physiological disturbances and physical factors F50–F59	0.17 (0.07–0.26)

'older' age range attended, but the most common age range for referral was 65–75, which made up almost 50 per cent of all referrals (30). NHS England continues to invest millions of pounds across various hospitals to achieve the core 24 service-level requirements, which include targeting 24/7 access to services, one-hour response time in EDs, and meeting the recommended staffing demands (31).

Prevalence of Common Psychiatric Disorders Seen in Acute General Hospitals

The prevalence of mental disorders is higher in acute hospitals than in community settings. However, published figures are rather variable, often have a wide range, and need to be considered in the context in which they were reported. For example, the prevalence of depression on a stroke ward or the prevalence of delirium on a surgical ward may be higher than the prevalence of either depression or delirium on wards that cover other specialties. Furthermore, on a medical ward such as an oncology patients may report depressive symptoms that are not unexpected in the context of their physical health challenges. Prevalence and incidence are also affected by recruitment times and worsened by the absence of standardised sampling methods (13).

Most liaison psychiatry teams offer training and advice to colleagues in acute specialties where possible. Liaison teams have expertise in delivering detailed, patient-centred psychosocial assessments that consider the strengths and needs of the patient as well as the risks (7). Most requests received by liaison psychiatry departments from acute wards are requests to review or discuss (in an advisory capacity) patients with pre-existing mental health conditions, new presentations, and age-related changes that may have a mental health dimension to them. It has been reported that 70–80 per cent of referrals are from medical departments, and around 5 per cent of patients go on to require in-patient treatment in a psychiatric hospital; a larger number (10–20 percent) are passed on to community teams (32).

Generally the 'three Ds' – depression, dementia, and delirium – account for over 80 per cent of the cases seen by the older people's liaison psychiatry team (6). The prevalence of the most common mental health conditions is highlighted in Table 2.3; more detailed information on each is available in subsequent chapters of this book.

A study reported by the Royal College of Psychiatry in 2005 (6) outlines the prevalence of a number of mental disorders in acute hospitals. These disorders showed

Table 2.3 The prevalence of mental disorders in community and hospital settings (6, 20)

Mental disorder	Community prevalence	Hospital prevalence
Depression	12%	29%
Dementia	5%	31%
Delirium	1–2%	20 % (20%–25%)
Anxiety disorders	3% (5–10%)	8%
Alcohol misuse	2% (0.51%–2.75%)	3%
Schizophrenia	0.1 (0.1%–0.5%)	0.4%
Bipolar affective disorder	0.1%	5–12%

a wide range, but when the mean was employed the most common diagnoses were dementia (31 per cent), depression (29 per cent), cognitive impairment (22 per cent), delirium (20 per cent), anxiety (8 per cent), alcohol misuse (3 per cent), and schizophrenia (1.4 per cent) (13). A more recent study, conducted in 2016 at the Addenbrookes Hospital in Cambridge, demonstrated a slightly different prevalence rate, with delirium at the top of the ladder. The study looked at the number of patients seen by the old age liaison psychiatry service over a one-year period. The most common conditions were, in decreasing order of frequency, delirium, dementia, depression, no active mental health problem, anxiety, alcohol-related disorder, schizophrenia, bipolar affective disorder, and adjustment disorders. These results differed from those of studies with working-age adults, in whom depression, schizophrenia, and bipolar affective disorders are the most prevalent. (18). This discrepancy further highlights the unique role of the old age liaison psychiatrist.

Mood disorders: Mood disorders are the most common mental health disorders in the United Kingdom, depression topping the list. The exact prevalence rates vary from one geographic area to another, depending on various factors (33). The statistics around the prevalence of **depression** in the elderly in acute hospitals vary depending on the source and have been summarised in Table 2.3. The Royal College of Psychiatry study referred to earlier places its prevalence at 29 per cent (6). Other sources quote a range between 10 and 12 per cent (34), with a wider interval of 3 to 52 per cent when the variations in specialties and diagnostic criteria are considered (18).

Dementia: The prevalence rates of dementia rise steeply with increasing age: a rate of less than 1 per cent in under-65s rises to 24–33 per cent in over-85s. In nonagerians who are being nursed in acute hospitals, these figures go up to 48.8 per cent in men and 75 per cent in women. The number of older people in the general population is increasing more rapidly than that of members of any other age group, and according to estimates the over-60s will reach about 2 billion by 2050 (35). The high and rising prevalence of dementia in the general hospital creates funding and care challenges related to this patient group (34). Some sources suggest an average prevalence of 31 per cent for the over-65s in hospital settings (6). The most widely accepted average prevalence of dementia among hospital residents over the age of 75 is 42.4 per cent; only half of these are diagnosed before admission (34).

Delirium: The prevalence rates for delirium vary widely across settings; thus rates of about 1 per cent in the community rise to about 25 per cent in acute hospitals, and up to a half of the hospitalised cases make a full recovery on discharge. The overlap of dementia and delirium is often missed by clinicians, who may suspect, for example, that the cause of a patient's worsening presentation is one of the behavioural and psychological symptoms of dementia (BPSDs) rather than a delirious process. In such cases they may prescribe psychotropic medications – for instance benzodiazepines, which can in principle worsen a delirium, prolonging the period of recovery and increasing the disease burden borne by the patient, the carers, and society at large (36). A qualitative study by Fick et al. (37) showed that family members could more readily spot the abrupt changes in the mental state of their loved ones when delirium coexisted with dementia. This highlights a worrying reality and shows how this potentially life-threatening condition may be underestimated by clinicians. A systemic review by Fick et al. (36) described how, in community and hospital populations, the prevalence of delirium superimposed on dementia in people older than 65 years ranged from 22 to 89 per cent. These rates were much higher in hospital studies with the three highest prevalence rates, from 76 to 89 per cent, and in most studies that showed a prevalence greater than 50 per cent (20).

Anxiety disorders: Generally the prevalence of anxiety disorders in older people in the community varies between 5 and 10 per cent. The variations are accounted for by the comorbid presentation of anxiety with other mental health disorders such as depression or disorders of cognition (20). A pooled meta-analysis of 32 studies showed a prevalence of 8 per cent for any anxiety disorder in in-patient general hospitals settings (6, 38).

Psychotic disorders: The community prevalence for schizophrenia is about 0.1–0.5 per cent, and 1–8 per cent (0.4%) in hospital settings for over-65s (6). In older persons, delusional disorders are prevalent in 0.04 per cent of the population. The prevalence for bipolar affective disorder is 0.1 per cent in over-65s, but this disorder accounts for about 5–12 per cent of in-patient admissions, despite its low prevalence in the community (18, 20).

Personality disorders (PDs): These sometimes coexist with other mental disorders and may in fact drive what cluster they fall into; for example, someone with a mood disorder in the background may present with more cluster C avoidant or dependent traits. The prevalence of PDs seems to vary across community (2.8–13 per cent), psychiatric outpatients (5–33 per cent), and psychiatric in-patient settings (7–61.5 per cent) and appears to be heavily dependent on the research methods used to determine them (20). There is generally a reported rise in the prevalence of obsessive–compulsive PD as people become older, and this may simply reflect failing powers to adapt to change rather than an intrinsic change in personality. As people get older, the traits and behaviours associated with PDs might improve, even though other comorbid disorders tend to enhance maladaptive coping skills (39).

Substance use disorders: Problems with substance use in the elderly can often go unnoticed. Alcohol is the most abused substance, while benzodiazepines are the commonest group of abuse in prescription medication, with a prevalence of 11 per cent (6). Although drinking patterns have often begun in earlier life, the amount consumed can increase as a result of adverse life events, loneliness, and cognitive problems (all common in older age). It is estimated that 10–15 per cent of over-65s consume quantities of alcohol over the recommended national limits in the community; the one-year prevalence for alcohol abuse and dependence ranges between 0.51 and 2.75 per cent (20). The prevalence in hospital settings is about 3 per cent (6). Rates of alcohol dependence are significantly higher in men than in women (20).

Other conditions: It is also important to consider other mental health conditions that affect older people who may be referred to a liaison psychiatrist. These include conditions such as sleep disorders, sexual disinhibition, behavioural disturbance, personality changes, forensic issues, and mental capacity or legal frameworks, as well as preexisting or acquired intellectual and cognitive problems. Although these conditions generally occur less frequently and are more likely to coexist with other mental and physical health conditions, it is crucial for healthcare professionals to maintain a high index of suspicion, if they don't want to miss them at the cost of worsening the morbidity burden. Some of these presentations are managed by the geriatricians and may not be referred to liaison services, unless there are other, 'more obvious' mental health problems (20).

The Influence of Coronavirus Disease 2019 (Covid-19) on the Prevalence of Mental Disorders in Acute Hospitals

The Covid-19 virus is a novel virus from a family similar to that of the severe acute respiratory syndrome (SARS) and of some types of common cold. It was first reported in Wuhan, China in December 2019 and later declared a global pandemic on March 11, 2020 (40). At the time of writing, there have been more than 546 million Covid-19 cases worldwide and well over 6.3 million deaths; countries such as the United States, Brazil, India, Russia, Mexico, and Peru top the mortality list. The United Kingdom currently ranks seventh on this list, with more than 22 million cases and well over 179,000 total deaths. Sadly, these figures continue to rise, albeit at a slower rate than when the pandemic first started, as the emergence of vaccines and greater medical knowledge played an important role (41, 42).

It is generally believed that older people are at higher risk of developing more severe and life-threatening forms of the Covid-19 infection – forms that require hospitalisation, ventilator support, or intensive care. They are also more likely to be hospitalised or die from Covid-19 when not vaccinated (34, 43, 44). Emerging evidence suggests that being fully vaccinated leads to a 94 per cent reduction in the risks of Covid-19-related hospital admissions and being partially vaccinated reduces the risk to 64 per cent (45). The risk of an adverse outcome increases with advancing age, the over 85s being the most likely to become very sick (40, 45). More than 80 per cent of Covid-19 deaths occur in people over the age of 65 (45).

Older people with physical health comorbidities, social inequalities, disabilities, and racial or ethnic differences have also played a role in both the mortality and the morbidity borne from Covid-19. The reasons for this are often complex and beyond the scope of this chapter, but the factors include social deprivation, chronic conditions, and various barriers to seeking health care (45). Alcohol has an interesting relationship with Covid-19, for example it increases the risk of contracting Covid-19 as a result of its impact on the immunity, existing liver disease, and inflammatory response. It also enhances susceptibility to and severity of Covid-19 and has led to an increase in acute presentations with alcohol-related emergencies such as suicide, methanol toxicity and alcohol withdrawal. The pandemic has also generated wider changes in drinking patterns. These have been affected by a number of determinants such as government policies and various social, economic, psychological, and biological factors (46).

During the pandemic there have been disruptions to critical mental health services in many countries; over 60 per cent of them reported major effects on services for vulnerable groups such as children and adolescents, older adults, and women requiring antenatal or postnatal services. The World Health Organisation (WHO) has issued guidelines and recommendations to various countries to limit the impact of the pandemic and to make plans for recovery. Poverty seems to be a major limiting factor; for example, 80 per cent of high-income countries used telemedicine and teletherapy to plug the mental health gaps compared to 50 per cent of low-income countries (47).

The Covid-19 pandemic has had a profound impact on the type and number of patients seen by liaison psychiatry, and the full impact is still yet to be realised. During the acute phases of illness, the number of people in hospital swelled, while the number of people using ED for psychiatric reasons fell (48, 49). Older people in hospital with Covid-19, especially those with dementia, were susceptible to delirium. The resulting combination was one of disorientation and fear, with resulting distress and secondary agitated behaviours, which led to people wanting to seek reassurance from staff or trying to leave wards. These behaviours were not compatible with social distancing.

Generally, the presentation and referrals to both mental and physical health services declined during lockdown, as changes were seen in service provision and in care-seeking behaviours. The changes in service delivery may have bridled access to mental health services, while the changes in patients' attempts to seek help could have been due to a reduction in need or to a lack of care seeking attributable to people's 'repressed' instincts (48). There has been a gradual return to activity as the lockdown has eased off and restrictive measures are being relaxed. An increase in demand was, however, noted for liaison services, except in eating disorders; and excess mortality was reported in the over-70s, especially those with severe mental illness (48). An observational study carried out in London by Sampson et al. (49) reviewed a new Mental Health Crisis Assessment Service created during the first wave of the pandemic in order to redirect people from EDs. It noted a fall in referrals during that first wave, but after the lockdown ended liaison psychiatrists saw an increase in the number of referrals from EDs by comparison to 2019.

A study by Varatharaj et al. (50) provided a bird's eye view of hospitalised patients with acute neurological or psychiatric complications associated with Covid-19. It demonstrated that about a third of patients presented with altered mental states, 92 per cent were new mental health-related diagnoses, 43 per cent had new-onset psychosis, 26 per cent had a neurocognitive (dementia-like) syndrome, and 17 per cent had an affective disorder. The altered mental state noticed in older patients may reflect hidden neurocognitive degenerative diseases or coexisting medical comorbidities. The study recognised a disproportionately larger number of neuropsychiatric presentations in younger-age groups (under 60 years) and more cerebrovascular complications in older patients, which may reflect the state of health of the cerebral vasculature and associated risk factors, exacerbated by critical illness in older patients. This was the first study of its kind; much larger and wider studies are needed to make conclusive statements. There are speculations about significant increases in mental health-related disorders in all age groups and genders, but more so in those with preexisting mental conditions, the young, women, and older people (51). It is also important to factor in the neurological and mental complications of Covid-19 such as delirium, stroke, and agitation, especially in the elderly. The presence of Covid-19 infections with co-morbid mental, neurological, or substance use disorders results in a greater risk of adverse untoward outcomes, including death (47).

At the onset of the pandemic, attention was focused on the immediate mental health consequences. However, as restrictions have eased and attempts are made to move towards some semblance of normality, systems and policies are required to deal with the after-effects of this global tsunami. As is often the case in times of crisis, communities pull cohesively together to fight against a common foe (48). It is, however, essential to remain vigilant about the long-term impact of such events when the natural fight or flight response may have waned. The effects on mental health are not always obvious or easily translated into concrete figures. There is nonetheless a need to emphasize the importance of people's overall mental well-being for the wider economic recovery and the cost implications, since this is often ignored. We all need to be mindful that further challenges lie ahead, both directly, from the virus (increased frailty and long Covid), and indirectly, through the impact of national lockdowns.

Older people in the United Kingdom have been isolated from family and social networks for long periods of time. They have had less access to support groups, community, and physical and mental health workers and fewer opportunities for physical exercise – for various reasons. Initial data are now emerging on the impact that this situation has had on the incidence of mental health problems and on the resulting harm to self and others. There isn't a large amount of information available yet; this remains a work in progress. Accurate and reliable figures about the impact of the pandemic on elderly patients are still being collated and interpreted.

Conclusion

This chapter has provided an overview of the prevalence of mental disorders in acute hospitals and in EDs. It has also highlighted the importance of liaison psychiatry departments in general hospitals. More research using larger studies is needed to better describe the prevalence of mental health conditions among older patients in acute settings.

Providing appropriate care for older people with mental illness in acute hospitals is a challenge, but one that can be overcome when carefully thought-out plans are implemented. Identifying the problems is the first step towards making the much needed change. It is therefore important that health and social service providers have an in-depth understanding of the guidelines and targets set by medical service chiefs and commissioners, if they are to grasp the role of professionals in liaison psychiatry who have the task of accomplishing these objectives (6). This requires a deliberate and conscientious attempt to bridge the gap between physical health and mental health care.

There is a need for better communication and collaborative work between the various professionals and services involved in the care of older patients (52). Much can be learnt from each other; this will allow us to build a better understanding and to adopt strategic processes to manage the emerging trends of diseases as well as the disease risk factors in this unique patient group (2). This is a clarion call to challenge current practice, to work synergistically with all stakeholders, and to embrace change.

References

1. Coggon, D., Rose, G., and Barker, D.J.P. What is epidemiology? In their *Epidemiology for the Uninitiated* (4th ed.), 1997. BMJ resources for readers. www.bmj.com/about-bmj/resources-readers/publications/epidemiology-uninitiated/1-what-epidemiology.

2. Minett, T., Brayne, C., and Stephan, B.C.M. Epidemiology of old age psychiatry: An overview of concepts and main studies. In Thomas, A. and Dening, T., *Oxford Textbook of Old Age Psychiatry* (3rd ed.). Oxford: Oxford University Press, 2020, pp. 45–76.

3. NHS England. Improving care for older people. NHS 75, n.d. www.england.nhs.uk/ourwork/clinical-policy/older-people/improving-care-for-older-people.

4. Goldie, I., Elliott, I., Regan, M. et al. *Mental Health and Prevention: Taking Local Action*. Policy report. London: Mental Health Foundation, 2016 (here pp. 1–41).

5. *The Five Year Forward View for Mental Health: A Report from the Independent Mental Health Taskforce to the NHS in England*. NHS, February 2016 (here pp. 4–32). www.england.nhs.uk/wp-content/uploads/2016/02/Mental-Health-Taskforce-FYFV-final.pdf.

6. Royal College of Psychiatrists. *Who Cares Wins: Improving the Outcome for Older People Admitted to the General Hospital:*

Guidelines for the Development of Liaison Mental Health Services for Older People. London: RCP, 2005 (here pp. 5–40). www .bgs.org.uk/sites/default/files/content/ resources/files/2018-05-18/ WhoCaresWins.pdf.

7. Parsonage, M., Fossey, M., and Tutty, C. Liaison Psychiatry in the Modern NHS. Report. London: Centre for Mental Health, 2012 (here pp. 3–4). www .centreformentalhealth.org.uk/sites/ default/files/2018-09/Liaison_psychiatry_ in_the_modern_NHS_2012_0.pdf.

8. Treat as One: Bridging the Gap between Mental and Physical Healthcare in General Hospitals. Report, National Confidential Enquiry into Patient Outcome and Death (NCEPOD), 2017 (here pp. 6–10). www.ncepod.org.uk/ 2017report1/downloads/TreatAsOne_ FullReport.pdf.

9. Department of Health. Annual Report of the Chief Medical Officer 2013: Public Mental Health Priorities: Investing in the Evidence. London: Department of Health and Social Care, 2014. assets.publishing .service.gov.uk/government/uploads/ system/uploads/attachment_data/file/ 413196/CMO_web_doc.pdf.

10. Naylor, V., Parsonage, M., McDaid, D. et al. Long-Term Conditions and Mental Health: The Cost of Co-Morbidities. London: Kings Fund Centre for Mental Health, 2012.

11. Singh, I., Ramakrishna, S., and Williamson, K. The rapid assessment interface and discharge service and its implications for patients with dementia. Clin Interv Aging 2013, 8: 1101–8.

12. Tadros,G., Salama, R.A., Kingston, P. et al. Impact of an integrated rapid response psychiatric liaison team on quality improvement and cost savings: The Birmingham RAID model. Psychiatrist 2013, 37: 4–10. doi: 10.1192/ pb.bp.111.037366.

13. Holmes, J. Liaison old age psychiatry. In Dening, T. and Thomas, A. (eds), Oxford Textbook of Old Age Psychiatry (2nd ed.). Oxford: Oxford University Press, 2013, pp. 325–34.

14. Royal College of Psychiatry. Liaison Psychiatry for Every Acute Hospital: Integrated Mental and Physical Healthcare. www.rcpsych.ac.uk/docs/ default-source/members/faculties/liaison-psychiatry/cr183liaisonpsych-every-acute-hospital.pdf?sfvrsn=26c57d4_2.

15. Burns, A., and Warner, J. Better access to mental health services for older people. Blog, 9 October 2015. www.england.nhs .uk/blog/mh-better-access.

16. Department of Health. National Service Framework for Older People. 2001, pp. 7–40. assets.publishing.service.gov .uk/government/uploads/system/uploads/ attachment_data/file/198033/National_ Service_Framework_for_Older_People .pdf.

17. Palmer, L., Hodge, S., Ryley, A. et al. Psychiatric Liaison Accreditation Network (PLAN): National Report 2012–2015. London: Royal College of Psychiatrists, 2016. www.rcpsych.ac.uk/docs/default-source/improving-care/ccqi/quality-networks/psychiatric-liaison-services-plan/plan-publications-and-links-national-report-2012-15.pdf?sfvrsn= 3814f12_2.

18. Thompson, F., and Baker-Glenn, E. Liaison old age psychiatry. In Dening, T. and Thomas, A. (eds), Oxford Textbook of Old Age Psychiatry (3rd ed.). Oxford: Oxford University Press, 2020, pp. 347–61.

19 Department of Health, Closing the gap: priorities for essential change in mental health, January 2014, https://assets .publishing.service.gov.uk/government/ uploads/system/uploads/attachment_ data/file/281250/Closing_the_gap_V2_-_ 17_Feb_2014.pdf.

20. NHS England, the National Collaborating Centre for Mental Health, and the National Institute for Health and Care Excellence. Achieving Better Access to 24/7 Urgent and Emergency Mental Health Care, Part 2: Implementing the Evidence-Based Treatment Pathway for Urgent and Emergency Liaison Mental Health Services for Adults and Older Adults: Guidance. NHS England Publications Gateway

Reference 05958. November 2016. www
.england.nhs.uk/wp-content/uploads/
2016/11/lmhs-guidance.pdf.

21. Rodda, J., Boyce, N., and Walker, Z. *The
Old Age Psychiatry Handbook: A Practical
Guide.* Hobocken, NJ: John Wiley & Sons
Ltd, 2008 (esp. pp. 23–244).

22. *Oxford Learner's Dictionaries.* Oxford:
Oxford University Press, 2021. www
.oxfordlearnersdictionaries.com.

23. Centres for Disease Control and
Prevention. *Epidemiology Glossary.* Data
and Statistics, n.d. www.cdc.gov/
reproductivehealth/data_stats/glossary
.html.

24. *Hospitals on the Edge? The Time for
Action: A Report by the Royal College of
Physicians.* September 2012. Download
from www.rcplondon.ac.uk/guidelines-
policy/hospitals-edge-time-action.

25. Imison, C., Poteliakhoff, E., and
Thompson, J. *Older People and
Emergency Bed Use. Exploring Variation.*
London: King's Fund, 2012.

26. Cassar, S., A. Hodgkiss, A., Ramirez, A.
et al. Mental health presentations to an
inner-city accident and emergency
department. *Psychiatric Bulletin* 2002, 26
(4): 134–6.

27. Javadi, S.M.H., and Nateghi, N. Covid-19
and its psychological effects on the elderly
population. *Disaster Medicine and Public
Health Preparedness* 2020 14(3): 40–1.

28. NHS England, Operational Information
for Commissioning. A & E attendances
and emergency admissions. Monthly
report, December 2016. www.england.nhs
.uk/statistics/wp-content/uploads/sites/2/
2016/06/Monthly-AE-Report-December-
16.pdf.

29. NHS digital. *Hospital Accident &
Emergency activity.* September 2020.
https://digital.nhs.uk/data-and-
information/publications/statistical/
hospital-accident–emergency-activity/
2019-20/further-information.

30. Crowther, G., Chinnasamy, M.,
Bradbury, S. et al. Trends in referrals to
liaison psychiatry teams from UK
emergency departments for patients over

65. *Int J Geriatr Psychiatry* 2021, 36(9):
1415–22. doi: 10.1002/gps.5547.

31. Healthcare Safety Investigation Branch.
Provision of mental health care to
patients presenting at the emergency
department. Investigations and Reports,
November 2018. www.hsib.org.uk/
investigations-and-reports/provision-
mental-health-care-patients-presenting-
emergency-department.

32. Anderson, D., and Ooman, S. Liaison
psychiatry and older people. In Guthrie,
E., Rao, S., and Temple, M. (eds),
Seminars in Liaison Psychiatry (2nd ed.),
London: Royal College of Psychiatrists,
2012, pp. 265–87.

33. Mental Health Foundation. Mental health
statistics: The most common mental
health problems. Mental Health Statistics,
2023. www.mentalhealth.org.uk/statistics/
mental-health-statistics-most-common-
mental-health-problems.

34. Sampson, E.L., Blanchard, M.R., Jones, L.
et al. Dementia in the acute hospital:
Prospective cohort study of prevalence
and mortality. *Br J Psychiatry* 2009, 195
(1): 61–6.

35. World Health Organization. Ageing and
health. Update of 4 October 2021. www
.who.int/news-room/fact-sheets/detail/
ageing-and-health.

36. Fick, D., Agostini, J., and Inouye, S.
Delirium superimposed on dementia:
A systematic review. *Journal of the
American* 2002, 50(10): 1723–32. doi.org/
10.1046/j.1532-5415.2002.50468.

37. Fick, D., and Foreman, M. Consequences
of not recognizing delirium
superimposed on dementia in
hospitalized elderly individuals.
J Gerontol Nurs 2000, 26: 30–40.

38. Walker, J., Niekerk, M., Hobbs, H. et al.
The prevalence of anxiety in general
hospital inpatients: A systematic review
and meta-analysis. *Gen Hosp Psychiatry*
2021, 72: 131–40.

39. Modekar, A., and Spence, S. Personality
disorder in older people: How common is
it and what can be done? *BJPsych
Advances* 2008, 14(1): 71–7.

40. Muller, A., McNamara, M., and Sinclair, D. Why does Covid-19 disproportionately affect older people? *Open-Access Impact Journal in Aging* 2020, 12(10): 9959–81.

41. Centres for Disease Control and Prevention. Covid data tracker. https://covid.cdc.gov/covid-data-tracker/#datatracker-home.

42. Worldometers. Covid-19 coronavirus pandemic. www.worldometers.info/coronavirus.

43. Dagan, N., Barda, N., Kepten, E. et al. BNT162b2 mRNA Covid-19 vaccine in a nationwide mass vaccination setting. *N Engl J Med.* 2021, 384(15): 1412–23.

44. Thompson, M.G., Burgess, J.L., Naleway, A.L. et al. Interim estimate of vaccine effectiveness of BNT162b2 and mRNA-1273 Covid-19 vaccines in preventing SARS-CoV-2 infection among health care personnel, first responders, and other essential and frontline workers, eight US locations, December 2020–March 2021. *Morbidity and Mortality Weekly Report (Weekly MMWR)* 2021, 70(13): 495–500.

45. Centres for Disease Control and Prevention. Covid-19 risks and information for older adults. https://www.cdc.gov/aging/covid19/index.html.

46. Murthy, P., and Narasimha, V.L. Effects of the Covid-19 pandemic and lockdown on alcohol use disorders and complications. *Current Opinion in Psychiatry* 2021, 34(4): 376–85.

47. WHO. Covid-19 disrupting mental health services in most countries: WHO survey. 5 October 2020, News release. https://bit.ly/3QghRzU.

48. Chen, S., Jones, P.B., Underwood, B.R. et al. The early impact of Covid-19 on mental health and community physical health services and their patients' mortality in Cambridgeshire and Peterborough, UK. *J Psychiatry Res* 2020, 131: 244–54.

49. Sampson, E., Wright, J., Dove, J. et al. Psychiatric liaison service referral patterns during the UK Covid-19 pandemic: An observational study. *Eur J Psychiatry* 2022, 36(1): 35–42.

50. Varatharaj, A., Thomas, N., Ellul, M. et al. Neurological and neuropsychiatric complications of Covid-19 in 153 patients: A UK-wide surveillance study. *Lancet Psychiatry* 2020, 7(10): 875–82.

51. McDaid, D. Viewpoint: Investing in strategies to support mental health recovery from the Covid-19 pandemic. *European Psychiatry* 2021, 64(1): e32.

52. Ruddy, R., and House, A. Meta-review of high-quality systematic reviews of interventions in key areas of liaison psychiatry. *Br J Psychiatry* 2005, 187: 109–20.

Elderly-Friendly Care Settings and Hospitals

Khalid Ali

Older People and Hospitalization

The rise in longevity is an emerging phenomenon across the world. Older people's life expectancy has risen dramatically over the past 50 years, the most prominent rise taking place in the oldest old (those over 80 years). The number of people over the age of 65 is projected to increase from 524 million in 2010 to almost 1.5 billion in 2050, the most prominent rise taking place in developing countries (1). In 2015, according to WHO statistics, it was estimated that there were 125 million people aged 80 years or more (2).

Older people are more likely to have multimorbidity and frailty and to be consumers of polypharmacy. They have a reduced functional reserve, which places them at an increased risk of hospitalization after an acute illness or a breakdown in their social support system in the community. Older people (over the age of 65) form the commonest age group admitted to hospital, namely 65 per cent of hospital bed days. There was a reported increase of 18 per cent in older people's emergency admission in the United Kingdom between 2010/11 and 2014/15 (3). Catering for the needs of an older population presents a significant challenge to acute hospitals. Hospitalization is a serious event for an older person, because it is associated with a series of complications such as malnutrition, delirium, falls, prolonged hospital stay, and a challenging post-discharge period (4–7). Following a hospital admission, a person with multiple chronic conditions is also at a higher risk of readmission (8).

The common entry pathway for older people to hospital admission via an emergency department (ED) is a daunting experience. If an ED is too fast-paced, too crowded, chaotic, poorly tailored to older people's needs, and poorly furnished, the result is unmet needs and subsequent frustration and angst among ED staff (9). There is a compelling demand to tailor hospital environments to the demands of a growing population of older people worldwide.

Elderly Friendly Hospitals

A commitment from senior hospital managers to make hospitals safe environments for older people is mandatory; and so are government-level initiatives with clearly defined policies dedicated to the same goal. The eldery-friendly hospitals initiative with an underpinning organization-wide framework was advocated in British Columbia, Canada in 1999 (10). Emphasis was placed on having a clear agenda on four specific domains: policies and procedures, care systems, social behavioural climate, and physical design (11). Similar high-level objectives and plans were explored in Taiwan (12) and in the United States (13); management structure, communication with stakeholders, adapted physical environment, trained and supported staff, interdisciplinary work ethics, and patient- and carer-centred care. The senior-friendly hospital (SFH) framework implemented in Ontario, Canada, was used in monitoring the performance of 155 acute hospitals, to identify gaps in the service and to implement changes towards delivering better targeted care for older people (14).

Elderly-friendly initiatives, coupled with service reorganization, staff training, interdisciplinary communication, early rehabilitation programs, and discharge planning in surgical wards, are being investigated in a robust research trial in order to develop new care models, informed by a sound evidence base (15).

Involving Older People in Decision-Making around Hospital Design

In planning appropriate and elderly-friendly environments, it is crucial to listen to the views of older people and to implement their preferences. The involvement of older people as 'patient advisors' in developing the acute care for elders (ACE) strategy has been a key element in the elder care improvement programs set up in Toronto, Canada (16).

A survey conducted among older hospitalised patients in the Royal Victoria Hospital in Edinburgh showed that patients preferred single rooms (17). The implementation of open visiting hours and care rounds reduced the feelings of isolation that can develop in single rooms. In this study, contrary to common beliefs, most patients preferred to eat their meals alone, by their bedside, rather than in a communal dining room. There are several advantages to single-room occupancy for older people, such as confidentiality during care consultations (18), maintaining dignity, quieter surroundings, and better sleep quality, as well as an improved hygiene and lower risk of hospital-acquired infections (19).

Meaningful Activities for Older People Tailored to Hospital Settings

In rehabilitation settings, the lack of meaningful activities, isolation, boredom, frustration, and disempowerment were highlighted as key factors that adversely affected an older person's experience during his or her stay (20).

The care of older people in end-of-life care settings also needs thoughtful consideration and research into what works best. In those environments older people value privacy, being close to their loved ones, proximity to their own homes, and being content with their current physical surroundings (21).

Integrating into acute care settings an arts-based program such as drawing, painting, listening to personalized music, and singing can create a stimulating environment with the potential to improve the patients' and their families' hospital experience (22). There is emerging evidence from systematic reviews that music and reminiscence therapy improve the well-being of older hospitalized people (23). However, the evidence from randomized controlled trials about the clinical effectiveness of dementia-friendly acute care settings (D-FAC) is limited (24).

Older People at Night: Health Hazards in Hospitals

In hospitals, older people are at an increased risk of delirium with serious complications such as falls, prolonged length of stay, discharge to a care home, and death (25–27).

Several strategies such as one-one care, anti-psychotic medications, and physical restraints have all being trialled in order to manage delirium in hospitalised patients. Evidence presented in clinical or cost effectiveness studies has shown their limitations (28–30).

Tailoring emergency departments to deliver senior-friendly interventions administered by trained staff – such as subdued lighting, thicker mattresses, medications reviews, and early screening for complications – has resulted in lower readmission rates (31). Poor sleep quality due to high levels of light and sound were reported in hospitalized older people (32).

Environmental Strategies Designed to Maintain Orientation

The Delirium Room Model

Purpose-built environments tailored to cater for the needs of hospitalized older people with delirium have been developed in various institutions around the world. One such model is the 'delirium room' at Saint Louis University Hospital, Missouri. The basic principles of the delirium room were avoiding physical restraints, adopting non-pharmacological approaches, and making close-by, continuous nursing observations. Nurses adopt a specific 'tolerate, anticipate, and don't agitate' (TADA) attitude towards confused patients. Longitudinal data collected from that unit over 13 years showed reduction in length of stay and mortality levels by comparison with data from older hospitalized patients without delirium (33). However, the authors acknowledge the limitation of their model, in that it was not subjected to a rigorous randomized controlled trial approach. In addition, it was not clear which components of the delirium room provided the key beneficial ingredient.

A personalized hospital environment (family photos in patients rooms) and colour-coded areas (different colours for rooms and dining areas) to make a ward more 'homely' are proposed with the aim of reducing challenging behavioural symptoms in people with dementia, for example wandering and restlessness (34).

Orientation Strategies

Orientation strategies by nursing staff have been recommended in some guidelines as a non-pharmacological approach to managing delirium in hospitalised older people. These strategies have been critiqued for being too dogmatic and leading to mistrust between care staff and patients' families (35).

However, practical environmental adaptations such as visible clocks and calendars are advocated, as they are believed to meet the needs of hospitalised older people (36).

Environmental Strategies to Enhance Safety

Lessons learnt from best practice, observational studies, and randomised controlled trials have stressed the need for older person-friendly hospital environments. Well-lit rooms, single occupancy, less noise, and comfort rounds are all crucial interventions. Trained specialist staff members who appreciate the complexity of caring for an older person are crucial to delivering a patient-centred service. Non-pharmacological measures such as the TADA approach are needed to enhance safety in hospitals. These features are summarised in Table 3.1.

Table 3.1 Features of elderly-friendly wards

Environment	Provision of	Advantage
Physical	Single rooms Quiet, well-lit rooms Clear signposts	Privacy, confidentiality Reduce disorientation Improve orientation, reduce risk of wandering and falls
Ward routines	Open visiting hours Comfort rounds	Reduce isolation Reduce malnutrition
Staff	Specialist, trained staff	Better hospital experience
Sensory stimulation: Arts and humanities	Meaningful activities such as singing, dancing, yoga, reminiscence therapy, and arts therapy	Mental stimulation and enhanced well-being
Spiritual	Quiet rooms for prayers	Enhance spiritual well-being and create better strategies for coping with illness

Essential Ingredients for Elderly-Friendly Hospitals

1. Commitment from senior hospital management to invest in high-quality services for old people and their families
2. Regular training and development of staff to recognize and manage promptly older people's afflictions, such as falls and delirium
3. Regular audit exercises and performance checks to ensure that an older person's hospital experience is a good one when bench-marked against the experience offered by top-performing elderly care units nationally and internationally
4. Rewarding good practice by offering incentives to promote excellence in clinical care
5. Recognising sub-optimal services and implementing adequate measures to improve standards
6. Meaningful integration of medical and social services at hospital level to support early safe discharge
7. Championing research in older people's health and well-being as an integral component of high-quality clinical service.

Top Qualities of the Good Elderly-Friendly Clinician

1. Knowledge and understanding of older people's common problems and atypical presentations
2. Good communication skills with patients and their families
3. Maintaining a holistic approach in exploring the physical, mental, and spiritual well-being of patients
4. Having keen observational skills to identify commonly missed problems, such as elder abuse
5. Team-player and team-leader skills in working with a multidisciplinary team with other specialists involved in an older person's care
6. Empathy in dealing with vulnerable, frail patients

7. Keeping an open mind and being ready to seek a second opinion, especially when dealing with complicated ethical decisions such as feeding decisions and end-of-life care

8. Adopting a scientific approach in practising evidence-base medicine and engaging with research in circumstances where evidence is evolving.

References

1. WHO, National Institute on Aging, and National Institute of Health. Global health and aging. WHO, National Health publication number 11-7737, October 2011. www.nia.nih.gov/sites/default/files/2017-06/global_health_aging.pdf.

2. WHO. Ageing and health. Fact sheet number 404. WHO, September 2015. www.who.int/news-room/fact-sheets/detail/ageing-and-health.

3. National Audit Office. *Discharging Older Patients from Hospital.* Report, NAO 2016. www.nao.org.uk/wp-content/uploads/2015/12/Discharging-older-patients-from-hospital.pdf.

4. Brennan, T.A., Leape, L.L., Laird, N.M. et al. Incidence of adverse events and negligence of hospitalized patients: Results of the Harvard Medical Practice Study 1. *N Engl J Med* 1991, 324: 370–6.

5. Covinsky, K. E., Pierluissi, E., and Johnston, C.B.. Hospitalization-associated disability: 'She was probably able to ambulate, but I'm not sure'. *JAMA* 2011, 306: 1782–93.

6. Murray, G.R., Cameron, I.D., and Cumming, R.G. The consequences of falls in acute and subacute hospitals in Australia that causes proximal femoral fractures. *J Am Geriatr Soc* 2007, 55: 577–82.

7. Covinsky, K.E. Malnutrition and bad outcomes. *J Gen Intern Med* 2002, 17: 956–7.

8. Berry, J.G., Gay, J.C., Maddox, K.J. et al. Age trends in 30 day hospital readmissions: US national retrospective analysis. *BMJ* 2018, 360: k497. doi: 10.1136/bmj.k497.

9. Kelly, M.L. Senior-friendly emergency department care: An environmental assessment. *Journal of Health Services Research and Policy* 2011, 16: 6–12.

10. Parke, B., and Stevenson, L. Creating an elder-friendly hospital. *Healthcare Manage Forum* 1999, 12: 45–8.

11. Parke, B., and Brand, P. An elder-friendly hospital: Translating a dream into reality. *Nurs Leadersh* 2004, 17: 62–76.

12. Chiou, S.T., and Chen, L.K. Towards age-friendly hospitals and health services. *Arch Gerontol Geriatr* 2009, 49S2: S3–S6.

13. Boltz, M., Capezuti, E., and Shabbat, N. Building a framework for geriatric acute care model. *Leadersh Health Serv* 2010, 23: 334–60.

14. Wong, K.S., Ryan, D.P., and Liu, B.A. A system-wide analysis using a senior-friendly hospital framework identifies current practices and opportunities for improvement in the care of hospitalized older adults. *JAGS* 2014, 62: 2163–70.

15. Khadaroo, R.G., Badawal, R.S., Wagg, A.S. et al. Optimising senior's surgical care: Elder-Friendly Approaches to the Surgical Environment (EASE): Rationale and objectives. *BMC Health Services Research* 2015, 15: 338. doi: 10.1186/s12913-015-1001-2.

16. Verma, J. Healthcare for the ageing citizen and the ageing citizen for healthcare: Involving patient advisors in elder-friendly care improvement. *Healthcare Quarterly (Toronto)* 2017, 20: 14–17.

17. Reid, J., Wilson, K., Anderson, K.E., Maguire, C.P.J. Older patients' room preference: Single versus shared accommodation. *Age and Ageing* 2015, 44: 331–3.

18. Van de Glind, I., Van Dulmen, S., and Goossensen, A. Physician–patient communication in single-bedded versus

four-bedded hospital rooms. *Patient Educ Couns* 2008, 73: 215–19.

19. Pennington, H., and Isles, C. Should hospitals provide all patients with single rooms? *BMJ* 2013, 347: f6333. doi: https://doi.org/10.1136/bmj.f5695.

20. Luker, J., Lynch, E., Bernhardsson, S. et al. Stroke survivors' experiences of physical rehabilitation: A systematic review of qualitative studies. *Arch Phsy Med Rehabil* 2015, 96: 1698–708.

21. Brereton, L., Gardiner, C., Gott, M., Ingelton, C., Barnes, S., and Carrroll, C. The hospital environment for end of life care of older adults and their families: An integrative review. *Journal of Advanced Nursing* 2011, 68: 981–93.

22. Ford, K., Tesch, L., Dawborn, J. et al. Art, music, story: The evaluation of a person-centred arts in health programme in an acute care older people's unit. *Int J Older People Nurs* 2018. doi: 10.1111/opn.12186.

23. Istvandity, L. Combining music and reminiscence therapy interventions for wellbeing in elderly populations: A systematic review. *Complement Ther Clin Pract* 2018, 28: 18–25.

24. Parke, B., Boltz, M., Hunter, K.F. et al. A scoping literature review of dementia-friendly hospital design. *Gerontologist* 2017, 57: e62–e74.

25. O'Keeffe, S., and Lavan, J. The prognostic significance of delirium in older hospital patients. *J Am Geriatr Soc* 1997, 45: 174–8.

26. Vazquez, F., O'Flaherty, M., Michelangelo, H. et al. Epidemiology of delirium in elderly inpatients. *Medicina* 2000, 60: 555–60.

27. Edlund, A., Lundstrom, M., Karlsson, S. et al. Delirium in older patients admitted to general internal medicine. *J Geriatr Psychiatry Neurol* 2006, 19: 83–90.

28. Campbell, N., Boustani, M.A., Ayub, A. et al. Pharmacological management of delirium in hospitalized adults-systematic evidence review. *J Gen Intern Med* 2009, 24: 848–53.

29. Lonergan, E., Britton, A.M., Luxenberg, J. et al. Antipsychotics for delirium. *Cochrane Database Syst Rev* 2007, 18: CD005594. doi: 10.1002/14651858. CD005594.pub2.

30. McCusker, J., Cole, M., and Abrahamowicz, M. Environmental risk factors for delirium in hospitalized older people. *J Am Geriatr Soc* 2001, 49: 1327–34.

31. Anon., E.D. Meet the needs of aging patients with a senior-friendly ED. *ED Management: The Monthly Update on Emergency Department Management* 2011, 23: 85–8.

32. Missildine, K. Sleep and the sleep environment of older adults in acute care settings. *Journal of Gerontological Nursing* 2008, 34: 15–21.

33. Flaherty, J.H., and Little, M.O. Matching the environment to patients with delirium: Lessons learned from the delirium room, a restraint-free environment for older hospitalized adults with delirium. *JAGS* 2011, 59: S295–S300.

34. Mazzei, F. Exploring the influence of environment on the spatial behaviour of older adults in a purpose-built acute care dementia unit. *American Journal of Alzheimer's Disease and Other Dementias* 2014, 4: 311–19.

35. Day, J., Higgins, I., and Keatinge, D. Orientation strategies during delirium: are they helpful? *Journal of Clinical Nursing* 2011, 20: 3285–94.

36. Anon. Specialised environments to meet the needs of older people. *Nursing Older People* 2007, 19: 39. Abstract at https://journals.rcni.com/doi/abs/10.7748/nop .19.2.39.s25.

Communication with Older People

Sarmishtha Bhattacharyya and Susan Benbow

It is believed that good communication is an important part of the healing process and lies at the heart of healthcare. It is key to preventing hospital admissions, providing appropriate treatment, and facilitating early discharge. Physical, physiological, sensory, psychological, and social changes associated with ageing impact on communication so that more time and patience may be needed in encounters with older adults.

This chapter explores factors affecting communication, namely factors related to the professional, the patient, the environment, the social context, and non-verbal communication. We examine the impact of increasing age and the needs of specific populations, such as people with protected characteristics and people with dementia. Language and communication are a major concern in providing services for black and minority ethnic elders. We explore the need to approach people with sensitivity and understanding.

Older people often present with multiple comorbidities. There is a dynamic interaction between physical and mental health, which may be impossible to separate. Integrated work and effective liaising between professionals and agencies facilitate person-centred care. As carers are in direct communication with older people and their family, their listening is as important as sharing information.

We present two reflective cases designed to aid personal learning and we conclude with tips for improving communication with older adults and with people with dementia.

Context: The Importance of Communication

The Oxford English Dictionary defines communication as 'the imparting or exchanging of information by speaking, writing, or using some other medium'. Good communication is person-centred and addresses clearly the needs of the individual. Person-centred care involves treating people with respect and dignity, and communication is fundamental to this: its goal is to hear what people say and to convey information to people clearly and simply, in a way that means that necessary things are understood and get done.

Good communication is an essential part of everyday healthcare practice and a teachable skill. Studies in the United States have reported that effective physician–patient communication has broader benefits: patients are more likely to adhere to treatment and health outcomes are better (1). Communication skills are indispensable to nursing care, as communicating effectively helps to reduce the risk of medical errors, ensures better patient outcomes, and nurtures patient satisfaction (2). A study of barriers to communication identified by nurses and patients found the most common barriers perceived by patients to be gender differences between nurse and patient; nurses' reluctance to communicate; a hectic ward environment; and anxiety, pain, and physical discomfort affecting the patient (3). The main factors identified from a nurse's perspective were differences in the language of nurses and patients, family interference, emergency admissions, and nurses being overworked. The authors concluded that it is essential to teach nurses communication skills and that there should be ongoing monitoring of such training. The study did not specifically focus on older adults, but the barriers identified, which were classified as nurse–patient, nurse-related, patient-related, and environmental, are applicable to communication with both younger and older adults and probably apply equally to healthcare professionals other than nurses.

Research shows that, even when older patients have appropriate access to medical services, they also need effective and empathic communication as an essential part of their treatment (4). This is even more so in older adults who are socially isolated, emotionally vulnerable, and economically disadvantaged, and therefore in need of the social, emotional, and practical support that sensitive provider–patient communication can provide.

Anecdotal evidence suggests that, in the past, older adults have held health professionals in high esteem and have been ready to accept advice. However, aging Baby Boomers are likely to take a more active and collaborative approach to managing their health care, and this will require partnership with healthcare professionals (5).

Basic Factors Affecting Communication

Table 4.1 sets out some of the important factors influencing communication and a few questions for healthcare professionals to consider. The factors are organised into the following categories: factors that affect the professional; factors that affect the patient; environmental factors; factors related to the social context; and factors of non-verbal communication.

The Healthcare Professional

Healthcare professionals are trained in communication skills, but when they are tired, stressed, or busy these skills may not be fully engaged. Under pressure, communication may be suboptimal, however highly qualified the professional.

Hospitals can be busy and confusing places. Patients are not only ill; they may be confused, frightened, and uncertain about what is happening to them. Modern healthcare involves a team of people whose roles patients may not fully understand, and these patients may have to get to know a number of new people who are all involved in their treatment. There have been campaigns to make sure that healthcare professionals introduce themselves to patients (visit e.g. https://hellomynameis.org.uk), but introduction may be needed on several occasions, or even every time, especially if people are confused or have a concurrent dementia. It is important to assume that, even if one is wearing a uniform and a name badge, introduction is still necessary, polite, and respectful.

Other healthcare professional factors influence communication, for example gender and age differences, cultural and religious differences, and different uses of language – all between the professional and the patient. Some of these differences may foster in both the patient and the health professional unhelpful assumptions about the other. The health professional may be influenced by stereotypes associated with particular patient

Table 4.1 Some important factors influencing communication and a few questions to consider

Category of factors	General points to consider	Points particularly relevant to older adults
The healthcare professional	Introduce yourself Explain your role Make sure tiredness, stress, and busyness are not affecting your approach Consider whether gender, age, cultural or other differences are influencing the conversational encounter Adjust your language to suit the patient (without patronising them)	Adjust your pace to suit the patient Make sure that the patient can see you clearly and that your speech is clearly enunciated You may need to wear clear masks and visors Be appropriately respectful towards an older person
The patient	Sensory impairments affecting communication Physical health issues affecting the conversation Medications affecting the conversation Psychological factors that may need to be addressed	This person has hearing aid This person is wearing glasses This person has false teeth: are they in place? Does this person need extra time for the encounter? Check that the patient has retained earlier information – or does it need to be repeated?
The environment	Minimise distractions (visual and auditory) Ensure privacy Consider whether the conversational topic is particularly sensitive Ensure that sufficient time is available to talk and allow for questions	If the patient is confused or very anxious, make sure they understand where they are and what is happening
The social context	Ask yourself whether you are being influenced by preconceptions or myths pertinent to this patient	Address the patient appropriately Having a relative present: does it help or hinder the assessment?
Non-verbal communication	Reflect on whether your non-verbal communications amplify your verbal communication Consider using other modalities (e.g. written material) for help	Use touch cue appropriately with the person in conversation

characteristics, and these stereotypes will serve only to impair conversational encounters even further. Such stereotypes may be related to age or to something completely different, for example the person's ethnicity, a learning disability, or alcohol or substance abuse.

When under pressure, professionals may need to slow down deliberately in order to accommodate the needs of an ill older person. Adjusting one's pace to the individual may be very helpful.

The Patient

Older people may have physical factors affecting communication. For example, they may have sensory impairments. Does the patient use a hearing aid? Have they got it with them? Is it working? Hearing difficulty may be exacerbated when the person talking with the patient speaks with an unfamiliar accent. The patient may have impaired vision: do they wear glasses? Have they got their glasses with them? Are the lenses clean enough to aid, rather than further impair, the person's vision?

Other physical factors may influence the encounter, too. Is the person in pain and unable to focus on the conversation? Are they on medications that make them drowsy and unable to concentrate? Is their mouth very dry (often a side-effect of drug treatment), which makes it more difficult for the person to enunciate words properly? Does the person usually wear false teeth? Do they have specific conditions that influence their ability to communicate, for example post-stroke dysphasia, dysarthria, or Parkinson's disease? Are they acutely or chronically confused, as this may influence their grasp of the situation?

Similarly, psychological factors may affect the encounter. If patients are depressed or anxious, they may not be able to concentrate on a conversation. Other people may be lacking in confidence, feeling vulnerable, or feeling disempowered. Being ill and lying in bed in nightclothes in an unfamiliar environment is not conducive to feeling an equal partner in conversation: some patients may react with anger and frustration, which may in turn impact on health professionals in a manner that irritates, frustrates, or antagonises them and further exacerbates difficulties. Others may feel that they are not being listened to and give up trying to express their needs and views.

The Environment

Hospitals are often noisy places with lots of activity and a myriad of people coming and going. Change of wards due to lack of beds may have a similar effect: as soon as a person gets to know the environment and the staff, he or she may be moved to another ward. The impact of a move will be greater if the person is confused. Being constantly distracted by auditory and visual stimuli can have a big effect on a person's ability to take part in communication. Lack of privacy may also influence what people are prepared to talk about; the person in the next bed could well have nothing to do but listen in to nearby conversations, and, if the topic is particularly sensitive, it will not help if people constantly interrupt. This is also the case when a professional is attempting cognitive testing with someone who is thought to be cognitively impaired.

From the professional's perspective, acutely ill patients and frequent new or emergency admissions may consume their attention and concern, cutting into the available time they have to communicate with other patients. It is important to be aware of patients who may not express their needs assertively and therefore risk being ignored.

The Social Context

To an elderly person, a doctor or a nurse may look surprisingly young (can they possibly be qualified, when they look just out of school?). An informal manner may appear disrespectful. How does this patient like to be addressed? We still sometimes meet elderly couples who, in conversation with a third party, refer to each other as 'Mr' and

'Mrs'. It may be safer to use Mr, Mrs, Miss or other appropriate mode of address, or to ask people how they prefer to be addressed.

Social barriers affect communication. For example, healthcare staff could make assumptions about patients on the basis of their age, culture, behaviour, or known disabilities, including sensory impairments or dementia. Communication with some of the staff members could be influenced by ageist preconceptions: they may believe, for example, that people with dementia cannot make decisions, or that older patients are of less worth than younger patients. This has certainly been revealed in palliative care (6, 7).

It is important not to stereotype older people. Communication will vary according to individual needs and behaviours, hence talking to a fit 90-year-old is different from talking to a frail 70-year-old. Moreover, some older adults find it discriminatory to be referred to as old or elderly, so choice of words needs consideration and care.

Tom Kitwood used the term 'malignant social psychology' to encompass the ways in which society and all of us in it can disempower and devalue people with dementia. Some of the behaviours that fall under Kitwood's umbrella term are relevant to communicating with ill older adults, for example outpacing them in conversation, not taking appropriate actions to help them to engage, intimidating frail people by pushing them to do things or take decisions that they might be uncomfortable with, or turning to family members for accounts of the older adult's experience and for answers to questions that the older adult should answer. The label 'malignant social psychology' is a salubrious reminder of how we can contribute, unthinkingly, to disempowering and excluding older people (8).

Non-Verbal Communication

While speech is an important mode of communication, non-verbal communication can also help or hinder a conversational encounter. Appropriate use of touch, provided that the patient is comfortable with it, may help that patient to focus on the communicator. For example, touching the person's arm when talking with them may cue them in to making eye contact with the speaker and to concentrating on the conversation; and eye contact itself is particularly important if the patient has hearing impairment and uses lip-reading skills. In addition, body language can amplify and extend what is being said: for example, the question 'Would you like to sit down?' may be accompanied by a gesture indicating a chair to sit in. Being with someone in silence may be a helpful and supportive way of communicating when that person is distressed. Listening and taking time are important aspects of communication that may be difficult to accomplish in busy environments.

Other means of communication may also be employed, either to extend or to replace communication that relies on speech. People with dementia may be able to sing despite having little speech. Drawing, painting, or other artistic expression may enable people to express how they are feeling. This might be of limited use in a busy hospital setting, but writing or drawing can be helpful in some circumstances, and with some patients picture charts can be used to good effect as communication aids.

Agitated people with dementia or confusional states sometimes find it easier to communicate while being active, for example while walking around when they can safely do so, or while having an aromatherapy massage.

The Covid-19 pandemic has made it compulsory for all to wear masks and for health and social care staff to wear personal protective equipment (PPE) such as masks or visors, to protect patients as well as themselves. However, some important aspects of communication remain non-verbal, for example eye contact, lip-reading, and matching speech with facial expression. This may be especially important for a person who is not able to hear well or is confused or unsure. PPE may also intimidate patients, in particular those who are confused and unable to understand the reason for its use. The use of PPE continues, but consideration needs to be given to its effect on communication in these circumstances.

Breaking Bad News

Breaking bad news well is an essential skill for doctors, but historically it has received little attention in medical training. Clinicians often deliver bad news, for example a difficult diagnosis or a poor prognosis, and this may occur most often in acute hospital settings (9). All the factors mentioned earlier need to be taken into account, but empathy, sensitivity, time, and listening skills are especially important when imparting unwelcome news (10). Poor communication, particularly with cancer patients, has been shown to be associated with worse clinical and psychosocial outcomes, worse adherence to treatment, confusion over prognosis, and dissatisfaction with not being involved in decision-making (11). If appropriate, a family member may be present together with an older person, to understand and support that person once confidentiality issues have been considered. An allocated quiet room and adequate time for questions explanations facilitate difficult conversations. These are examples of good practice.

Communication Barriers in Older People

With advancing age, people may accumulate age-related barriers to communication. Ageing is accompanied by physiological changes in speech, hearing, and vision, all of which may contribute to difficulties in a conversational encounter, particularly in an unfamiliar environment and when engaging with unfamiliar people at a time of increased anxiety.

Alongside physiological changes, physical conditions such as stroke, Parkinson's disease, and dementia may have a long-term and serious direct effects on communication. Thus older persons' communication may be impaired in a number of ways. For example, they may experience word-finding problems and talk around the word in a manner that makes them appear more confused; may use repetitive words or phrases; may confuse semantically related words such as 'he' and 'she', 'wife' and 'mother'; may suffer loss of fluency; may have difficulty comprehending complex speech or sentences; may get stuck and come to a full stop; or may lose track of what they want to say.

Other physical conditions can indirectly affect communication. People with severe kyphoscoliosis sometimes have difficulty making eye contact during conversation with others and, if they lipread, this will exacerbate communication difficulties. Impaired mobility may affect patients' ability to position themselves optimally in relation to conversational partners.

Older people may have multiple comorbidities, and there is often a dynamic inter-action between physical and mental health conditions, which are closely intertwined. Communication is likely to require sensitivity, time, and patience when there is a combination of these factors.

Ageist stereotypes may influence the patient as well as the health professional. For example, a person who sees her- or himself as old and approaching the end of life may be less likely to advocate active treatment of conditions that she or he consider to be part of getting older, or may regard deteriorating health as only to be expected and not something that is worth seeking advice for or treatment of. Ageist preconceptions on behalf of the patient and the professional may influence their encounter in terms of both what is communicated and how it is communicated.

Research on communication with residents in long-term care (LTC) settings has identified 'elderspeak' (12), which has been defined as an

> intergenerational communication style that is common in interactions between staff and residents in LTC settings. Elderspeak (i.e. infantilization, or secondary baby talk) features simplistic vocabulary and grammar, shortened sentences, slowed speech, elevated pitch and volume, and inappropriately intimate terms of endearment.
>
> ((12), p. 12)

The authors found that elderspeak contributes to behavioural and psychological symp-toms of dementia and resistance to care. While elderspeak may be more commonly employed in communication with people with dementia, some components of it may be used with older people generally, especially if a communicator is influenced by ageist stereotypes. It is important for health professionals to tailor their communication to their conversational partner, but at the same time to avoid patronizing and disrespectful language and approaches.

Protected Characteristics

Black and minority ethnic (BME) groups make up just under 20 per cent of the population of England and Wales, and 8 per cent of the BME population in England and Wales is aged 60 and over (13). The use of interpreters in such population groups may enhance or diminish good communication. Language and communication form a major area of concern in improving BME elders' access to healthcare services. There is a need for sensitivity in approaching BME elders in order to ensure patient dignity and to promote person-centred care.

Similarly, people who identify as lesbian, gay, bisexual, transgender, gender-variant, gender-non-conforming, or intersex may not share information relevant to their health and well-being unless they are approached in a sensitive and respectful manner, which avoids preconceptions and leaves space for them to disclose. Disability is another protected characteristic and encompasses physical and mental disabilities, including significant intellectual disabilities in people who also need a sensitive, tailored approach – particularly when the intellectual disability is compli-cated by ageing or dementia (or both). Unconditionally positive regard for others and a non-judgemental approach are essential qualities in those who provide care to a diverse population.

Use of Interpreters

Lack of appropriate communication between healthcare professionals and BME elders can undermine trust and increase the risks to patient safety (14). Myths about these communities, their engagement with professionals, and access to services remain influential (15).

An European study found that the type of interpreter (professional or non-professional) was decided by professionals in everyday healthcare (16). Professional interpreters were used for medical issues and care planning issues, and non-professional interpreters (such as bilingual healthcare staff and family members) were used for everyday caring issues and for unpredictable issues that come up at short notice.

Interpreting services may be inadequate and rely too heavily and inappropriately on family and friends (17). This can have implications for the patient, as the family may collude with patients or be too anxious to give adequate and appropriate information. One study showed that the content of advice and guidance on critical matters such as compliance with treatment regimes might not be fully understood; psychological support for patients and carers may be limited; and privacy and confidentiality may be compromised (17).

Another study highlighted a lack of awareness of interpreting services among members of BME community groups, and difficulty communicating in English meant that they were unable to articulate their needs to the health professionals with whom they had contact. They lacked a voice and relied on primary care nurses to provide them with the opportunity to access an interpreter. The limited knowledge that some nurses had about interpreting services meant that they were not in a position to enable community participants to make informed choices as to whether they preferred an interpreter or a family member (18). Interpretation by family members can be influenced by their own views. In some situations in hospital care, it is necessary for healthcare practitioners to involve a professional interpreter in order to get responses uninfluenced by family relationships.

Box 4.1 sets out a case vignette involving the use of an interpreter.

Box 4.1 A reflective case designed to illustrate the use of family as interpreters

Mrs Singh, 70, widowed, presents to a memory clinic with self-neglect, apathy, and some confusion. Her son is present and says that she understands English, but the clinician is unable to make out what she is saying. The son starts to act as an interpreter.

The son reports that his mother is fine and, although she sits in a corner most of the day, she is no different from what she was a year ago. She has never taken much interest in housework or finances, and all the daily chores are done by her daughter-in-law. The son is angry that the GP has referred his mum for a possible diagnosis of dementia, as he feels that his mother is just 'old' and fine.

It appears to the clinician that he is answering questions for her.

- How would you handle this situation?
- Is the son best placed to act as an interpreter?
- What options are there for managing the situation?
- How would you decide what is in Mrs Singh's best interests?
- What would you consider when engaging an interpreter from outside the family? Would a female interpreter from the same community help?
- How would you respond if family members want to be present during the assessment?

Communication with People with Dementia

Communication with people with dementia requires paying attention to the same principles as those involved in communication with people of all ages. It is important to avoid using 'elderspeak', although people who are confused, distracted, and struggling to concentrate may benefit from shorter, simpler sentences and a slower pace. Speech needs to be tailored to the conversational partner. Time, patience, and empathy are essential in such situations.

When someone is known to have memory problems, it may be even more important to supplement verbal communication with written materials that this person and the family can take away and study at leisure, in a less stressful environment. Copying letters to patients was an initiative introduced by the Department of Health some years ago, and can contribute to achieving a clear communication with both a person with dementia and the family (19). Repetition will also be important in communicating with people with dementia, as they may not recall previous conversations.

The key principles of the Mental Capacity Act 2005 guide us to presume capacity. For someone to demonstrate that they have the capacity to make a specific decision, they need to understand, retain, weigh in the balance, arrive at a decision, and communicate that decision. Hence all avenues to enhance communication need to be explored in order to exchange information about a particular decision that is to be made. For example, written documents or pictures may be required in order for the person to understand the context. Moreover, if the person cannot see or hear, other means of communication will be necessary. Until and unless all avenues have been explored, one should not presume incapacity. Even in the case of those people who are proved to lack the capacity to make particular decisions, it is important that the relevant decisions are communicated to them in an appropriate way and that they are involved as far as they are able.

One of the tricky topics often raised in the context of communication with people with dementia is so-called therapeutic lying. For example, a person with dementia is likely to ask where their deceased spouse or parent is, and may be distressed or shocked if told that the spouse or parent in question died some years ago. This may prompt those around to take the view that it would be 'kinder' to tell a 'little white lie', for example by saying that the spouse or parent is out and will be back later (or something similar). The term 'therapeutic lying' has been used in this context, and guidelines for therapeutic lies have been suggested. Such guidelines suggest that lies should be told only in the best interest of the patient, after assessment of mental capacity. The lie would need to be agreed upon, documented, and used consistently across all settings, as a way of enhancing well-being after considering the potential risks and benefits of using this lie. It should not lead to a situation where the person with dementia is disrespected. Is this practice ethical? Professionals may take differing positions on this question and other ways of managing the situation should always be considered, as so-called therapeutic lies may have unintended consequences.

People with dementia have been studied for their views on the use of lies in dementia care, and the acceptability of lies and deception in this field has been found to vary according to whether or not the lie is in the person's best interest (20). Three themes were found to be relevant to the best interest decision: the person with dementia who is being lied to; the people who do the lying; and the nature of the lie itself. Figure 4.1 is adapted from Day et al.'s paper and illustrates the complex relationship between these themes when it comes to the acceptability of using lies in dementia care. Box 4.2 illustrates the complexity of lying to people with dementia and, to preserve anonymity, is based on an amalgam of real cases.

Box 4.2   A reflective case to illustrate the use of so-called therapeutic lying

Harry has Alzheimer's disease complicated by several chronic physical illnesses, such that his wife, Gladys, who has her own health problems, is unable to continue to care for him in their home. He moves into care and for a long time she visits him regularly, several times a week.

She then has a stroke, is admitted to hospital, and dies shortly afterwards. Their son, David, contacts the home to say that under no circumstances should Harry be told that Gladys has died, as he would get very upset. The staff members looking after Harry feel uncomfortable about this and are not sure what to do.

- How would you handle this situation?
- Is David the sole arbiter of the decision?
- What options are there for managing the situation?
- How would you decide what is in Harry's best interests? And what factors would you want to take into account?
- What are the potential consequences of telling Harry that Gladys has died?
- What are the potential consequences of keeping Gladys's death from Harry?

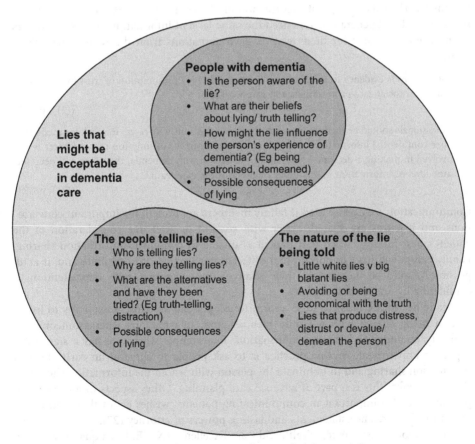

Figure 4.1 Perspectives of people with dementia regarding so-called therapeutic lies (adapted from (20))

Communication with Family and Family Carers

Being in hospital is stressful not just for the patient but also for carers and families. In many situations family members may be able to support communication between staff members and the patient, as they know the patient well. In some situations, however, family members may exacerbate the communication problems, for example by repeatedly jumping in and answering for the patient and not allowing the patient to relate his or her experiences and give his or her own views. This is often a result of anxiety on the part of the carer or family member. It may be anxiety that the patient would not give an accurate account of his or her illness; it may be anxiety that the carer would be unable to pass on to the health professional the relevant information or ask the questions that the carer or family member feels are important. Thus it may be helpful to explain the importance of hearing from the patient and to ask the carer not to interrupt, making it clear that the carer will have the opportunity to share his or her account, information, or questions later. In particularly difficult situations, it may be necessary to kindly but firmly ask the relative to leave in order to allow the patient to talk unattended.

With respect to people who may be unable to consent to aspects of their care and treatment, a report entitled *Dementia: Ethical Issues*, by the Nuffield Council on Bioethics (21), makes the point that the notion of 'best interest' is often interpreted too narrowly and that generally carers need the same level of information as other members of the team that cares for their relative. Two quotations from the report make these points:

> Unless there is evidence to the contrary, there should be a presumption of trust in carers by health and social care professionals and care workers.
>
> ((21), p. 120)

> Professionals should be made aware of the legitimate reasons why carers may ask for medical or other confidential information, and ordinarily start from the assumption that if a carer is involved in making a decision on behalf of the person with dementia, then they will need the same level of information as any other member of the care team.
>
> ((21), p. 121)

Communication may be assisted if family members are present for important conversations and if letters are shared, either with consent or after due consideration of the patient's best interest, when that patient is unable to consent to information sharing. Family carers will have important and different perspectives to contribute and, if at all possible, should be included in their relative's care planning, with due attention to confidentiality and mental capacity.

Many healthcare providers use a form to ask patients to consent explicitly to information being shared with a family member and, in situations where someone has difficulty retaining and sharing information, for example when one has a significant cognitive impairment, routine practice is to ask people to agree at an early stage to information sharing and to nominate the person with whom the information should be shared. In effect this is a part of advance care planning. Other aspects of advance care planning are also important in communicating patients' wishes about their end-of-life care, including advance statements and lasting powers of attorney (22).

The National Institute for Health and Care Excellence (NICE) has a quality standard on advocacy for people with dementia that requires that people with dementia be enabled, with the involvement of their carers, to access independent advocacy services (23). The Covid-19 pandemic led to restrictions on hospital visits that reduced carers' ability to communicate with loved ones and with healthcare professionals. In these difficult circumstances, the safe use of video calls can be helpful and comforting. It is also important to ensure that regular telephone contact between healthcare professionals and families continues, in order to keep family members updated and involved in decision-making. This may create a new challenge to future communication channels between older adults, their carers, and professionals during hospital admissions.

There remains nonetheless a myth around older adults and their inability to use remote devices for assessment. We should not automatically presume that technological devices cannot be used as a way of communication; rather we should offer our older patients the opportunity to use them, should they wish to do so.

Communication between Health Professionals

Communication between health professionals and between health and social care is often important in ensuring joined-up care of people with multiple comorbidities and with complex physical and mental health conditions. Older adults and their families can be kept in the loop, if letters are copied to them – provided that the patient consents or that this is in the patient's best interest when he or she is unable to make a decision about information sharing (19). General practitioners are often key to patient care, and information needs to be shared appropriately with them. Some healthcare professionals have experimented with carer-held records for people with dementia (24) as a way of improving information sharing when a number of practitioners are involved with one patient; but a systematic review of the use of patient-held records for patients living with chronic disease concluded that it did not clearly benefit care or improve patient satisfaction (25).

Integrated work and good communication among various professionals and agencies, as well as between the older person and his or her carers, can provide good person-centred care. General practitioners and social services have an important role to play in the care of older people. Communication with them is therefore vital to improving patient care and safety in older adults. Services aim to be person-centred but should be equally relationship-centred, which means involving the families and ensuring continuity of care (26).

Care plans should be developed collaboratively and communicated clearly to those who provide care. In practice, this should mean that the nurse and the medic or named consultant draft the plan together with the carer or the family. They should also work with social care staff members, families, and carers to ensure and support the discharge planning upon admission.

Some hospitals use visual signals such as the Butterfly Scheme (butterflyscheme.org. uk) to communicate to staff that a person has dementia. A national audit on dementia (27) reported that just over 40 per cent of hospitals had a system in place to make staff aware of a person's dementia, and of these hospitals just over 60 per cent used a visual symbol or an indicator to impart this information. The scheme is intended to avoid stigmatising people with dementia, but some might argue that, by identifying people by a special symbol, it risks doing the reverse.

Alzheimer's Society has developed a useful leaflet titled 'This is me', which aims to assist in gathering and sharing personal lifestory information and to support person-centred care (28).

How to Improve Communication with Older Adults

Communication is a multidimensional and multifactorial phenomenon, which is affected by extrinsic and intrinsic factors. Box 4.3 lists some general tips for improving communication and Box 4.4 lists tips for improving communication with people living with dementia.

It is important to acknowledge that there is no one-size-fits-all approach to giving information to patients, and physicians must gauge the appropriate amount of information for each patient and the best way in which to convey it, for example by using more than one modality – say, written materials, drawings, websites, experts by experience, audiotapes, or videos – to supplement speech. Too much information can overwhelm some patients, while too little may leave others distressed and confused (4). Appropriate information transfer for each patient is central to a strong and effective therapeutic relationship and has important implications for patients' health. Above all this, as healthcare professionals, we must listen to our patients and their families and try

---

Box 4.3 Ten tips to improve communication with older adults

- Remember that older adults, just like younger people, are diverse and unique: one approach does not fit all.
- Introduce yourself and explain your role – they may not remember meeting you before.
- Use a respectful form of address, say, 'Mr Smith' not just 'John' – unless they give you permission to address them by their first name.
- Show respect.
- Establish rapport; this may need more time.
- Be aware of sensory difficulties: check if hearing aid or glasses are needed and in place.
- Try to understand what the person is going though.
- Practise active listening.
- Avoid jargon.
- Ensure privacy for confidential or sensitive matters.

Box 4.4 Ten tips to improve communication with people with dementia

- Be seen.
- Minimise distractions.
- Think about your body language.
- Make eye contact.
- Speak clearly, calmly, simply, avoid complexity.
- Think about the NOW.
- Go slowly.
- LISTEN – and try to get 'in their shoes'.
- Show interest and get to know the person.
- Use memory aids.

to understand their perspectives, experiences, and wishes, if we are to provide them with care that meets their needs.

References

1. National Institute on Aging. Tips for communicating with older patients. NIH, Talking with your older patients, 2017. www.nia.nih.gov/health/tips-improving-communication-older-patients.

2. Lang, E.V. A better patient experience through better communication. *Journal of Radiology Nursing* 2012, 31(4): 114–19.

3. Norouzinia, R., Aghabarari, M., Shiri, M., Karimi, M., and Samami, E. Communication barriers perceived by nurses and patients. *Global Journal of Health Science* 2016, 8(6): 65–74.

4. Williams, S.L., Haskard, K.B., and DiMatteo, M.R. The therapeutic effects of the physician-older patient relationship: Effective communication with vulnerable older patients. *Clin Interv Aging* 2007, 2 (3): 453–67.

5. National Institute on Aging. Providing care to a diverse older adult population. NIH, 2017. www.nia.nih.gov/health/providing-care-diverse-older-adult-population.

6. Lloyd, A., Kendall, M., Carduff, E., Cavers, D., Kimbell, B., and Murray, S.A. Why do older people get less palliative care than younger people? *European Journal of Palliative Care* 2016, 23(3): 132–7.

7. Macmillan Cancer Support. *The Age Old Excuse: The Under Treatment of Older Cancer Patients.* 2012. www.macmillan .org.uk/documents/getinvolved/campaigns/ageoldexcuse/ageoldexcusereport-macmillancancersupport.pdf.

8. Kitwood, T. *Dementia Reconsidered: The Person Comes First.* Buckingham: Open University Press, 1997.

9. Schildmann, J., Cushing, A., Doyal, L. et al. Breaking bad news: Experiences, views and difficulties of pre-registration house officers. *Palliative Medicine* 2005, 19(2): 93–8.

10. General Medical Council. *Good Medical Practice.* 2013. http://www.gmc-uk.org/guidance/good_medical_practice.asp.

11. Hanratty, B., Lowson, E., Holmes, L. et al. Breaking bad news sensitively: What is important to patients in their last year of life? *BMJ Support Palliat Care* 2012, 2(1): 24–8.

12. Williams, K.N., Herman, R., Gajweski, B., and Wilson, K. Elderspeak communication: Impact on dementia care. *Am J Alzheimers Dis Other Demen* 2009, 24(1): 11–20.

13. Office for National Statistics. Population estimates by ethnic group (experimental), Mid-2009. WHO, 18 May 2011. http://www.ons.gov.uk/ons/rel/peeg/population-estimates-by-ethnic-group-experimental-/current-estimates/index .html.

14. Divi, C., Koss, R., Schmaltz, S., and Loeb, J. Language proficiency and adverse events in US hospitals: a pilot study *Int J Qual Health Care* 2007, 19(2): 60–7.

15. Bhattacharyya, S., and Benbow, S.M. Mental health services for black and minority ethnic elders in the United Kingdom: A systematic review of innovative practice with service provision and policy implications. *International Psychogeriatrics* 2013, 25(03): 359–73.

16. Hadziabdic, E., Lundin, C., and Hjelm, K. Boundaries and conditions of interpretation in multilingual and multicultural elderly healthcare. *BMC Health Services Research* 2015, 15: 458.

17. Gerrish, K. The nature and effect of communication difficulties arising from interactions between district nurses and South Asian patients and their carers. *Journal of Advanced Nursing* 2001, 33: 566–74.

18. Gerrish, K., Chau, R., Sobowale, E., and Birks, E. Bridging the language barrier: The use of interpreters in primary care

nursing. *Health and Social Care in the Community* 2004, 12(5): 407–13.

19. Clark, M., Benbow, S., Scott, V., Moreland, N., and Jolley, D. Copying letters to older people in mental health services: Policy with unfulfilled potential. Quality in Ageing and Older Adults 2008, 9(3): 31–8.

20. Day, A.M., James, I.A., Meyer, T.D., and Lee, D.R. Do people with dementia find lies and deception in dementia care acceptable? *Aging and Mental Health* 2011, 15: 822–9.

21. Nuffield Council on Bioethics. The needs of carers. In Nuffield Council on Bioethics, *Dementia: Ethical Issues.* Cambridge, 2009, pp. 114–25. http://nuffieldbioethics.org/wp-content/uploads/Dementia-Chapter-7-The-needs-of-carers.pdf.

22. Henry, C., and Seymour, J. Advance care planning: A guide for health and social care staff. NHS, 2008. www.ncpc.org.uk/sites/default/files/AdvanceCarePlanning.pdf.

23. National Institute for Health and Care Excellence. *Dementia: Independence and Wellbeing: Quality Standard.* QS30, 2013. www.nice.org.uk/guidance/qs184/documents/previous-version-of-quality-standard-2.

24. Sato, S., Kazui, H., Shimizu, Y., Yoshida, T., Yoshiyama, K., Kanemoto, H. et al. Usefulness of carer-held records to support informal caregivers of patients with dementia who live at home. *Psychogeriatrics* 2018, 18(3): 166–74.

25. Ko, H., Turner, T., Jones, C., and Hill, C. Patient-held medical records for patients with chronic disease: A systematic review. *Quality and Safety in Health Care* 2010, 19(5): e41.

26. Benbow, S.M., and Bhattacharyya, S. Older peoples' mental health and wellbeing. Paper 3 in Growing Older in the UK: A Series of Briefings on Ageing and Health. *BMA, London, 2016. www.bma.org.uk/media/2105/supporting-healthy-ageing-briefings-final.pdf.*

27. Royal College of Psychiatrists. *National Audit of Dementia Care in General Hospitals 2012–13: Second Round Audit Report and Update.* London: Healthcare Quality Improvement Partnership, 2013. www.rcpsych.ac.uk/pdf/NAD%20NATIONAL%20REPORT%202013%20reports%20page.pdf.

28. Alzheimer's Society UK. This is me: A support tool to enable person-centred care. 2018. www.alzheimers.org.uk/get-support/publications-factsheets/this-is-me.

Privacy and Dignity in Acute Hospitals

Eve Braithwaite and Sean Ninan

Introduction

Age discrimination is one the most common forms of discrimination in the United Kingdom. The most common representation of older people is one of biological, physical, and mental decline, and society views an ageing population negatively, as an ageing tsunami or a demographic time bomb (1). It is a curious sort of discrimination, which betrays a lack of empathy, from the young and the middle aged, towards their future selves, almost denying the fact that it cannot be avoided without prematurely dying.

> 'What folly made young people, even those in middle age, think they were immortal? How much better, their lives, if they could remember the end. Carrying your death with you every day would make it hard to waste time on unkindness and anger and bitterness, on anything petty. That was the secret: remembering your dying time, in order to keep the stupid and the ugly out of your living time' (2).

This is, unfortunately, reflected in the way we care for older people, as numerous reports highlight deficiencies in care (3–9). The Francis Report laid bare inadequacies in the provision of nutrition and hydration, deficiencies in supplying personal hygiene care, and a lack of person-centred care – all of which meant that patients were not treated with dignity and respect.

Witness statements included reports of patients left unwashed, lying in a soiled bed as a result of not being taken to the toilet, and reports of patients who were not given assistance to eat when they were unable to feed themselves.

> The ward was noisy and chaotic and the patient was so distressed by other patients that he was unable to sleep. Water and food were left on his table, but he could not reach them and when a family friend questioned the nurse in charge she responded that she 'was only a bank nurse' and was 'too busy' to answer questions. On one occasion the patient told his daughter that he was afraid to spill his drink, as if he did his sheets would not be changed and he would stay in dirty, wet ones (9).

The report discusses a culture in which individuals do not take responsibility for reporting issues or for addressing them as they happen. People considered issues not to be their own personal responsibility. Additionally, tolerating poor care was accepted either for fear that it would be too difficult to change or on the grounds that it could be perceived as 'normal' within hospital. Apart from personal responsibility, it was noted that management failed to recognise and respond appropriately to concerns raised by staff and to complaints submitted by patients. In his report, Sir Robert Francis made

290 recommendations for changes designed to reduce poor care as seen at Mid Stafford Trust. It was recommended clear that standards of care should be set by the government, by clinical commissioning groups, and by professional bodies. At the centre of these recommendations was ensuring that patients' safety and well-being is the first priority. But there was a strong focus on dignity too, particularly for older people, who may be most at risk of receiving substandard care; and there was an even greater focus on quality, as well as on saving money and being financially frugal (10).

Older people may have surprisingly low expectations of what constitutes acceptable care; there are accounts of undignified care being tolerated with an attitude of reluctance to complain or gratitude for having a national health service (11). A study titled *Dignity in Practice* that explores dignified care in hospitals identified conflicts of interest between the priorities of hospital organisations, members of staff, and patients that came out in the Francis Report. Components of dignified care were considered to be

- respectful communication;
- respecting privacy;
- promoting autonomy and a sense of control;
- addressing basic human needs such as nutrition, elimination, and personal hygiene or appearance in a respective and sensitive manner;
- being inclusive and encouraging participation;
- promoting identity;
- focusing on the individual;
- recognising human rights such as equality, respect, and autonomy (11).

The study highlighted how dignity can be compromised as a result of tensions between priorities. Organisations have been accused of focusing on external targets – 'what matters is what is measured', so that performance targets such as infection control were prioritised above other matters. Managing risk can have unintentional consequences for dignified care, for example the fear of litigation or the pressure to avoid falls and to keep waiting times low could have knock-on effects on the unmeasured activity of dignified care. Moving patients around the organisation in order to 'make beds' can produce loss of continuity and situations in which the patient is considered to be 'in the wrong place' despite the fact that most adult wards contain a high proportion of older people. Therefore the 'system' of care in the hospital could itself undermine dignity, as patients are subject to the rules and policies of an organisation, and those rules and policies are extended to routines and procedures. This could mean that getting enough sleep, meeting nutritional needs, being washed and dressed, and getting to the toilet have to fit around the priorities of staff and systems rather than around the priorities of the individual. Rules of visiting reduced personal contact and the potential for greater advocacy for the patient's interests. A picture is built of a system that needs to get its work done 'safely' and free of blame and that doesn't always promote dignity – something that those of us with experience in health care as providers or consumers may recognise.

Older people in hospital were also often seen as being somehow in the 'wrong place', and there was a general view that people could be cared for better 'somewhere else'. Such a view is reflected in policies that aim to keep older people out of hospital and to move them on as soon as possible. Looking after older people in the hospital has traditionally been an unglamorous area of work; it lacks prestige and compares unfavourably in status with looking after other patient groups, apparently with more 'specialist' needs. This contradicts the fact that geriatric medicine is the largest medical specialty in hospitals and that people admitted to hospital with frailty syndromes do better on specialist elderly medicine wards, receiving multicomponent care known as 'comprehensive geriatric assessment' (12, 13) (for more details, see Chapter 19).

'The 10-point dignity challenge', now known as 'the 10 dignity do's', describes what high-quality services should do to respect a person's dignity (14):

1. Have a zero tolerance of all forms of abuse.
2. Support people with the same respect you would want for yourself or a member of your family.
3. Treat each person as an individual by offering a personalised service.
4. Enable people to maintain the maximum possible level of independence, choice, and control.
5. Listen and support people to express their needs and wants, including cultural, religious, and personal needs.
6. Respect people's right to privacy.
7. Ensure people feel able to complain without fear of retribution.
8. Engage with family members and carers as care partners.
9. Assist people to maintain confidence and positive self-esteem.
10. Act to alleviate people's loneliness and isolation.

Concepts of Dignity

While it is easy for most of us to describe what must be done to maintain dignity, the concept of dignity has actually been the subject of much discussion in healthcare philosophy and deserves a more detailed discussion.

The word 'dignity' comes from the Latin *dignitas* ('merit', 'worth'), a noun derived from the adjective *dignus* ('worthy', 'deserving', 'proper'). The Oxford English dictionary defines it as the quality of being worthy of honour and respect, of being honourable, or of holding an honourable office (15). Immanuel Kant contended that all human beings, regardless of position in society, have an intrinsic worth or dignity that they are born with and cannot forfeit, although he tied this dignity to an understanding that human beings have a 'rational nature' that enabled them to act autonomously. This view may cause problems insofar as it fails to acknowledge that individuals who lack the capacity to act autonomously may still have dignity.

Our modern understanding of dignity, particularly in relation to older people, is influenced heavily by the work of Lennart Nordenfelt, who categorised dignity into four subtypes (16):

Human dignity – the dignity that each individual has as an essential component of being a human being. This is universal and inherent and exists to the same degree within each one of us. The term *Menschenwurde* is widely used to describe it and has no exact English equivalent.

Dignity of personal identity – the dignity that humans have through their ability to have self-respect, their autonomy and their biography, the fact that they are people with a past and a future who relate to other human beings. This dignity can be affected by a changes in a person's body and mind and by the actions of others. It encompasses integrity, a state of being whole and undamaged, entirely oneself.

Dignity of merit – the honour and rights one receives as a result of one's rank in society, whether inherited or made. This is the sort of dignity that a bishop or a doctor or a cabinet minister may possess by virtue of the rights that are attached to their various positions. It is very unevenly distributed among human beings. It exists in degrees, and can come and go. People may be promoted, but also demoted.

Dignity of moral stature – the respect from others and from oneself that comes as a result of one's own actions and attitudes. This kind of dignity can be gained and lost through deeds. It refers to the concept of dignity's being linked to both character and virtue; and it is required if one is to have self-respect.

All older people have an inherent personal dignity that gives them worth and cannot be taken away from them. This is their *Menschenwurde*, otherwise referred to as 'human dignity' (17). Nordenfelt also asserts that older people are particularly worthy of a special type of dignity, which is attached to them by virtue of their having lived a long life, having experienced both more suffering and more blessings than younger people, and having come to understand life itself better, through experience. All of this attaches to them, a particular dignity of merit – wisdom – that comes with having more practical experience and knowledge of what to do in a particular situation. Nordenfelt does not claim that all older people have the dignity of merit or wisdom, as it is clear that not everyone has accumulated the same intellectual and emotional intelligence; nor has everyone gained a wide range of experiences. However, as a group, they have this *typical* virtue of being wise.

Other forms of dignity can be promoted or diminished. There is a possibility that older people in hospital have less *dignity of merit* because of their position in society, but this is not a foregone conclusion and may vary across societies. The demotion of one's dignity of merit can happen through systems that prioritise the elective care of younger people with diseases in hospital specialties such as cancer care or the treatment of heart attacks, which attract more funding and prestige, over the treatment of older people with multimorbidity, frailty, and related syndromes in less glamorous areas of the hospital. It can also happen during personal interactions, if older people are treated rudely, brusquely, or pejoratively termed 'bed blockers' or 'acopic'.

Older people are particularly susceptible to the violation of their *dignity of personal identity* as a result of their potential vulnerability in hospital, where they are subject to the rules, routines, and systems that the organisation may impose on them. When people are unwell and potentially dependent on others for food, medical treatment, and personal care, there is an asymmetry of power and resources that, if combined with antipathy – say, when others are prejudiced, hostile, arrogant, or impatient – can end up in a violation of dignity (18). Acts of care are inherently personal and private, and a failure to promote autonomy and provide compassionate care can lead to undignified care.

Dignity can be promoted when older people are in a position of confidence – they have a sense of self-assurance and self-esteem – and when those who care for them are in a position of compassion – they are kind, open-minded, and honest and act with good intentions. Where the relationship with older people has reciprocity, rapport, empathy, and trust, dignity is also promoted.

Dignity and the Environment

The physical environment can promote or suppress dignity. An environment that promotes privacy through the use of single rooms or through adequate physical barriers that maintain privacy during personal care or during consultation is a key component of dignified care. Yet reports of patient's experience note:

- lack of physical distance between bedspaces,
- transparent or poorly fitted curtains,
- conversations taking place within the earshot of others,
- lack of privacy during personal care or toileting,
- poor aesthetics, older people's wards sometimes being poorly decorated with low-quality furnishings,
- lack of spaces in which to socialise,
- mixed-sex accommodation.

Beside the physical environment, the environment of care is also important, and previous reports have raised concerns around (8, 11).

- responsiveness to patient requests for basic needs such as toileting, nutrition, and hydration,
- staff speaking in raised voices,
- staff talking over patients,
- failure to request permission before entering doors or curtains,
- attitudes towards older people,
- the priority of the care of older people within organisations.

Older people living with dementia are particularly vulnerable to a poorly designed environment. Designing wards to be 'dementia-friendly' (19) can help to orient patients, encourage regular sleep patterns, and empower patients to be more independent. There are many things to consider when designing the space; a few examples are presented in what follows.

Adequate Lighting

As people age, they need more light to interpret the environment with clarity. Ensuring good even lighting throughout the ward can help patients move safely around the ward. Having good natural light promotes a healthy sleep–wake cycle.

Clear Signage

People who have dementia may easily become lost and disorientated. Clear signage for toilets, shower rooms, and day rooms can improve independence around the ward and reduce the anxiety associated with becoming lost.

Contrasting Colours

Clearly contrasting colours can make it easier for people to find doors, chairs, or toilets. Minimising things such as sliding doors, which may be confusing, can make moving around the ward easier.

Floor

High-shine floors can be interpreted by someone with delirium or dementia as being wet. Highly patterned floors may be taken to be littered, while dark spots can be interpreted as holes and can be distressing.

Clocks and Photographs

Clocks should be visible from every bedspace, helping to orient patients. Photographs of local landmarks around the ward can also help in this regard, as well as providing a more homely and welcoming environment.

Reducing Noise

People with dementia can become very sensitive to noise and find noisy environments distracting and distressing. Keeping the noise to a minimum, especially overnight, would reduce this risk and improve sleep. Quiet spaces dedicated to time away from the bedside can be useful.

Day Rooms and Communal Eating Areas

Having a place to eat meals away from the bedside can improve oral intake and nutrition. It also gives carers a space where they can assist with feeding and, for those patients who want to socialise, it allows them to do so in a friendly space.

Empowering independence is important for all older people (with or without dementia) admitted to acute hospitals. Not only does it promote faster recovery, but many people associate becoming more dependent with loss of dignity.

In addition to changes to the physical environment, allowing flexible visits to the ward from loved ones who care for their relative is thought to be beneficial to patients. John's campaign was set up as a movement towards welcoming to the ward carers of people who have dementia, to support their loved one through the admission (20). Carers can help to reorient patients; they can act as their advocates, sharing stories that promote the dignity of personal identity and support personalised care.

Dignity and Staff Interaction

If we were to imagine staff providing dignified encounters in health care, we would envision the staff member

- having personal relationships formed through continuity of staff;
- providing information on how care will be provided ('We will bring you breakfast at 08.00 and the doctors will see you between 09.00 and 12.00');
- knocking on a patient's door before entering and introducing oneself;
- making sure the patient's room is clearly marked as 'engaged' for an encounter;
- asking the patient how they would like to be addressed;
- providing clear communication, tailored to the patient;
- promoting autonomy and choice;
- having interactions that demonstrate sensitivity, empathy, and kindness;
- demonstrating careful listening;
- allowing adequate time for the encounter;
- allowing time for general conversation as well as for task-centred communication;
- asking permission before examinations or acts of personal care;
- before leaving, returning any furniture to its previous place and ensuring that the call bell is in easy reach.

Unfortunately, this ideal may not be reached. Nursing shifts are often 13 hours long, resulting in fewer days worked in succession. Staff shortages, the training, the organisational culture, the lack of time, the lack of education, and the lack of robust systems that promote patient-centred care can act as barriers to dignified care.

Healthcare staff members have been reported to communicate with older people, unintentionally, in a patronising manner, using what is known as 'elderspeak'. This is a form of infantilising communication whereby healthcare staff members talk to patients in short sentences, with a simplified vocabulary and grammar, in slowed speech and high pitch. Inappropriate terms of endearment may be used such as 'darling' or 'dear'. Elderspeak is analogous to the kind of communication that adults use with infants, and it implies a lower capability that older people can find patronising. The matter is complicated because, for some people with significant cognitive impairment, some aspects of elderspeak can be useful, for example a simplified grammar, but the whole mode of address is often patronising and can sometimes hinder communication and understanding. Some older people who are the target of elderspeak and find it demeaning may have their dignity of personal identity violated and become more isolated as a result. This is a complex area, as this violation of dignity may result either from attitudes towards older people or just from thoughtlessness and lack of communication skills.

In the context of people living with dementia, elderspeak has also been associated with increased resistiveness to care: patients may resist acts involving personal care and display behaviour associated with distress.

To fully respect individuals' need for dignity, it is best to ascertain their communication preferences and level of understanding and to tailor the communication to the needs of individual patients.

Nutrition

The most basic standard of care, providing adequate food and water to vulnerable older people, was highlighted in the Francis Report and led to the development of the Malnutrition Task Force. Older people should not go hungry. They need a choice of food, adequate access to foods and fluids, and assistance with eating and drinking, when they are not able to meet this fundamental need independently.

Personal Hygiene

A person's physical appearance is an important part of their self-respect. Being clean and well groomed and sitting out of bed in one's own clothes impacts on how people feel about themselves and on how others react to them. Older people may need assistance with personal hygiene, either because they are unable or because the routines of the hospital rob them of their independence and autonomy. Wherever possible, independence and autonomy should be maintained; but assistance, when it is required, needs to be provided in a respectful and person-centred way, with consideration for gender preference, timing, and cultural issues and beliefs.

Person-Centred Care

Person-centred care is a legal requirement under Regulation 9 of the Health and Social Care Act 2008 (Regulated Activities) Regulations 2014 (21). People using a service should have care or treatment that is specifically personalised to them, on the basis of an assessment of their preferences, needs, and values.

For acute trusts, this means

- carrying out collaboratively, with the relevant person, an assessment of the service user's needs and preferences for care and treatment;
- designing the care or treatment with a view to achieving service users' preferences and ensuring that their needs are met;
- enabling and supporting relevant persons to understand the care or treatment choices available to the service user and to discuss, with a competent health care professional or other competent person, the balance of risks and benefits involved in any particular course of treatment;
- providing opportunities for relevant persons to manage the service user's care or treatment;
- involving relevant persons in decisions related to the way in which the regulated activity is conducted, insofar as it relates to the service user's care or treatment;
- making reasonable adjustments to enable the service user to receive his or her care or treatment;
- when meeting a service user's nutritional and hydration needs, having regard for his or her well-being, so that people are offered a choice over what they eat and drink.

It is important that person-centred treatment includes valid consent and that, when people lack the capacity to make decisions about their care, relevant others are involved, including lasting powers of attorney – when relevant. Person-centred care enhances the person's dignity by putting the needs of that person before the needs of the service. Patients have their own views on what is best for them, and their priorities may differ from those of healthcare staff. Dignity can be promoted by considering patients to be equal partners in their own care, so that healthcare staff take into account what people want when they plan and deliver care. To enable genuinely shared decision-making, the use of patient decision aids is desirable, along with access to personal health records. Training is required so that staff members develop the skills that enable them to participate as equal partners in decision-making; and the clear communication of risk is one of these skills. The model recognises staff members as people, too; and it also recognises their need to be themselves engaged, if they are to be able to deliver a more personalised approach. The principle here should be: 'What matters to you?'

For true person-centred care that enhances dignity, older people need to be recognised as individuals, people with a history, values, a set of beliefs, cultural differences, and personal relationships. They are people who were once young, at stages in life similar to those of the healthcare staff members who care now for them; and understanding this is key to maintaining their dignity and personal identity.

This is particularly relevant for people living with dementia. The work of Tom Kitwood has been crucial in developing our understanding of dementia as more than a biological disease – as a complex interplay between neurological impairment, personal health and fitness, one's personal life story, personality, and social psychology (22). People living with dementia have fundamental psychological needs of comfort, attachment, inclusion, occupation, and identity.

Comfort includes being well nourished and hydrated, being clean and free of pain and restraint. When caregivers provide comfort, the person who receives care benefits from a feeling of closeness and being able to bond with others. Attachment refers to the feeling of connectedness to the surrounding environment, which can be so important to the person with dementia brought to an unfamiliar place. The need to be included requires effort from those around. People with dementia may lose track of conversations or may be spoken over. Meaningful occupation is important too, in a way that reflects the person's current and previous life, while caregivers need to understand the person's narrative and identity.

Recording biographical details alongside the preferences and values of patients and subsequently integrating them into how these patients are cared for can dramatically alter how both patients and healthcare workers experience interactions. For example, imagine Walter, a man with Alzheimer's disease who resists attempts to help him, getting washed and dressed and constantly trying to get up and leave the ward: the healthcare staff exhorts him to sit down and brings him back to his chair, and this results in what is labelled as 'aggression'.

A holistic approach may use information recorded in a document such as 'This is me', produced by Alzheimer's Society (23). Walter used to run his own business and was very much used to being in charge. He found being cared for demeaning, but was particularly uncomfortable about receiving personal care from female staff and did not enjoy terms like 'dear' or 'pet'. He was an avid walker, not used to sitting still. Having this information, the ward tries to use male staff to provide personal care, and staff members talk to Walter with respect, asking about his business and his hobbies. He is encouraged to walk with a member of staff when he gets up, and his 'aggression' subsides.

End-of-Life Care

Dying will come to us all with even greater certainty than old age, and most people who are dying will not be looked after by specialists in palliative care. Although most people indicate a preference to die at home, around 80 per cent of those older than 75 die in hospital, by comparison with 34 per cent of people aged 15–64 (24). Older people's preferences at the end of life include (25):

- being free from pain or suffering;
- maintaining one's cognitive awareness and identity;
- enjoying and maintaining one's independence;
- having a choice as to where they live;
- being clean and having good personal and nursing care without feeling like they are a burden;
- being loved and having good relationships;
- being supported when needed by people who care about them.

Menschenwurde, the dignity that each individual has as an essential component of being a human being, means that all older people have a right to respect and dignity when dying. Even when we are dying, we should be afforded respect for our lives, and we should be protected from the humiliation of being unclean, of suffering unnecessarily, and of losing our autonomy. Suffering is a particular concern in the process of dying and, for many, a dignified death could be described as one that happens quickly, without pain or ugliness.

The idealised death scenario might place us in our own home, surrounded by loved ones, with autonomy and self-respect. Perhaps we might share stories of a life lived, summing up our personal history and experiences as we write a final chapter, so that we may be remembered. There might be an opportunity to explore guilt or remorse, to reconcile, to finalise stories, and to explore religious expression and ritual. For others, death may be a private event, an afterword, following an epilogue that is firmly in the state of living. Affording older people the autonomy to choose their circumstances in this regard is an important part of preserving their dignity – which may be facilitated only by eliciting their preferences. These conscious attempts to maintain one's dignity of personal identity may require courage and more searching and enquiries from healthcare practitioners, who could be tempted to ask superficial questions such as 'Where is your preferred place of care?'. This individualised level of care and support in dying shows respect for the person's narrative and may be even more important when there has not been a chance to explore the person's wishes. In these cases, understanding how someone lived their life and what was important to them enables healthcare workers to share this narrative with relatives or carers and to ensure that a person's death is as dignified as possible.

References

1. Centre for Ageing Better. Doddery but dear? Examining age-related stereotypes. 2020. www.ageing-better.org.uk/sites/default/files/2020-03/Doddery-but-dear.pdf.

2. Mistry, R. *Family Matters*. London: Faber, 2001.

3. National Dignity Council. The Dignity in Care campaign. About page, 2023. www.dignityincare.org.uk/About/Dignity_in_Care_campaign.

4. Health Service Ombudsman. Care and compassion: Report of the Health Service Ombudsman on ten investigations into NHS care of older people. Parliamentary and Health Service Ombudsman, 2011. www.ombudsman.org.uk/publications/care-and-compassion.

5. Centre for Policy on Ageing. *Ageism and Age Discrimination in Secondary Health Care in the United Kingdom*. Centre for Policy on Ageing, 2009. www.cpa.org.uk/information/reviews/CPA-ageism_and_age_discrimination_in_secondary_health_care-report.pdf.

6. Care Quality Commission. *Dignity and Nutrition Inspection Programme: National Overview*. Care Quality Commission, October 2011. www.cqc.org.uk/sites/default/files/documents/20111007_dignity_and_nutrition_inspection_report_final_update.pdf.

7. The All-Party Parliamentary Group. Inquiry into human rights and older people: Protecting our rights as we age. Age UK, 2018. www.ageuk.org.uk/globalassets/age-uk/documents/reports-and-publications/appg/appg_ageingandolderpeople_humanrights_jun18.pdf.

8. Alzheimer's Society. *Counting the Cost: Caring for People with dementia on Hospital Wards*. Alzheimer's Society, 2009. www.alzheimers.org.uk/sites/default/files/2018-05/Counting_the_cost_report.pdf.

9. Francis, R. *Report of the Mid Staffordshire NHS Foundation Trust Public Inquiry*. London: The Stationery Office, 2013. assets.publishing.service.gov.uk/government/uploads/system/uploads/attachment_data/file/279124/0947.pdf.

10. Department of Health. *Patients First and Foremost: The Initial Government Response to the Report of the Mid Staffordshire NHS Foundation Trust Public Inquiry*. 2013. assets.publishing.service.gov.uk/government/uploads/system/uploads/attachment_data/file/170701/Patients_First_and_Foremost.pdf.

11. Tadd, W., Hillman, A., Calnan, M., et al. *Dignity in Practice: An Exploration of the Care of Older Adults in Acute NHS Trusts*. Cardiff University and Kent University,

2011. www.netscc.ac.uk/hsdr/files/ project/SDO_FR_08-1819-218_V02.pdf.

12. Ellis, G., Gardner, M., Tsiachristas, A., et al. Comprehensive geriatric assessment for older adults admitted to hospital. *Cochrane Database Syst Rev* 2017, 9: CD006211. doi: 10.1002/14651858. CD006211.pub3.

13. Ellis, G., and Langhorne, P. Comprehensive geriatric assessment for older hospital patients. *Br Med Bull* 2004, 71: 45–59. doi: 10.1093/bmb/ldh033.

14. National Dignity Council. The 10 dignity do's. About page, 2009. www .dignityincare.org.uk/About/The_10_ Point_Dignity_Challenge.

15. Oxford English Dictionary, s.v. 'dignity'. Oxford: Oxford University Press.

16. Nordenfelt, L. *Dignity in Care for Older People*. Oxford: Wiley Blackwell, 2009, here p. 00.

17. Jacobson, N. Dignity and health: A review. *Soc Sci Med* 2007, 64(2): 292–302. doi: 10.1016/j. socscimed.2006.08.039.

18. Jacobson, N. A taxonomy of dignity: A grounded theory study. *BMC International Health and Human Rights* 2009, 9(1): 3. doi: 10.1186/1472-698X-9-3.

19. The Kings Fund. Is your ward dementia friendly? EHE environmental assessment tool. 2014. www.kingsfund.org.uk/sites/ default/files/EHE-dementia-assessment-tool.pdf.

20. John's Campaign. About. https:// johnscampaign.org.uk/about.

21. The Health and Social Care Act 2008 (Regulated Activities) Regulations 2014. legislation.gov.uk, 2014. www.legislation .gov.uk/uksi/2014/2936/regulation/9/made.

22. Kitwood, T.M. *Dementia Reconsidered: The Person Comes First*. Buckingham: Open University Press, 1997.

23. Alzheimer's Society. This is me: A support tool to enable person-centred care. Alzheimer's Society, 2020. www .alzheimers.org.uk/get-support/ publications-factsheets/this-is-me.

24. Age UK. End of life care (England). Policy position paper. Age UK, 2019. www .ageuk.org.uk/globalassets/age-uk/ documents/policy-positions/care-and-support/ppp_end_of_life_care_en.pdf.

25. Sutton, E.J., and Coast, J. Development of a supportive care measure for economic evaluation of end-of-life care using qualitative methods. *Palliative Medicine* 2014, 28(2): 151–7. doi: 10.1177/ 0269216313489368.

Liaison Psychiatry and Law

Hugh Series

Introduction

This chapter focuses on aspects of mental health law that are of particular relevance to psychiatrists working in general hospitals. The law is described as it stands in England and Wales on 1 August 2021, where the Mental Health Act (MHA) 1983 (amended in 2007) regulates the treatment of people with mental disorders and the Mental Capacity Act 2005 is intended to empower and protect people who lack the capacity to make decisions. Many countries have similar arrangements for mental health, particularly those in common law jurisdictions such as the United States, Canada, Australia, and New Zealand. Mental capacity law is more diverse across jurisdictions. A few jurisdictions, for instance Northern Ireland, have introduced legislation that fuses mental health and mental capacity, although it has not yet been implemented.

The convention is adopted here that the patient is referred to using male pronouns, but the chapter refers equally to all patients.

Capacity and Consent

Mental capacity and consent are concepts that underlie almost all medical practice. Treatment given without valid consent could amount to the criminal offence of battery, and valid consent cannot be given by a patient unless he has the mental capacity to give it.

The Mental Capacity Act 2005 (MCA) (1) puts into statute the previous common law definition of capacity. The Act states that a person lacks capacity to make a decision if, as a result of a disorder of, or an impairment in the functioning of, the mind or brain, he is unable to make the decision because he is unable to understand the relevant information, retain it, use or weigh it, or communicate his decision. Capacity is time- and decision-specific. A failure in any one of the four elements of decision-making renders the person unable to make the decision and therefore lacking in capacity with respect to that particular decision at that time. The Act is underpinned by five principles:

- a person must be assumed to have capacity unless it is established otherwise;
- a person is not be treated as unable to make a decision unless all practicable steps to help him in this regard have been taken without success;
- a person is not to be treated as unable to make a decision merely because he makes an unwise decision;
- an act done or a decision made under the Act for a person who lacks capacity must be done or made in his best interest;

- before the act is done or the decision made, it must be considered whether that purpose can be achieved in a less restrictive way.

The Act itself is accompanied by a Code of Practice (2), which is an extremely practical and helpful document.

In its regular inspections, the Care Quality Commission frequently comments, on the poor understanding and recording of mental capacity in clinical notes. Courts regularly consider cases in which highly significant decisions, be they on medical treatments or on placement, were made for people where the assessment of the person's capacity and best interest was absent or inadequate. There is a sense of proportionality here. A minor or relatively inconsequential decision does not require a lengthy or detailed assessment of capacity, but major decisions do. One might suggest that the more significant the decision in terms of its potential impact on the patient, the more attention should be given to the assessment and recording of capacity, especially if any disagreement about what should be done arises among any of those involved in the case.

The logical sequence is that, first, the decision or act in question needs to be identified. It could be, for example, about a medical or surgical procedure, or about a future placement. Second, in the case of medical or surgical treatment, a careful attempt should be made to inform and discuss with the patient the risks and benefits of each treatment option or of having no treatment at all, and the patient should be invited to decide which option he prefers and to give his consent to it. If the patient has capacity according to the definition given in MCA and consents, his decision should be recorded, and the treatment can go ahead. If he has capacity but refuses, then, in general, the treatment may not go ahead. If the discussion with the patient suggests that he could lack capacity, then an assessment of capacity needs to take place. There is no legal requirement for this assessment to be carried out by a doctor. It is for the person providing the treatment to satisfy himself that an adequate assessment of capacity has been conducted, either by himself or by someone else, appropriately qualified. If the patient has capacity and refuses, then the treatment cannot go ahead – unless it is treatment for mental disorder and the patient is detained under the MHA 1983. (Even then, a detained patient who has capacity may refuse non-urgent electroconvulsive therapy.)

If the patient lacks capacity, then all practicable efforts must be made to involve him in the decision, for example by ensuring that he is able to see and hear adequately, by spending time to give the information in a simple and straightforward way, and by involving others who may be able to help via discussion with the patient.

If, despite those efforts, the patient still lacks capacity to make the decision, a consideration of his best interest must come into play. There is no legal requirement about how a best interest decision should be arrived at and no legal definition of 'best interest', but section 4 of the MCA explains what factors should be taken into account in making a best interest decision. In complex or contentious cases, it is often helpful to have a formal best interest meeting, but this is not a legal requirement. The Act says that the person making a best interest decision must not do so merely on the basis of the person's age, appearance, or condition or on the basis of an aspect of behaviour that may lead to unjustified assumptions about what could be in his best interest. The decision maker must consider all the relevant circumstances, in particular whether it is likely that the patient would at some time have capacity in relation to the matter of interest and, if so, whether it is practicable to postpone the decision until then. He must do what is reasonably feasible to encourage the person to participate as fully as possible in the decision (even if the person lacks capacity). Where the matter relates to life-sustaining treatment, he must not be motivated by a desire to bring about the person's death. He must consider:

- the person's past and present wishes and feelings;
- any relevant written statement made by the person when he had capacity;
- the beliefs and values that would be likely to influence the person's decision if he had capacity; and
- any other factors that the person would be likely to consider if he were able to do so.

He must take into account the views of the following people, if it is practicable and appropriate to consult them:

- anyone named by the person as someone to be consulted;
- anyone engaged in caring for the person or with a personal interest in his welfare;
- any donee with a lasting power of attorney (LPA) granted by the person; and
- any deputy appointed by the court.

This can be quite a long and detailed list, and decision makers should give thought to whether they have complied with the law in this respect before they proceed to put into effect a best interest decision (3). If a best interest meeting is held, it should be chaired carefully, the chair should explain to those present what is meant by capacity and best interest, and each person should be given an opportunity to hear the evidence of others and to give their own views. An attempt should be made to reach a consensus, but if this is not possible the Code of Practice states that for most day-to-day decisions the decision maker will be the carer most directly involved with the person at the time, and that, where the decision involves the provision of medical treatment, the doctor or some other member of healthcare staff responsible for carrying out the particular treatment or procedure is the decision maker. When nursing or paid care is provided, the nurse or the paid carer will be the decision maker for decisions about that care. If a relevant LPA has been made and registered, or if a deputy has been appointed under a court order, the attorney or the deputy would be the decision maker for decisions that fall within the scope of that authority (Code of Practice, paragraph 5.8). A careful record of the capacity assessment and best interest meeting should be kept that should explain why each decision was arrived at and by whom – not simply that it was decided.

Section 5 of the MCA means that, provided that the person carrying out an act of care or treatment on behalf of someone who lacks capacity 'reasonably believes' that the person lacks capacity and that it is in his best interest that the act be done, then the legal effect is that it will be as if the patient had given valid consent for the act to be done. This means that the person who administers the treatment would have a legal defence against a charge of assault. However, the legal protection offered by section 5 operates only if the person has taken reasonable steps to assess capacity and to determine best interest. A health professional who failed to take these steps would not be protected under section 5.

In English law, no one can consent to treatment on behalf of an adult patient, except an attorney under a LPA for health and welfare (on which more later) or a court-appointed deputy. The practice of inviting the next of kin to sign a consent form on behalf of a patient who is unable to do so has no basis in law. With the exception of the

MHA, which gives a precise definition of 'nearest relative', there is no legal definition of 'next of kin'. Even if a next of kin could be clearly identified, such a person has no authority to make decisions on behalf of the patient. This is something that many relatives or spouses may find surprising. Although asking a relative to sign a consent form could provide evidence that the doctor has discussed the matter with the relative, it does not give legal authority. A consent form signed by anyone but a mentally competent adult patient, an attorney named under a care and welfare LPA, or a court-appointed deputy does not in itself provide authority to treat. Treatment given would need to be on the basis of lack of capacity and best interests determined as described above.

An area of law that changed in 2015 is the nature of the information that should be provided to a patient in order to allow him to make a valid decision as to whether to consent to treatment. In the past, the legal test of how much information was sufficient was determined on the basis of what a reasonable doctor who offered the treatment thought was reasonable (the Bolam test). However, after the *Montgomery* ruling, a doctor must disclose to the patient any material risks involved in the proposed treatment and any reasonable alternative treatments (4). A risk is material if, in the circumstances of the case, a reasonable person in the patient's position would be likely to attach significance to the risk, or the doctor is or should be aware that the particular patient would be likely to attach significance to it. This is not a matter of percentages: the significance of a risk will be affected by many factors specific to each patient. A doctor can withhold information from the patient if he reasonably considers that its disclosure would be seriously detrimental to the patient's health, but this 'therapeutic exception' must not be abused.

Restraint

The MCA is very helpful in setting out the extent to which restraining a person is lawful. This is dealt with in section 6, where restraint is defined as the use or threat of force to do something that the patient is resisting, or the restriction of the patient's liberty of movement. Restraint is lawful provided that the person doing it 'reasonably believes that it is necessary to do the act in order to prevent harm to P' ('P' is used in MCA to describe the person lacking capacity) and that the act is a proportionate response to the likelihood of P's suffering harm and to the seriousness of that harm. 'Proportionate' means that the restraint must be the minimum necessary to achieve the end.

The legal protection afforded by the Act in section 5 concerns only harm to the patient. In some circumstances it may be necessary to restrain a patient in order to prevent harm to others. It is arguable that, if the patient is threatening other people, it may be necessary to restrain him in order to protect him from the consequences of his harming those others (e.g. retaliation or legal repercussions). If the situation develops in a hospital, then the hospital is likely to owe a duty of care to others present, and hospital staff may be entitled, or may have a duty under common law, to do what is necessary to ensure the safety of other people.

Lasting Power of Attorney

The MCA provides for two types of LPA (5). The first deals with property and finances (PF) and the second deals with care and welfare (CW), also referred to as health and welfare (HW). They are distinct documents, and an attorney named under one type does not thereby have authority to make decisions under the other type. Before accepting an attorney's decision about medical treatment or care, the doctor should satisfy himself that the person is a care and welfare attorney, not just a property and finances attorney. If the matter is significant, it may be wise to ask to see a copy of the LPA document itself, as attorneys do not always understand the limits of their authority. It is not unusual for an attorney under an LPA–PF to believe, albeit incorrectly, that he has authority to make care and welfare decisions.

An LPA must be executed when the donor still has capacity to make it. The document itself sets out the name of the person who makes the LPA (the donor) and the name of the person or persons appointed as attorneys (donees). If more than one person is appointed as an attorney, the appointment can be joint or several – where 'several' means that any one of the attorneys can make a decision on behalf of the donor and 'joint' means that all the attorneys must agree on every decision made. The document must be signed by the donor, and also by a person known as a certificate provider, who either has relevant professional skills to confirm the donor's capacity or has known the donor for at least two years. An LPA form must be sent to the Office of the Public Guardian (OPG) for registration before it is legally effective, and this is usually done as soon it has been signed. An LPA–CW has effect in relation to a particular decision only when the donor has lost the capacity to make that decision. Capacity, as always, is specific to each decision made at a particular time, and the meaning of 'capacity' is as defined in MCA, sections 2 and 3, described above. The LPA–CW form specifically requires the donor to make a decision as to whether he wishes the attorney to have authority to refuse life-sustaining treatment on his behalf. This is another reason for the doctor to ask to see the LPA form itself: he must see it in order to clarify whether the attorney has authority to make such a decision. Even if the attorney is not authorised to decide to refuse life-sustaining treatment, it may still be appropriate for the doctor to consult him on a decision of this kind because, if the donor asked that person to be his attorney, it is likely that he is someone whom the donor would wish to be consulted.

In the event of a dispute about an LPA or about the actions of a court-appointed deputy, the matter can be referred to the Court of Protection for a decision. Although the Court is under great pressure and may take a long time to hear non-urgent decisions, there is a mechanism for obtaining an urgent decision, if necessary, by phoning the Court office at the Royal Courts of Justice in London, even out of hours. The same is true for urgent decisions required for matters outside the Court of Protection's jurisdiction, for example a decision on urgent treatment in relation to a child (the MCA applies only to people of 18 years or older). The High Court has an inherent jurisdiction under which it may make decisions for a person who is vulnerable but still has capacity, and is therefore outside the remit of the MCA.

In order to be valid, an LPA must be registered with the OPG. It is possible to telephone the office to confirm whether an LPA has been registered in the name of the person concerned.

The law on LPAs came into effect on 1 October 2007. Before that date, a person could make an enduring power of attorney (EPA), which was limited to decisions about property and financial affairs. There was no previous equivalent of the LPA–CW. EPAs made before that date, once registered, are still legally valid, but only for decisions about property and affairs. Therefore a person appointed under an EPA is not entitled to make healthcare decisions. However, he would be entitled to make financial decisions, such as those required to fund care in a care home, which could have an impact on the available care options.

Court-Appointed Deputy

The MCA allows the Court of Protection to appoint a deputy to make a decision or a class of decisions on behalf of a person who lacks capacity. The deputy must abide by the five principles that underlie all decision-making under the MCA and must act in the best interest of the patient; but, within that framework and within the limitations on the scope of his decision-making set by the Court, a deputy has the same authority to make decisions as the patient himself.

Advance Decisions

An advance decision enables a person aged 18 or over, who has capacity, to refuse a specific medical treatment for some future occasion(s) when he may lack the capacity to consent to or refuse that treatment. It has the same effect as a decision made by the person at the relevant time to refuse the treatment, and is therefore binding on healthcare professionals (6).

There is no specific document or form of words for making an advance decision, although a number of organisations have drafted forms of words that can be used. Some people seek legal advice for preparing an advance decision, but this is not a requirement. In the MCA, the only requirement is that, if the decision is to refuse life-sustaining treatment, it must be presented in writing, signed by the person himself, and witnessed, and it must state clearly that the decision applies even if life is at risk.

In order to be effective, an advance decision must be valid and applicable. It will not be valid if the person making it has done anything that clearly goes against the advance decision in the intervening time, if he has withdrawn it, if he has subsequently conferred the power to make that decision on an attorney under an LPA, or if he would have changed his decision had he known more about the current circumstances (e.g. if a new form of treatment is now available that was not available at the time when the LPA was signed and that the donor might have considered). It will not be applicable if the terms of the advance decision do not cover the current situation, about which a treatment decision is to be made.

As noted, an advance decision does not have to be written, unless it is a decision to refuse life-sustaining treatment. However, it is very difficult for a healthcare professional to know exactly what the advance decision covered if the only account of it is oral. This is really a question of evidence; if the decision is a significant one and the doctor believes that to follow an oral advance decision, as reported to him, would be against the patient's best interest, then it would be wise to seek legal advice about what to do.

Unlike in the case of LPAs, there is no register of advance decisions. It would be sensible for a person making an advance decision to ensure that copies of it are available to healthcare professionals who might be asked to provide treatment in future. This could mean ensuring that close friends or relatives have copies and that there is a copy in the person's GP records.

Advocates

The MCA creates a new independent mental capacity advocate (IMCA) service. Its purpose is to help particularly vulnerable people, who lack the capacity to make important decisions about serious medical treatment and changes of accommodation and who have no family or friends to consult about those decisions, as would be appropriate. IMCAs will work with and support people who lack capacity and will represent their views to those who try to work out their best interest.

The MCA states that an IMCA *must* be instructed and consulted in the case of people lacking capacity who have no one else to support them (except for paid staff) whenever an NHS body or a local authority is proposing to provide serious medical treatment, care in a hospital for longer than 28 days, or care in a care home for longer than eight weeks (7). 'Serious medical treatment' is defined as treatment for both mental and physical conditions where there is a fine balance between likely benefits and burdens and risks, the choice of treatments is finely balanced, or what is proposed is likely to have serious consequences for the patient (8). 'Serious consequences' may include serious and prolonged pain, distress, or side-effects; stopping life-sustaining treatment; having heart surgery; or consequences with a serious impact on the patient's future life choices. A few examples of serious medical treatments given in the Code of Practice (paragraph 10.45) are chemotherapy and surgery for cancer, electroconvulsive therapy, therapeutic sterilisation, major surgery such as open-heart surgery and neurosurgery, major amputations such as loss of an arm or leg, treatments that result in permanent loss of hearing or sight, withholding or stopping artificial nutrition and hydration, and termination of pregnancy.

An IMCA *may* be instructed to support someone who lacks capacity to make decisions concerning care reviews and, in adult protection cases, where there is no other unpaid person available to support that person.

The only situation in which the duty to instruct an IMCA need not be followed is when an urgent decision, for example to save a person's life, is needed. However, referral for an IMCA will still be required for any serious treatment that follows the emergency treatment.

Accident and Emergency

Unless there is a clear advance decision or a decision by an attorney under an LPA–CW to the contrary, it will almost always be in the best interest of a person who lacks capacity to be given urgent treatment without delay. In cases of doubt, for example where it is suggested that a patient lacking capacity might wish to refuse treatment, it would be wise to seek an urgent second opinion from a senior colleague or from the hospital's legal services, especially if withholding urgent treatment could result in death or serious harm to the patient.

In the case of a patient attending an accident and emergency department after serious self-harm, if the patient refuses treatment, it will be necessary to carry out an assessment of whether the patient has capacity to refuse treatment. This can be extremely difficult under emergency conditions, especially where there is a lack of knowledge about the patient and his psychiatric history. In essence, the decision for the clinical team is between withholding potentially life-saving treatment on the grounds that the patient has capacity and refuses this treatment and giving potentially life-saving treatment on the grounds that the patient may lack capacity and that it is not in the patient's best interest to delay treatment pending a fuller assessment of capacity. In the view of the present author, although the MCA requires a person who assesses capacity to assume that the patient has capacity until shown otherwise, if delay in giving treatment could result in serious harm, there will be a very strong presumption that treatment should be given. It will require extremely robust evidence that the patient has capacity to refuse life-saving treatment to overturn the normal presumption that it will be in a patient's best interest to preserve his life. An argument may be made that physical treatment after deliberate self-harm could be given under the MHA where it is thought that the self-harm results from mental disorder such as depression. While this could be argued, and one (very controversial) court decision even found that it was lawful to carry out a caesarean section under the MHA (9), it would be a very unusual approach, given that the MHA may be used only for the treatment of mental disorder. The key legal issue here would be whether the physical treatment proposed could properly be seen as a treatment for mental disorder that falls within the scope of treatment that can be authorised under MHA.

Deprivation of Liberty

The law on deprivation of liberty has gone through a profound transformation in the past 20 years. The story begins in 1953, with the coming into force of the European Convention on Human Rights (ECHR) signed by the 47 member states of the Council of Europe, including the United Kingdom. The context at that time was the terrible events of the Second World War. Article 5 of the Convention limits the circumstances under which a person may properly be deprived of liberty, one of which is that the person is of unsound mind. Anyone who is deprived of his liberty has a right under ECHR to speedy access to a court capable of ordering his discharge. Patients with mental disorder who required treatment in hospital could be detained under the MHA 1983, which automatically gives patients the right to appeal to a tribunal, satisfying the article 5 requirement. Until 1997, if a person lacked capacity to consent to treatment and did not appear to be objecting, he was usually admitted to hospital informally and treated on the basis of the doctrine of necessity, which stipulated that it was in his best interests to receive treatment. However, the landmark case of Bournewood (*HL* v *United Kingdom*) challenged that position by asserting that it was a breach of article 5 to hold in hospital a person lacking capacity, on the grounds that that was necessary and in his best interests, and without further authorisation. The case went through the English courts to the House of Lords, as it then was, and was then appealed to the European Court of Human Rights, which found that there had been a breach of article 5 in those circumstances because there was no mechanism by which the person deprived of liberty could speedily appeal to a court (10). The government responded in 2007 by bringing in the Deprivation of Liberty Safeguards (DOLS), which are set out in schedules 1A and A1 of the MCA, together with a Code of Practice (11). Under these procedures, the ward manager (for patients in hospital) or the care home manager (for people in care homes) of anyone who lacks capacity and is deprived of liberty must seek authorisation for the deprivation. The ward manager can authorise urgent deprivation for up to 14 days, while an application to the local authority is made for authorisation of the deprivation of liberty for longer periods. The local authority must send two assessors, one of whom must be a doctor, to investigate whether six qualifying requirements are met. These requirements are that the person is aged 18 or older, lacks capacity, and has a mental disorder; that there are no relevant objections; that the deprivation is in the patient's best interest; and that the person is 'not ineligible' for detention under MHA. At the time when these procedures were introduced, it was anticipated that there would not be very many applications. However, after the landmark judgement in *Cheshire West* (12), where 'deprivation of liberty' was clarified as meaning that the patient is in a state of continuous supervision and control and is not free to leave, the number of applications for DOLS authorisations escalated to a point where local authorities across the country were (and are) unable to respond to all the requests, with the result that the statutory time limits for authorisation cannot be met and large numbers of people in hospitals, care homes, and elsewhere are, strictly speaking, being deprived of their liberty unlawfully. The government accepted that this was an unworkable position and the Mental Capacity (Amendment) Act 2019 has been passed with the aim of simplifying and streamlining the process. This Act replaces DOLS with Liberty Protection Safeguards (LPS), although these have not yet been introduced, and a new Code of Practice is awaited.

At the time of writing (September 2021), the position is that hundreds of thousands of people in England and Wales are being unlawfully deprived of their liberty; many of them are in general hospitals, where the legal position is particularly difficult. Patients who lack capacity because of delirium or other medical causes (probably a very large group), those under general anaesthetics, and the majority of those in intensive care units would appear to be being deprived of their liberty, and very few of them have had their deprivation authorised in the prescribed way. At present, people who die while subject to a deprivation of liberty authorisation are considered to have died in state detention, and their death must be referred to the coroner regardless of the views or feelings of the family. The *Ferreira* case concerned a woman who had died while being intubated in ICU (13). Although she had not had a deprivation of her liberty authorised under the procedures in the MCA and was not detained under the MHA, it was argued that, since she had died in state detention, her death should be reported to the coroner for an inquest. However, the Court of Appeal found that her loss of liberty was due to her physical condition and to the life-saving treatment that she required, rather than being imputable to the state; therefore she had not been in 'state detention' and her death did not have to be referred to the coroner. This case is widely seen as setting an important precedent.

The LPS introduce a number of changes from DOLS. The responsible body that authorises deprivation of liberty will become the body that commissions or provides the care (under DOLS, all deprivations are authorised by the local authority); for a patient in hospital, this would be the NHS Trust or the relevant clinical commissioning group (CCG). There will no longer need to be a new medical assessment in every case; it will be possible to rely on the evidence of mental disorder recorded previously for other reasons. There will no longer be a best interest assessment, although there will be a requirement to show that the deprivation is necessary and proportionate. The LPS will apply to people aged 16 or older (at present DOLS applies only to those aged 18 or older). At the time of writing, the LPS is scheduled to be implemented on 1 April 2022.

Under LPS it remains difficult to determine whether DOLS/LPS or MHA is more appropriate for patients who are compliant with admission and treatment but lack capacity to consent. The Wessely independent review of the MHA suggested that the choice of route should be based on whether the patient was objecting, but this proposal has not been accepted by the government so far.

Although the LPS have not yet been introduced in England and Wales, the Mental Capacity (Amendment) Act passed into law in 2019, and this provides a legal basis for the LPS. This Act allows a person to be deprived of liberty in an emergency, for the purpose of receiving life-sustaining treatment or doing a vital act (one that is necessary to prevent a serious deterioration in P's condition). This would appear to provide a legal basis for depriving a person of liberty in an accident and emergency department in order to give him life-sustaining or vital treatment.

Children and Young People

In law, a 'child' is any person under the age of 18. The Family Law Reform Act 1969 states that a child aged 16 or 17 can consent to treatment in the same way as an adult. If the child is under 16, he can consent if he can show that he is 'Gillick competent'. This means that the child has 'sufficient understanding and intelligence to enable him/her to understand fully what is proposed' (14). The child must understand the medical issues: the proposed treatment, the consequences of not having it, and the effects of having it. The more complex the medical procedure, the harder it will be for a child to show that he is competent. The child must understand the moral family issues involved. The child needs to have the maturity required to consent only to the specific treatment involved in his care, not a more complex one. Where there is fluctuation in capacity, the child should be treated as lacking capacity. The child's decision should be an independent one, not simply a repetition of the views of his parents or guardians.

The MCA does not generally apply to people under the age of 16. Most of the Act applies to people aged 16 and older who lack the capacity to make decisions. Exceptions are that only a person aged 18 or over can make an LPA or an advanced decision to refuse treatment, and the rules on DOLS apply only to those aged 18 or over.

Mental Health Act 1983

There will be occasions on which people with mental disorder need treatment in the general hospital. This could be because they have a physical disorder that gives rise to a mental disorder, or because they have a mental disorder that has physical consequences in need of treatment (e.g. severe dehydration or malnutrition in a person with depression or dementia). Or it may be that the person is being treated for mental disorder under the MHA, but a new, unrelated physical problem arises that requires transfer to a general hospital for its treatment.

If the patient has capacity to consent to the proposed treatment for the physical disorder, then the treatment can go ahead, on the usual basis of valid consent. However, there will be many occasions on which a person lacks capacity, for example because of severe mental disorder. It can be difficult to decide whether treatment, together with any associated deprivation of liberty, should be provided under the MCA (including DOLS/LPS) or the MHA.

In cases where the patient has been detained under the MHA for the treatment of his mental disorder, the MHA itself authorises both the deprivation of liberty and the treatment of the mental disorder.

A common situation is that a patient has been detained in a psychiatric hospital under MHA but needs to be transferred to the general hospital for some kind of physical treatment. The patient can be put on leave (section 17 of MHA) to the general hospital, and the treatment for the mental disorder can be given to a patient on leave in the same way as if he were still in the detaining psychiatric hospital. There will need to be a clear decision about who is the responsible clinician (RC) during the period of leave. It could be the RC at the psychiatric hospital, provided that that person is in a position to continue to supervise the psychiatric treatment, or it could be an appropriately qualified clinician at the general hospital (usually this will be a psychiatrist). As discussed earlier in relation to the case of a person presenting at the accident and emergency department after deliberate self-harm, if the patient lacks the capacity to consent to physical treatment, a decision will have to be made as to whether the treatment for the physical disorder is provided on the basis of the best interest principle under MCA, or whether it is considered that the physical treatment is an aspect of the treatment for mental disorder authorised under MHA. While this question is important, it is suggested that concern about how to resolve it should not delay urgent treatment.

Covert Medication

On occasion, there may be reason to consider giving medication to a patient covertly, that is, without the patient's knowledge or consent. The medication may be added to food or drink or, in hospital, to an intravenous infusion. In a care home study by Treloar, 71 per cent of the nursing homes under study reported that medicines were 'sometimes given covertly' (15). In general hospitals, medications are occasionally given covertly, namely in situations where the patient lacks capacity to consent, for example because of a mental disorder such as dementia or delirium. When drugs are being given, while the patient is under a general anaesthetic, the administration is covered by his prior consent to the procedure, if he had capacity to give it.

If the patient lacks capacity, medication can be given on the basis of best interest, whether covertly or otherwise. A number of professional bodies have given guidance on the administration of covert medication. The Care Quality Commission states that there should be evidence that the organisation providing the care has a policy on covert administration, that staff have been trained in the relevant issues, that medication is given covertly only to those lacking capacity, and that there should be a best interests meeting and an agreed management plan covering the administration (16). In 2004 the Royal College of Psychiatrists published (pre-MCA) guidance, which stated that covert medication should be exceptional and should be given only to those who lack capacity (unless the patient is detained under MHA); an attempt should be made to give them medication openly first, and there should be discussion with a relative, carer, any nominated representative, pharmacist, and GP. The guidance states that covert medication should not be given in a situation in which it is likely that the patient recovers capacity (although the guidance does not seem to have envisaged a situation where covert medication would have to be given because of delirium in a general hospital, where it is likely that the patient would recover capacity after the delirium had resolved). Where a patient is subject to DOLS, case law has established that the use of covert medication is a matter that would be of relevance to the best interest assessor and should be communicated to the relevant person's representative and supervisory body.

Providing Reports

Occasionally liaison psychiatrists may be asked to provide opinions and reports on other areas of legal decision-making, for example on whether a patient in hospital has capacity to make or revoke a will or a lasting power of attorney. This is outside the scope the present chapter, but the interested reader is referred to the excellent guide to assessment edited by Keene (17). A doctor should not provide an opinion that falls outside the scope of his knowledge or expertise. The General Medical Council (GMC) gives guidance on acting as a witness in legal proceedings (18). The Royal College of Psychiatrists has published a report titled 'Responsibilities of psychiatrists who provide expert opinion to courts and tribunals' (19).

MHA Reform

After the Wessely review of the MHA 1983, the government has published a White Paper and completed a consultation about reform of the MHA, addressing particularly the need to strengthen patients' rights and making the criteria for detention more rigorous. At the time of writing, a bill has not yet been put before parliament.

References

1. Mental Capacity Act 2005. www.legislation.gov.uk/ukpga/2005/9/contents.

2. Mental Capacity Act Code of Practice. GOV.UK, Office of the Public Guardian, 22 July 2013. www.gov.uk/government/publications/mental-capacity-act-code-of-practice.

3. Mental Capacity Act (MCA) Code of Practice.

4. Hughes, J., Crepaz-Keay, D., Emmett C., and Fulford, K. The Montgomery ruling, individual values and shared decision-making in psychiatry. *BJPsych Advances* 2018, 24(2): 93–100. For the case itself, see *Montgomery v Lanarkshire Health Board* [2015] UKSC 11. See also *Bolam v Friern Hospital Management Committee* [1957] 1 WLR 582.

5. MCA, sections 9–14.

6. MCA, sections 24–26.

7. MCA, sections 36–39.

8. MCA Code of Practice, paragraphs 10.42–10.50.

9. Dolan, B. Caesarean section: Treatment of mental disorder? *Tameside & Glossop Acute Services Unit v CH (a patient)* [1996] 1 FLR 762. *BMJ* 1997, 314: 1183.

10. *HL v The United Kingdom* 45508/99 [2004] ECHR 720 (5 October 2004).

11. *Deprivation of Liberty Safeguards: Code of Practice to Supplement the Main Mental Capacity Act 2005 Code of Practice.* London: TSO, 2008. www.cqc.org.uk/sites/default/files/Deprivation%20of%20liberty%20safeguards%20code%20of%20practice.pdf.

12. *P v Cheshire West and P and Q v Surrey County Council* [2014] UKSC 19.

13. *Regina (Ferreira) v Inner South London Senior Coroner* [2017] EWCA Civ 31.

14. *Gillick v West Norfolk and Wisbech Area Health Authority* [1985] 3 All ER 402, at 423, *per* Lord Scarman.

15. Treloar, A., Philpot M., and Beats, B. Concealing medication in patients' food. *Lancet* 2001, 357: 62–4.

16. Care Quality Commission. Brief guide: Covert medication in mental health services. April 2018. www.cqc.org.uk/sites/default/files/20180406_9001398_briefguide-covert_medication_mental_health_v2.pdf.

17. Ruck Keene, A. (ed.). *Assessment of Mental Capacity* (4th ed.). London: Law Society/British Medical Association, 2015.

18. General Medical Council. Acting as a witness in legal proceedings. April 2013. www.gmc-uk.org/ethical-guidance/ethical-guidance-for-doctors/acting-as-a-witness/acting-as-a-witness-in-legal-proceedings.

19. Rix, K., Eastman, N., and Adshead, G., on behalf of the Special Committee for Professional Practice and Ethics. Responsibilities of psychiatrists who provide expert opinion to courts and tribunals. CR193. Royal College of Psychiatrists, 2015. www.rcpsych.ac.uk/docs/default-source/improving-care/better-mh-policy/college-reports/college-report-cr193.pdf?sfvrsn=c0381b24_2.

Safeguarding Adults

Sarah Murphy and Sabeena Pheerunggee

Introduction

The present chapter is intended to be an outline of the key elements of safeguarding adults and a tool to assist you in your work in acute hospitals and to make you confident about identifying and acting on abuse and neglect, including self-neglect.

What Is Adult Safeguarding?

Safeguarding means protecting the health, well-being, and human rights of vulnerable adults and enabling them to live safely, free from abuse and neglect. It also means making sure that the well-being of adults is supported and that their views, wishes, feelings, and beliefs are respected when they agree on any action.

Statutory Responsibilities

Statutory responsibilities for the integration of care and support between health and local authorities are set out in the Care Act 2014 in England and in the Social Services and Well-Being Act 2014 in Wales. Although local authorities have statutory authority, NHS England, clinical commissioning groups (CCGs), integrated care systems (ICSs), and their equivalents must work in partnership with local social care services to ensure the safety and well-being of all patients who receive health services. Please note that while we make reference to the laws for England and Wales, there may be nuanced differences in the legislation in your area – for example, between the Adult Support and Protection (Scotland) Act 2007 in Scotland and the Protection of Children and Vulnerable Adults (2003) Order in Northern Ireland. But the core principles of safeguarding should remain the same.

Safeguarding legislation defines the responsibilities of local authorities and partner organisations, including the NHS, towards adults who have care and support needs and who may be at risk of abuse or neglect. Central to the Act is a 'well-being' principle with a clear focus on interventions that prioritise the well-being of individuals.

Duty of Care

We all have a duty of care in accordance with our professional bodies' codes of practice, for example the General Medical Council (GMC), the National Midwifery Council (NMC), and the Health Care Professional (HCP). This duty is not limited to the service user but encompasses your employer, your colleagues, and the public, as well as yourself.

Responses should be structured to give people more control over their lives so that they remain independent, in line with the Making Safeguarding Personal (MSP) initiative and approach.

Safeguarding Adults Principles

The safeguarding principles central to the Care Act (1, 2) and the proactive interventions are set out in Figure 7.1.

Types of Abuse and Neglect

Table 7.1 presents a list of what is often deemed to be the most common types of abuse and neglect. There may be other indicators that are not listed here but are relevant. These can be seen in the clinical setting, but do remember to look out for them also on home visits, where they may be even more apparent.

- *Empowerment*

People are supported and encouraged to make their own decisions and informed consent.

"I am asked what I want as the outcomes from the safeguarding process and this directly inform what happens."

- *Prevention*

It is better to take action before harm occurs.

"I receive clear and simple information about what abuse is. I know how to recognise the signs, and I know what I can do to seek help."

- *Proportionality*

The least intrusive response appropriate to the risk presented.

"I am sure that the professionals will work in my interest and they will only get involved as much as is necessary."

- *Protection*

Support and representation for those in greatest need.

"I get help and support to report abuse and neglect. I get help so that I am able to take part in the safeguarding process to the extent to which I want."

- *Partnership*

Services offer local solutions through working closely with their communities. Communities have a part to play in preventing, detecting and reporting neglect and abuse.

"I know that staff treat any personal and sensitive information in confidence, only sharing what is helpful and necessary. I am confident that professionals will work together and with me to get the best result for me."

- *Accountability*

Accountability and transparency in delivering safeguarding.

"I understand the role of everyone involved in my life and so do they."

Figure 7.1 The safeguarding principles and proactive interventions

Table 7.1 Common types of abuse and neglect

Types of abuse	Indicators	Examples
Physical	• marks • bruising • guarded/fearful • appearing to be in pain • drowsy/disoriented	• hitting • slapping • female genital mutilation (FGM) • restraint, including chemical and physical restraint
Sexual	• bleeding • bruising • guarded/fearful • genito-urinary infection • medically unexplained symptoms • deliberate self-harm • alcohol/substance misuse	• rape / sexual assault • indecent exposure • sexual harassment • being made a subject of imagery (photo and video) or • forced to view it
Psychological	• timid • confused • forgetful • low self-esteem • anxious +/−depressed • no voice (another speaks on their behalf) • medically unexplained symptoms • deliberate self-harm / suicide attempt • alcohol/substance misuse	• humiliation/shaming • blaming • belittling • control / coercive control • verbal abuse • bullying • intimidation • forced isolation • gaslighting (3) Please remember that many of these can also take place online
Financial/ material	• anxious • self-neglecting • cuckooing (4) • hoarding	• scams: door/phone/Internet i.e. financial affairs related to wills, pensions, life insurance, property • fraud: bank / stolen identity • being used for benefit fraud • misuse of power regarding the lasting power attorney (LPA) for financial affairs • theft (maybe committed by someone they know and let into the house)

	• delayed presentation • appearing malnourished • withdrawn • anxious • tired • poor recall • genito-urinary infection • no access to finances – reliant on others • partial or total disengagement from services	• forced labour • domestic servitude • sex work • organ harvesting
Domestic abuse *violence or abuse among 16-plus-year-olds who are or have been intimate partners or family members, regardless of gender or sexuality	• guarded/fearful • anxious/depressed • low self-esteem • no access to finances – reliant on others • withdrawn • no voice (someone else speaks on their behalf) • bruising • medically unexplained symptoms • substance/alcohol misuse • gambling addictions Remember: it takes up to 35 encounters to obtain a disclosure.	• controlling behaviour • coercive behaviour • misuse of LPA for health and welfare and for financial affairs • threatening Can also encompass (but is not limited to): • psychological abuse • sexual abuse • financial abuse • emotional abuse • 'honour'-based violence • forced marriage • faith or cultural practices
Self-neglect	• malodorous • dishevelled • dental/facial pain complaints • malnourished: underweight or obese • uncontrolled chronic illness • partial or total disengagement from services • substance misuse • alcohol misuse Home visit indicators: • hoarding • cold environment • empty fridge • unkempt environment	• neglecting personal hygiene (including oral hygiene) • poor concordance with medication • recurrent hospital admissions • physical environment risks (e.g. trip and fire hazards)

Table 7.1 (cont.)

Types of abuse	Indicators	Examples
Neglect and acts of omission	<ul><li>malodorous</li><li>dishevelled</li><li>dental/facial pain complaints</li><li>malnourished</li><li>skin breakdown, including pressure sores</li><li>fearful</li><li>reluctant to share information</li><li>no access to finances – reliant on others</li><li>withdrawn</li><li>no voice (someone else speaks on their behalf)</li><li>uncontrolled chronic illness</li><li>delayed presentation for acute illness</li><li>partial or total disengagement from services</li></ul>Home visit indicators:<ul><li>hoarding</li><li>cold environment</li><li>restricted access to fridge</li><li>unkempt environment</li></ul>	Family/partner/carer/person in a position of trust ignoring/ withholding:<ul><li>medical care needs (medication/appointments)</li><li>emotional needs</li><li>physical needs</li><li>nutritional needs</li><li>warm safe residence requirement</li><li>appropriate clothing requirement</li><li>independent translation +/– advocacy services</li></ul>Can also include failure to intervene in situations that are dangerous to the person concerned or to others, particularly where the adult at risk lacks the mental capacity to assess risk for themselves.
Organisational *within an institution or a specific care setting such as a hospital or care home, or in relation to care provided in one's own home	<ul><li>dehydration</li><li>malnourishment</li><li>skin breakdown, including pressure sores</li><li>bruises</li><li>fractures</li><li>fearful/guarded/withdrawn</li><li>hygiene deterioration</li><li>keeping visitors away (during a pandemic this could be amplified)</li></ul>Visits to care settings or supported/sheltered accommodation<ul><li>call bells not accessible or answered</li><li>unclean environment</li><li>no refreshments</li><li>use of bedrails</li></ul>	<ul><li>neglect</li><li>restraint (chemical/physical)</li><li>poor care / poor professional practice</li><li>significant event</li><li>never event</li></ul>Can also include:<ul><li>physical</li><li>sexual</li><li>psychological</li><li>emotional</li></ul>High profile cases, e.g.<ul><li>the Winterbourne view</li><li>Mid-Staffordshire, the Francis Inquiry (5)</li></ul>both pre-Care Act 2014

Discriminatory	Related to:
• loss of confidence	• race
• lack of the person's voice	• gender and gender identity
• belittled	• sexual orientation
• submissive	• religion
• signs of inequality and inequity	• disability (including mental health diagnosis)
• signs of cultural appropriation	Resulting in:
	• bullying and harassment (slurs, hate mail, undermining behaviour)
	• exclusion due to protected characteristics
	• denial of basic rights, e.g. access to independent interpreting and translation (including British Sign Language (BSL) and Easy Read format) and to advocacy
	• denial of education
	• denial of health care
	• criminal justice in relation to protected characteristics
	• substandard service provision vis-à-vis protected characteristics

Radicalisation

Although radicalisation is not a category of abuse or neglect, it is important to remember that vulnerable adults may be subjected to it. This is a process through which people come to support increasingly extreme political, religious, or other ideals. Radicalisation can push them to support violent extremism and terrorism.

People can also self-radicalise by reading or listening to extremist literature or speakers. More commonly, there will be an individual or group actively seeking to persuade others to adopt their views. It is important to ensure that you have had your preventive training and are familiar with your organisation's policy.

Who Commits Abuse and Neglect?

The answer is that anyone can carry out abuse or neglect:

- spouses and partners,
- other family members,
- neighbours,
- friends,
- acquaintances,
- local residents,
- people who deliberately exploit adults whom they perceive to be vulnerable to abuse,
- paid staff or professionals,
- volunteers and strangers including in faith sectors.

Where Do Abuse and Neglect Take Place?

Abuse and neglect can happen anywhere: in someone's own home, in a public place, in the hospital, in a care home, or in an educational establishment. It can occur when an adult lives alone or with others.

Who Is Most Vulnerable and Why?

The following are factors that can make individuals more vulnerable to abuse or neglect (or both):

- absent or fluctuating capacity, which impaires one's ability to consent;
- having a mental health diagnosis or learning disabilities (or both);
- being physically dependent on others for assistance, especially for financial matters and personal care;
- low self-esteem;
- previous history of abuse;
- negative experiences of disclosing abuse;
- communication issues (e.g. language problems, speech impairment, sensory impairment);
- advancing age;
- social isolation;

- poor mobility;
- lack of access to health and social services or high-quality information;
- receiving care in one's own home;
- experiencing discrimination (e.g. hate crime) (6).

Potential Barriers to Disclosure

It is possible that older people are less likely to disclose information, and this is due to some of the following reasons:

- a poor understanding of what constitutes abuse and neglect, as a result of which they are unsure what abuse actually is and when to report it;
- the fact that older, more vulnerable adults do not understand their rights and therefore do not know that they can report abuse;
- reluctance to report abuse for fear of reprisal or out of shame.

Reasons can also be more specific, as in these examples:

- Older people who are being abused by their adult children may be reticent to seek help for fear of adverse consequences for their adult child and for themselves.
- A parental bond may prevent adults from speaking to others, asking for help, or enacting advice they receive.
- The reporting of adult abuse committed by adult children is surrounded by shame and stigma.
- Older people may need practical support to take action or to report abuse when there is less likelihood of adverse consequences.
- Older people may have language or physical–intellectual disabilities that make reporting difficult.
- Some interpreters would be reluctant to convey the full message because of cultural values or lack of training.
- Anxiety related to finances, housing, or lack of recourse to public funds can be a barrier to reporting.
- There may be poor or inappropriate documentation around abusive incidents, and some individuals may not understand the approaches that would be taken by the organisations to whom they report abuse.
- Older people may feel rushed during an appointment or a consultation and would not want to 'waste' a professional's time.
- The perpetrator is present, hence the vulnerable adult does not have an opportunity to speak freely.
- Older people may find it difficult to talk about the abuse.
- Vulnerable older people may worry about not being believed.
- The false belief that no good outcome could happen (no one would care) can be an obstacle.
- Existing gaps in the system when it comes to responding to abuse may put people off.

Professional Barriers

Diagnostic overshadowing has been noted in many safeguarding adults' reviews (7), especially in the context of adults with learning disabilities. So what is diagnostic overshadowing and how does it relate to adult safeguarding?

Diagnostic overshadowing is a situation in which professionals make the assumption that the behaviour of a person with learning disabilities, cognitive impairment, mental health, or behavioural diagnosis is part of that person's condition without exploring other factors, organic and inorganic. Therefore it is pertinent to explore a holistic approach, which takes into account physiological and pathological determinants of behavioural changes as well wider environmental factors.

Some of the signs that could lend themselves to diagnostic overshadowing are:

- being quiet and withdrawn;
- showing aggression and anger for no obvious reason;
- being subject to sudden character changes such as appearing helpless, tearful, depressed.

A fuller list of signs and symptoms of abuse can be found in Table 7.1, which outlines types of abuse and neglect. Remember that safeguarding concerns can be encountered anywhere, which is key to contextual safeguarding. Contextual safeguarding looks at how professionals can best understand the risks, engage with the person, and help to keep the person safe. As they do all this, professionals must also be mindful of cultural sensitivities and recognise and address unconscious bias, which could act as a barrier to the recognition of safeguarding risk(s) .

Making Safeguarding Personal (MSP)

Making Safeguarding Personal (8) constitutes a safeguarding culture that focuses on personalised outcomes desired by people with care and support needs. It reflects the six core principles of the Care Act 2014. The embedding of this approach enables professionals to give the consultation or exchange process the best possible chance.

This initiative can be supported by making reasonable adjustments such as asking for an independent translation (e.g. into British Sign Language) and for advocacy, ensuring hearing aids, asking whether it would be helpful to wear a transparent mask to enable lip-reading, and adopting large fonts and Easy Read material.

People in Positions of Trust (PiPoT)

The Care Act 2014 outlines the requirements of safeguarding adult boards to establish and agree a framework and a process for organisations to respond to allegations about anyone who works with adults who have care and support needs. This is the equivalent of the local authority designated officer (LADO) in children safeguarding. You may find that, thanks to evolving governance processes in adult safeguarding, some areas have a joint LADO/ PiPoT post.

Both the designated lead officer and the arrangements for managing issues related to people in positions of trust can vary from area to area, but the designated professional for safeguarding in your organisation should be cited in your local process and procedure.

Your Role When Detecting a Safeguarding Risk

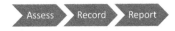

Assessment and Supporting Disclosure

If the individual is accompanied by someone, best practice is to ask the person to leave, so as to offer the individual a safe space for sharing any concerns in confidence.

If translation is required, an independent translator should be used. If no onsite translator is available or it has not been possible to arrange for one in time for the encounter, all trusts should have access to a phone translation service. It may be culturally sensitive and appropriate to consider asking whether there is a gender preference related to the translator, as sometimes the nature of the problem may give preference to one gender over the other.

Establish the principles of confidentiality and consent. It is important to be open and transparent with the person (with or without family and carers) from the outset. As one applies these principles, one should remember that any third party accompanying the person may perpetrate abuse and that, by sharing your intentions with them, you could increase the risk to the victim. It is important to remember that consent is not a barrier to information sharing. This idea is supported in the safeguarding principles of the GMC (9) and NMC (10).

What to do and not to do around disclosures is summarized in the following box:

Do	Do not
• Listen carefully.	• Do not show shock or disbelief.
• Offer reassurance.	• Do not ask leading questions.
• Keep good records (verbatim).	• Do not promise confidentiality, even if the adult asks you.
• Refer to or seek advice.	• Do not confront the source of risk.
• Be transparent about what you intend to do with the information.	
• Ask open questions (what, who, where, when, how).	
• Consider the person's immediate safety.	
• Make sure that the consultation environment is deemed, by the patient, safe for talking.	

What to Do If You Are Concerned and What to Expect from a Referral

1. Document factually and clearly, in the patient's records, the date and time and the full name and designation of everyone present. Record what you have advised the patient regarding the next steps and whether you have sought and gained consent. If you have not obtained consent and intend to share information, state clearly why.
2. Complete a risk assessment to establish the level of danger; see Figure 7.2.

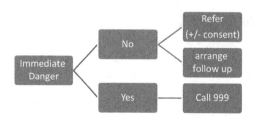

Figure 7.2 Risk assessment decision tree

Is the person in front of you in immediate danger? If so, you may need to call 999. If not, you may need to arrange a follow-up. This could take place via phone or video call or in a face-to-face appointment. It would not be appropriate to simply signpost back to the GP.

In the context of domestic abuse, there is a domestic abuse, stalking, harassment, and honour-based violence assessment (DASH) risk assessment tool that is used to assess the level of risk and intervention required.

Reporting

- Consult your organisation's safeguarding policy and procedures.
- You may also wish to seek advice from the safeguarding lead in your organisation, for support and clarity regarding local processes.
- It is important to be open and honest with the person.
- Use the adult multiagency safeguarding referral form for your area, to make a timely referral.
- On your referral form, state clearly what you are concerned about and provide as much information as possible. This will assist the adult social care team in understanding the reasons for referral and its priority.
- If you have discussed with the safeguarding lead in your organisation, please also indicate what conversation you have carried out.
- You may also need to share your concerns with the person's GP; this can be done in a phone call and followed up in writing.
- Once you have made the referral and coded it on your clinical system, set a date and time for you, your administrator, or a colleague to follow up the outcome and update the records.
- When working with domestic abuse, you may need to consider a referral to the Multi-Agency Risk Assessment Conference (MARAC). A MARAC (11) is a meeting where information on the highest-risk domestic abuse cases is shared between representatives of local police, health, child protection, adult social care, housing practitioners, independent domestic violence advisors (IDVAs), probation officers, and other specialists from the statutory and voluntary sectors. It is important to note that, while consent is always preferable, it is not essential for a referral.

What Will Happen Once You Have Made the Referral

The possibilities are:

- an information gathering process,
- a possible Section 42 enquiry (12) to which you would most likely be asked to contribute, and
- a multi-agency meeting with all those involved in the case, that is, the team around the person.

There may be a number of outcomes, depending on the enquiry or investigation carried out; and such outcomes may include criminal prosecution, if abuse and neglect are proven. Additional care and support needs may be identified, and it could take wider multi-agency involvement to implement or add to existing care and support plans the measures that these needs demand. All assessment and all decisions will take place in liaison with the concerned adult or their representative (an independent mental care advocate (IMCA) if that person lacks capacity).

Information Sharing

The challenges of working within the boundaries of confidentiality should not prevent anyone from taking appropriate action. Whenever possible, informed consent to the sharing of information should be obtained. However, there are a few caveats.

- Emergency or life-threatening situations may warrant the sharing of relevant information with the relevant emergency services without consent.
- The law does not prevent the sharing of sensitive, personal information within organisations. If the information is confidential, but there is a safeguarding concern, sharing it may be justified.
- The law does not prevent the sharing of sensitive, personal information between organisations when the public interest served this way outweighs the public interest served by protecting confidentiality – for example, when a serious crime may be prevented.

Whether the information is shared with or without consent from the adult at risk, the information-sharing process should fall within the parameters of the General Data Protection Regulation (GDPR) and the Data Protection Act 2018. GDPR and the Data Protection Act 2018 should not be a barrier to sharing information. They provide a framework for ensuring that personal information about living persons is shared appropriately.

Sharing the right information at the right time with the right people is fundamental to good safeguarding practice, but has been highlighted as a difficult area of practice. Section 45 of the Care Act 2014, concerning the 'supply of information' duty, covers the responsibilities of others to comply with requests for information. Sharing information between organisations as part of day-to-day safeguarding practice is covered by the common law duty of confidentiality, the GDPR, the Data Protection Act 2018, the Human Rights Act 1998 and the Crime and Disorder Act 1998.

The legislation allows us to share information without consent in certain circumstances. If it is deemed to be in the public interest (13), data may be collected, processed, shared, and stored. It may also be stored for longer periods if this is in the public interest and in order to safeguard the rights and freedoms of individuals.

Vital interests (14) are a lawful basis for sharing personal data to protect someone's life, but you must check whether there is a less intrusive way to protect the person's life. Always document and justify your decisions.

Carers

Carers can be both formal and informal, with a range of roles in relation to safeguarding.

Anyone can be an informal carer, including children and adults who look after a family member, partner, or friend who needs help because of illness, frailty, disability, a mental health problem, or an addiction and cannot cope without their support. The care they give is unpaid. Formal carers are paid for the care they provide.

Informal carers often do not regard themselves as carers, and it can be difficult for them to see their caring role as separate from the relationship they have with the person for whom they care, whether that be as a parent, child, sibling, partner, or friend.

In older adult care, carers can often be older adults themselves, for instance spouses or children, and may or may not have their own care and support needs, or other care-taking responsibilities.

They may find it hard to recognise they are not coping or may require additional support in their care-taking role. This can result in difficult or even confrontational conversations with professionals.

It is important to remember that carers can be the persons who raise a safeguarding concern. They themselves can be vulnerable to abuse and harm, or they could be perpetrating abuse and neglect. Therefore, it is important to hear not only the service user's or the patient's voice (with all reasonable adjustments in place), but also the carer's voice (again, with all reasonable adjustments in place); and it is also important to share openly your concerns and risk assessment, so that a safe plan of action may be put in place.

Safeguarding Adults Boards

Safeguarding Adult Boards are statutory multi-agency boards that are committed to protecting an adult's right to live in safety, free from abuse and neglect. It has overall responsibility for co-ordinating safeguarding adult matters and for ensuring that partner agencies carry out safeguarding adults work. Safeguarding Adult Boards are responsible for commissioning safeguarding adult reviews in their locality. Safeguarding multi-agency arrangements can vary according to your locality.

Conclusion

As highlighted throughout this chapter, the effective safeguarding of adults requires professional curiosity backed up by prompt, person-centred, and responsive action. Central to good safeguarding work is knowing how to access safeguarding support. Safeguarding training is part of a mandatory continuous professional development. It should be reviewed annually, as part of staff appraisal, in conjunction with individual learning and development plans and triennial refresher training. Your designated safeguarding leads will follow the intercollegiate guidance (15) to advise you about training requirements.

We end with a list of relevant UK telephone numbers.

National helpline numbers:

MIND – tel: 0300 123 3393
Age UK – tel: 0800 678 1602

Domestic Violence:

National Helpline – tel: 0808 2000 247
Victim support – tel: 0808 1689 111
SafeLives: www.safelives.org.uk

References

1. Care Act 2014. www.legislation.gov.uk/ukpga/2014/23/contents/enacted.

2. Guidance: Care Act factsheets. GOV.UK, 19 April 2016. www.gov.uk/government/publications/care-act-2014-part-1-factsheets/care-act-factsheets.

3. 'Gaslighting' is a term that refers to trying to convince someone that they are wrong about something even when they are not. Browse Gaslighting — what are the signs and how can it be addressed? | Relate.

4. Cuckooing is a practice in which people take over a person's home and use the property to facilitate exploitation. It takes the name from cuckoos, who take over the nests of other birds. Visit the site What is cuckooing | Cuckooing | Oxford City Council.

5. The Francis Report was published on the basis of a public inquiry into poor care at the Mid Staffordshire NHS Foundation Trust. The report examined what led to poor standards of care and unnecessary patient deaths at the hospital, and why the warning signs of serious failings were not recognised.

6. A hate crime is defined as '[a]ny criminal offence which is perceived by the victim or any other person, to be motivated by hostility or prejudice based on a person's race or perceived race; religion or perceived religion; sexual orientation or perceived sexual orientation; disability or perceived disability and any crime motivated by hostility or prejudice against a person who is transgender or perceived to be transgender'

(Metropolitan Police definition, as quoted at www.cps.gov.uk/crime-info/hate-crime).

7. Browse Safeguarding Adults Reviews (SARs) - SCIE.

8. Browse Making Safeguarding Personal (MSP) – SCIE.

9. Browse Information sharing principles – the purpose and context – GMC (gmc-uk.org).

10. Browse nmc-code.pdf.

11. Browse https://safelives.org.uk.

12. The Care Act 2014, Section 42 requires that each local authority make enquiries or cause others to do so, if it believes that an adult is experiencing, or is at risk of, abuse or neglect. An enquiry should establish whether any action needs to be taken to prevent or stop abuse or neglect, and if so, by whom.

13. An item of 'overriding public interest' refers to a situation where it is essential to share information in order to prevent a crime or to protect others from harm (e.g. hate crime, which we have a statutory responsibility to report). This definition is supported by the Crime and Disorder Act 1998.

14. The term 'vital interests' is intended to cover only interests that are essential for someone's life. So this concept's lawful basis is very limited in scope; generally it applies only to matters of life and death.

15. Browse Adult Safeguarding: Roles and Competencies for Health Care Staff | Royal College of Nursing (rcn.org.uk).

Chapter 8

Carers' Needs before, during, and after Hospital Admissions

David Jolley, Brenda Roe, and Caroline Sutcliffe

Informal carers of people with dementia work with the person with dementia and professionals to form a secure triangle of care (see Figure 8.1). They make a huge contribution to the health and well-being of individuals and to the economics of care. They have rights recognised in legislation.

Unfortunately they are often dismayed by the care received by individuals with dementia when admission to a general hospital becomes necessary. This can be avoided and much better outcomes achieved for all concerned if professionals work with informal carers throughout the process of considering admission, effecting it, and living through it to discharge or death. Informal carers do not constitute a homogenous group: they have a range of characteristics, strengths, and needs.

Some are old and many have pathologies of their own and multiple responsibilities. They require to be listened to and to be respected.

Informal carers, who are often family carers, form a triangle of support and knowledge with the individual who is in need and with the professionals who give their expertise and time to understanding and resolving their difficulties.

Working together these elements of the triangle makes for strength, as depicted in Figure 8.1. Lack of trust or respect between any of two them can be damaging.

Who Are the Carers of Older People Who Are Admitted to General Hospital Wards in the United Kingdom?

While 95 per cent of people in the United Kingdom designated 'old' by virtue of a cut at 65 years live in ordinary housing, on their own or with a partner or other relatives, the very old (85 plus) are more likely to be using specialised supportive accommodation, including care homes or nursing homes. Many in their sixties and seventies, and even beyond, remain entirely robust and independent. They are able to look after themselves and are engaged in creative and leisure activities, often providing help to others of similar age or to younger people – family or otherwise. When people lose their abilities, members of family, especially live-in partners, simply fill in their needs without question and without recognising themselves as 'carers'. It has been estimated that in the United Kingdom informal carers devote 1.34 billion hours of time to helping others each year: this is valued at £11.6 billion, if provided by paid professionals. Almost 60 per cent of carers are women. Twenty percent of people aged 50–64 are providing care for another adult; even among 85-year-olds, 10 per cent are active in a caring role. Some carers are young, about 700,000 are of school age, and increasing awareness is beginning to address the special needs of children and adolescents who devote much of their lives to caring for their parents or grandparents (1, 2, 3, 4, 5).

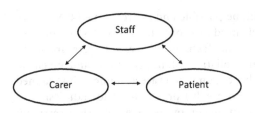

Figure 8.1 The triangle of care

Carers Have Rights, Which Are Specified in the Carers Act 2014 (6, 7)

'Section 10: Where it appears to a local authority that a carer may have needs for support (whether currently or in the future), the authority must assess whether the carer does have needs for support (or is likely to do so in the future), and what those needs are (or are likely to be in the future). ...

"Carer" means an adult who provides or intends to provide care for another adult. The duty to carry out a carer's assessment applies regardless of the level of the carer's needs for support, or the level of the carer's financial resources or of those of the adult needing care.

A carer's assessment must include an assessment of whether the carer is able, and is likely to continue to be able, to provide care for the adult needing care, whether the carer is willing, and is likely to continue to be willing, to do so, the outcomes that the carer wishes to achieve in day-to-day life, and whether, and to what extent, the provision of support could contribute to the achievement of those outcomes.'

The assessment must involve the carer and any person whom the carer asks the authority to involve.

Thus the provision of an assessment is a statutory and mandatory duty of a local authority. It is expected that plans for the future will include agreement if and when needs will be reviewed.

Carers' Needs before Admission

There are instances in which individuals find themselves in a carer–cared-for relationship as a result of an illness or injury that requires hospital admission, when previously these individuals were independent. Among older people, however, hospital admission is often sought because of a surge in the needs of someone who is already known to have limitations due to pathologies and impairments, but who has been coping, hopefully thriving, thanks to the help of others. When people move into supervised care or care homes, some of the responsibilities of family carers are taken on by professional carers, but family carers continue to have a role and ultimate responsibilities. The work of family and friends may be supplemented by regular contributions by professional staff from health and social care organisations or commercial care agencies. In addition, voluntary organisations may have a part in the matrix of care. Any or all of those providing care may notice changes that require additional help.

It may be immediately obvious that hospital care and treatment is the only option, for example in the case of a fall and fracture. There are many instances, however, in which careful assessment by medical or nursing staff members who know the patient in primary care will be essential. It may be concluded that additional care and treatment, at home or in a care home, will be possible and is preferable (4, 8, 9, 10). In making a decision in this regard, people need to know what resources and options are available locally, from social services and from health care. Carers are to be respected, involved in the collection and collation of information, and given all necessary information for the next stage, be it augmented care at home (with planned regular review of success or of need for more help) or a request for admission to hospital. This approach is well established within comprehensive geriatric assessment (see Chapter 19).

Transition to Hospital

Removal from home to hospital is a potentially traumatic life event. Transfer may be in a family vehicle, but more often will be by ambulance, after an assessment by paramedics. Paramedics have rightly become highly respected figures in the community. They represent the friendly, competent face of the hospital in people's own homes and in the streets. They will work with the patients, their carers, and others in assessing and balancing existing needs and in making the decision to admit or to continue the care at home.

Matters may be complicated if the unwell individual is confused and lacks the capacity to understand what is happening to him or her or what will be the best way of dealing with his or her difficulties. In cases where individuals have lost capacity over a period of time because of dementia or similar disorders, this may have been formally acknowledged. Lasting power of attorney may rest on a carer, and it may cover decisions on health care and welfare (11, 12). Some individuals will have completed an advance directive or an advance care plan (13), in anticipation of such situations and in the event of their losing capacity. Carers are the likely custodians of such information, which will help and inform decisions.

If it is possible for a carer to accompany the patient to hospital, this will always be helpful; it will provide a degree of reassurance through familiarity and will allow the carer to be part of the venture, steer it to a degree, and report on it to others who need to know.

The removal of one vulnerable older person from home may leave alone another, who has helped or been helped – alone and also fearful of what has become of their partner, and perhaps in need of extra support themselves. There may be cats, dogs, or other smaller dependents who should not be forgotten: one needs to make sure that they are safely provided for and that their owner has peace of mind on this subject.

Carers' Needs during the Period in Which the Person They Care for Is in Hospital

First impressions: In many instances patients will be 'processed' via an Accident and Emergency Department (A&E), then by an Admission or Assessment Unit (14). Neither of these environments is famed for its calm or its perceived friendliness (15, 16). Clissett quotes an observation: 'A & E was seen as a chaotic place' (15, p. 2710).

For some, this will be the first experience of the hospital; for others, it will be a return to sites that may carry legacies of good or not so good experiences. Transfer from ambulance or other transport ought not to be delayed, for the safety, comfort, and reassurance of both patient and carers. Anxiety will be running high and symptoms may be worsened.

The process of registration is crucial to progress. Members of A&E staff will always do their best to be welcoming, calm, and informative. Their task is not eased by the pressure of referrals at some times of the day and night, and it certain to get even more complicated if there is antisocial behaviour among patients and their associates.

Approaches to calmness: Older patients are likely to be fearful, and some will be confused. In the potential chaos, the staff has to give priority to people who require most immediate attention, and this means that some will have to wait.

The presence of one or more carers is helpful in that it provides reassurance and, when the registration and assessment can proceed, these people contribute key information on the development of symptoms and difficulties; they also represent points of contact with this and other agencies from the recent and less recent past. They may carry medication or relevant documents that bring clarification and facilitate decision-making. To optimise their contribution, carers need to be involved in the process, listened to, and their needs for comfort and understanding acknowledged. Their presence at the initial examination of the physical and mental state of the patient may be appropriate and welcomed by the patient – but the patient needs to be asked.

When the examination is followed by investigations, the process can take quite a long time. While investigations are conducted and results awaited, carers will help by offering support, but will require the availability of food and drink, toilet, and basic necessities. They and the patient will need to have a clear understanding of what is going on and who will let them know when results are available and decisions can be made. They will want to be able to communicate with others to inform them of progress or to ask for key information or resources that they have not brought with them. This will often be possible by mobile phone, used with consideration.

Both patient and carer, then, need a clear account of what has been found by the doctors and nurses and a provisional interpretation of what this means and what will be done. What will be done includes the decision to offer admission, along with a discussion of alternatives.

Admission: This is likely to be in the first instance to an assessment ward. Here the emphasis is usually on intensive investigation of physical ill-health – more clinical examinations, blood tests, urine tests, and maybe x-rays, scans, ultrasounds, or ECGs and monitoring. Space is often limited, members of staff move about with urgency, and there may be visits from any number of clinical teams and experts; noise is distracting and can be oppressive. It is desirable that space be provided for carers to be with or near the person they care for. They should be made welcome and assured that their knowledge and views will be fully respected and acted upon. Carers, in response, are to be expected to contribute reasonably – there should be a maximum of two carers in attendance for one patient at any one time. They will need to understand that the staff has to care for, and respond to, all patients and families and cannot be with everyone at the same time.

It will be helpful if a named individual in the clinical team is identified in each shift as the source of information and support for each patient and his or her carers. An area that offers time and space for carers to discuss matters with staff members in quiet and privacy should be available. Access to toilet facilities, refreshments, and modes of communication with others are requirements. Some carers who have travelled from afar will be pleased to be given information about local shops, accommodation, buses, trams, trains, and other facilities. Safe car parking at modest tariff is a must.

Carers and patients will contribute to the history of the present complaint. They should be made aware of what clinical examinations and investigations are being done and why. It is good practice for one member of family to be identified as the 'scribe'; this member should be asked to keep notes of the main points in such discussions and to check with the informant that they have understood the communication correctly and recorded it accurately. Their notes can be updated as new information, the results of investigations, their interpretation, and the resulting plans become available. All this knowledge can be shared with others on a need-to-know basis, to reduce anxiety about the unknown and to keeping the channels open for sharing more relevant observations and ideas.

Mental disorders: Although the main reason for hospitalisation relates to a change in physical health, this is often complicated by the presence of altered mental function. Such alteration may be something that was evident, recognised, and established before admission, but could emerge as a component of the multidimensional decompensation that has determined that admission is appropriate.

The common mental disorders that affect older people admitted to the general hospital wards are dementia, delirium, and depression (see Chapters 9, 11, and 12). The individuals involved and their family carers may be well aware of these conditions and confident in their knowledge of them, but, for many, this will be a first encounter with or first awareness of them. It will be important for staff in the assessment unit, directly or with help from others, to be able to explain these conditions to family carers. It will be helpful if verbal explanations can be backed up with suitable written material and references to easily available, trusted Internet resources (17, 18, 19).

Mental Capacity: Any severe mental disorder can impair individuals' competence to comprehend their situation and circumstances and their ability to make valid decisions about what is to happen to them. This is most regularly so when individuals have dementia or delirium. In the event of someone losing the capacity to speak for themselves, additional responsibilities fall upon the hospital staff and upon family carers. The Mental Capacity Act (12) clarifies the concepts of mental capacity and loss of mental capacity. Where loss of capacity is confirmed, current legislation requires that Deprivation of Liberty Safeguards (DoLS) be invoked (see Chapter 6 for details) (20). Completion of this procedure allows the hospital to care for the individual and to undertake appropriate treatment, which should be informed by considering that person's best interest. This may be a new world of experience and legislation for family carers. It is important that staff members on the ward feel adequately trained to introduce and discuss these matters, either directly or via easy access to knowledgeable people. It will be important to have written material on the ward for carers to read and take way, together with references to the relevant websites. DoLS are part of the Mental Capacity Act 2005 and have come to be seen by some as an expensive bureaucratic process, which delivers few clinical benefits and can be distressing. A reform of all mental health legislation is under consideration. The Law Commission has produced an inspirational report, which recommends better alternatives to DoLS (21).

Relocation within the hospital: Some patients' hospital experience will end in death or in discharge home from the assessment unit. The remainder will move to a ward that is best equipped to deal with the illness identified as their main problem at the time. The process of progressive patient care, which sees patients transferred from A&E to the assessment unit and from there to the final ward, has its advantages, but means that patients and family carers have to cope with three transitions before they can settle into receiving treatment and getting better. There are many advantages when patients and carers find themselves in a familiar ward, among staff they know. Multiple admissions are not uncommon for frail older people. Systems that are designed to place them in the same ward will maximise the therapeutic potential of shared knowledge and respect between members of staff, patients, and carers.

Unfortunately, pressure on beds and 'on take' arrangements often means that this continuity does not happen. The shift system ensures that staff members often receive information via notes rather than carrying personal knowledge from one day to the next; and something like 'I have been off for a week', followed by reference to a slip of paper, does not endear the communicant to an anxious family or to other professionals.

There are particular problems for patients who have become confused through either a symptomatic delirium or established dementia, for they cannot complete the narrative themselves. The task of helping them to understand where they are and what is going on can benefit from the involvement of family carers.

Dissonance: The fact that carers often feel excluded and ignored can become the basis of what Jurgens has termed 'the cycle of discontent' (16). Carers find themselves in an alien environment. They are the people who know the patient best. Every day they have probably devoted hours to caring at home, and have given up only in the face of increasing problems – but with an expectation that the hospital and its staff can reverse the difficulties. Thus sensitised, carers become anxious and are easily angered if they find themselves and their knowledge dismissed rather than included. When they see needs and problems that pass unnoticed by staff, or when they do not receive an appropriate response in reasonable time, their energies are likely to get diverted and channelled towards hypervigilant querulousness and complaints.

Their suspicions are well founded:

> 'It is everybody's experience, that staff do not really know their patients and often fail to provide even the basics of care.' This from a consultant psychiatrist who is often called to help when there are problems on a general hospital ward. Nicci Gerrard and her friend Julia Jones were so devastated by the treatment received by Nicci's doctor father, when he was admitted to a hospital, that they have established 'John's Campaign' to alert everyone to the hazards, and in the belief that things can be better.
>
> (22)

Barbara Hodkinson was similarly motivated by the care that her mother required, and thus she established the Butterfly Scheme (23). There are any number of reports and publications that document failings and their consequences. These include reports from the Ombudsman and from the Care Quality Commission and other inquiries (24, 25, 26). This is not to say that there are not carers and visitors who are unreasonable or vexatious. It is important to be aware and beware of such, but they are rare in comparison with the many who are rightly concerned and would wish to be constructive.

Good Practice

Provide time and space for the task of making carers welcome.

- Listen to their comments and their wisdom about what works best when it comes to reassuring and settling their relative. Make sure staff members in all shifts are aware of these pieces of advice and use them in their caring.

- If the patient is muddled or lacks the confidence or ability to communicate, supplement the knowledge about him or her with the help of cue lists such as 'This is me' (27); consider using the Butterfly Scheme or something similar for a discrete identification of patients who need special understanding.
- Take care to acknowledge difference – in culture, sexual orientation, educational achievements or limitations – and act accordingly.
- Provide education and training for staff on the hospital ward, and do it with the involvement of carers.
- Celebrate good news stories, so that they may be used as models.
- Nurture an open and caring attitude of mind.
- When families have limited English, identify their preferred language of communication. Obtain the help of a competent translator in order to gather information from them, to explain to them what is being done, and to convey to them the findings and the interpretation of examinations and investigations, as well as the proposed plans of action.
- Strong support for patients' families will often come from in local communities and faith organisations.
- Be culturally sensitive, because beliefs about altered mental function differ greatly across cultures and the stigma associated with mental disorder can be very strong (28). This means that in such cultures appreciating and accepting the presence of dementia, delirium, or depression is even more difficult and requires extremely sensitive communication and explanation.

Progress within the ward: During their relatives' hospital stay, some carers will wish to give them time beyond the limited visiting hours. They may help with meal times. This is particularly helpful when patients are confused or impaired by dementia; it reduces the risk that food and drink are not taken because the patient fails to recognise the need, or to recognise nutrition for what it is, or to coordinate the sequences needed to achieve consumption. Carers may be able to help with toileting or alerting staff to the need, thus avoiding incontinence, distress, and the requirement for additional change of clothing or bedding. They may be able to support their relative and the staff when these attend investigations done by other units in the hospital. Journeys through corridors and lifts to strange places can be alarming and compound patients' confusion. The presence of a carer provides continuity for the patient and is often helpful to staff members of the special unit, who cannot always be easily aware of every aspect of the patient's difficulties. There may be situations in which a relative's involvement at bath time can turn a trial into a cooperative pleasure.

Carer initiatives: Some wards will organise carer groups or will encourage carers to form such a group. This has the potential to facilitate communication and discussion with carers collectively as well as individually. Members will share thoughts and experiences and will help one another in practical ways. Such groups can develop a life of their own, and people will continue to be involved beyond the time of admission. Some groups will organise activities, raise funds, improve standards, and make representations to the hospital hierarchy (29).

Diagnosis and prognosis: The hope is that treatable conditions will be identified and will respond to therapy. Carers will want to know what has been discovered, what treatment is being undertaken, and what the likely outcome would be. They will want to know these things in order to counter their own anxieties and fears and those of the patient and so they can make plans to continue their support. Yet the sharing of such privileged information has to respect the privacy and confidentiality of the patient. In many instances a competent patient will agree to share information with key carers. When patients are severely unwell and their competence is impaired, staff members must make a best interest judgement about sharing with key carers their knowledge and their anticipation of future needs. There must be clear advice on limitations – that is, on limiting how this information can be used.

Resolution: The time course over which symptoms resolve is variable. In cases where symptomatic confusion or delirium has complicated a physical illness, the confusion often persists for days after other markers such as temperature and blood tests have returned to normal. Carers as well as staff have to be aware of this and encouraged to remain expectant and optimistic of recovery. It is important not to make plans on the basis of a partial recovery, as they prove to be unnecessarily restrictive and expensive in the goodness of time.

Persisting or progressive symptoms: There are instances in which it becomes clear that the illness is such that it is not responsive to treatment in the short run and will end in death in hospital. In others it may be possible to achieve resolution for the immediate problems, but the underlying and perhaps progressive pathology will persist and require additional help and therapy in the future.

Death: Death in the hospital is not an outcome that is welcomed. The hospital is a place where most deaths in the United Kingdom occur, yet surveys repeatedly find that people prefer the prospect of dying at home, or maybe in a hospice (30). Very old people, particularly those with established dementia, increasingly find death in a care home (31).

People fear death in hospital because they doubt that the ward would look on the process positively and make proper provision for the comfort and dignity of patients (32, 33, 34). This fear and the potential for distress and anger are felt most acutely by carers who are closest.

Once the proximity of death is identified, it is essential that it be shared with the patient and with key carers. This has to be done carefully, with sensitivity, by a senior member of the ward team, in a situation of privacy, and with time for emotions, contemplation, and discussion. Some will wish to include a chaplain or a faith leader. Others will wish to consider returning home or being transferred to a hospice. But, for many, the only practical and realistic option is death in the hospital. This requires that the ward adopts a palliative mode, which is at odds with the mode that informs its dominant image of recovery. The Gold Standards Framework for End of Life Care in the United Kingdom provides useful guidance, tools, and training specifically for the event of dying (35).

Carers will be grateful for a private place and for the option to be present in reasonable numbers at all hours of the day and night and to be updated on progress and plans. Their needs for rest, refreshments, and means of communication should be met as far as is possible. They may spend time alone with their loved one, but will value regular and frequent interactions with staff.

After the death, carers will continue to need time and space to come to terms with what has happened and to make plans for the next move. They will return later to deal with the practicalities of receiving the death certificate, registering the death, and making arrangements for a funeral. For some families, their faith with have particular requirements as to how the death and its aftermath are to be handled. It is essential that the ward is aware of these and is able to respect them.

When the process of dying and death are handled well, families are grateful. When there are problems and disharmony, the pain of loss is compounded, so that both feelings for and memories of the hospital will be adverse.

The death of a loved one, even a person with severe dementia, is something that few can take in their stride. It is even more difficult when people are changed by mental disorder during the dying time, as family members have to struggle to maintain some sort of contact and communication, sometimes having to deal with fierce and alien behaviour. Having this as a final memory is hard indeed after many years of life together, especially a life blessed with peace and harmony. Extra time and extra supportive counselling may be needed.

Specialist services relating to older people with altered mental function: Issues of mental health, particularly dementia, delirium, and depression, are so common that many general hospitals now arrange their own services to deal positively and effectively with these conditions. There are good arguments for developing one ward that has a special interest and expertise in the assessment, care, and treatment of patients with the most complex and challenging mix of physical and mental health problems. This ward will accommodate those in the greatest difficulty, but will also act as a base for outreach and for the support of other wards, with the help of nurses and others who have expertise (29).

Specialist dementia nurses may work without having the advantage of a specialised ward. In addition, mental health services will provide a liaison service. Liaison services constitute a more effective and less costly option than employed guards (36). When staff on a ward considers asking for help from a mental health liaison team or specialist nurse, family carers should be made aware of this and consulted on their views. They should be invited to attend when the specialist nurse or the liaison team makes contact with the patient for the first time. They can then share their knowledge and thoughts with the team and contribute to plans. This may be the beginning of continued involvement with specialist mental health services, or the team's advice may be of use to the ward team or to primary care when the patient leaves hospital.

Transition from Hospital and Carers Needs Thereafter

When plans are made for individual patients to leave hospital, they may be taken to their own home, where they were living prior to admission; but the move can also be to a more supported accommodation or a care home. In the series described by Clissett and colleagues, only six out of sixteen people living alone returned home, while eight went into care. Out of eleven people living with family members, five returned home and four went into care. Four of the seven who previously lived in care returned to be in care (15). This means that, for many, the setting after hospital will be different from the one they had before. Carers and patients should be included in the multidisciplinary, multi-agency meetings that decide upon placement and upon the support to be made available from the moment of discharge. These are major decisions, stressful to all parties. Carers are likely to be heavily involved in identifying a care home placement. They need to have information about the availability of homes and access to reports of their characteristics and to Care Quality Commission ratings. They will visit homes with the patient and contribute to discussions with staff from potential placements, at the hospital. When patients have limited or lost mental capacity, carers will play a large role in determining best interest for them. They will also be key to a successful transition into the new world of life in a care home. They will reassure and confirm the identity of the individual who moves into care; they are the main continuity factor for this person, as they carry his or her culture from home as was to home as is and will be. They will weigh staff and regimes and encourage and contribute to good practice. At a basic level, they will make sure that the practicalities of taking appropriate clothes and other belongings to the home are achieved, that the new doctor becomes known, and that therapy begun in hospital is continued as planned.

When it is felt that return home is feasible, there will be expectations from carers that they return to their caring role – sometimes with added responsibilities. Expectations should not be unreasonably demanding. In many instances it will be possible to complement the informal care at home with expertise and dedicated time from healthcare or social care professionals. The care plan should be written and approved with the involvement of the patient and main carers. An individual or a role designation should be identified as the point of reference (single point of access or contact with a telephone number), which can be contacted if modifications are needed in the light of experience, or to avoid a potential crisis. A key component of a successful discharge home is communication with the primary care team and its agreement and involvement in continuing therapy. Medication may differ from the regular prescription prior to admission. Carers can play a role in communicating with primary care. They will also be involved in follow-up arrangements made by specialist services.

The Health of Carers

Carers are not a homogeneous group; some are young, though of them many are old. Women constitute the majority, but many men take willingly to the task. Many are retired from paid work, some are still employed. Differences in faith, culture, language, and sexual orientation may mark individuals and couples as 'minorities' within the wider population.

But all carers have it in common that they are exposed to stress and to various constraints on their personal freedom.

Among older carers, physical illness, disability, and symptoms are common: arthritis, joint problems, back problems, heart disease, cancer, pain or discomfort, and depression are often found in surveys (2, 35). When individuals are caring for more than one dependent, the logistics of how to make the time and effort equate with the needs are more challenging and the stress greater. Requests for care may come from younger members of family as well as from the older generations. Carers who are aged over 75, who are disturbed at night, who provide heavy physical care, or who have to cope with challenging behaviour usually are the ones most at risk of becoming unwell and of finding themselves feeling burdened and overwhelmed. Lack of support from other members of the family, or narrow insistence, from the patient, that all care must come from one carer are other factors that push people beyond what they can do.

There may be marked differences of view between family members. These possibly have their roots in long-established mutual hostilities or reflect different readings of what is best for the member who is in need of help. It is not unusual for carers' loyalties to be strained as a result of calls upon them from more than one family member in need. All these difficulties compound the stress and may lead to decompensation. They (or some of them) may emerge as issues during the time in hospital, perhaps most acutely when carers are planning their next move.

Some carers continue to work and have a professional life, but others sacrifice their careers in order to make time to be carers. Finances are often severely squeezed, benefits may not be accessed for lack of knowledge or out of pride and, even when they are, they rarely compensate fully for carers' loss of earnings. Carers usually give up hobbies and withdraw from social and other voluntary activities. This leaves them isolated and lonely, vulnerable to depression, loss of sleep and appetite, and further deterioration of their own health.

Abuse does occur in care situations. This is something that services must be sensitive to. Abuse may emerge when a carer is overstressed and can find no way to escape unbearable and unremitting expectations of them. Carers may be agents of abuse, but sometimes they are victims (37).

Factors that mitigate the stresses of caring include the timely and reliable provision of help from services: aids and adaptations, help with the basics of care for the patient and the home, time for oneself by way of a respite – someone to share the care with, maybe attendance at a day centre, or a respite admission. Education and training in techniques of lifting, or dealing with, behavioural change have their place. Just having someone to talk to who will listen non-judgementally is therapeutic in itself, though some will find advantage in talking therapies or peer group meetings and discussion with others in similar positions. Admiral Nurses were created in response to a family's declaration that they needed help themselves, as they struggled with the physical and emotional strains of living with their father's progressive dementia (38). Yet out of the struggle came insights and knowledge that can now be usefully shared with others. TIDE (together in dementia everyday) is an organisation that offers carers support and training to share their stories in order to educate professionals, commissioners, politicians, and others who should know (39).

Studies confirm that all these approaches reduce measures of stress, improve measures of help among carers, and reduce the likelihood of repeated admission to hospital (40–46).

Summary in a Box: The essentials for carers

- respect
- information
- to be listened to
- to be involved
- to be understood
- to be offered help with stress and illness
- to be offered education and maybe training
- to be offered regular respite breaks if required
- single point of contact or person / phone number

Covid-19 and Its Impact on the Experience of People with Dementia and Their Family Carers in the Course of Hospitalisation in the United Kingdom, 2020–1

The Covid-19 pandemic has had a massive impact on the lives of people in the United Kingdom and on the healthcare and social care services. Hospital wards have been closed to routine and non-emergency admissions, to make it possible for beds to be used for cases of Covid-19. Staff has been redeployed from its usual roles and made to care for people with Covid.

People with dementia who had become ill enough to qualify for hospital admission were told, like everyone else, that they could not receive visitors. This strategy, introduced in order to reduce the spread of the virus, has been particularly difficult for people with dementia and their family carers. Patients are often unable to understand what is happening; they cannot comprehend why their family has deserted them. They become distressed, and their illness is compounded. Families were distraught as a result of being separated from the loved one whom they had been caring for at this frightening time. Deaths have occurred in great numbers among people with dementia; for many, the death has followed a period of enforced isolation from their family.

The interpretation of this policy has varied across hospitals. Some hospitals have allowed visits from a named carer, especially when the end of life was seen to be approaching. Balancing the advantages of visits with the risks of infection and the emotional stress to patients, families, and professionals is recognised to have been extremely difficult.

Approaches designed to allow some form of contact during hospital stays have included the use of mobile phones and video links via the Internet. Although there is no effective replacement of the reassurance of face-to-face contact, which was supplanted by the power of touch, there has been some beneficial learning to come from these necessities (45-49).

Acknowledgement

The ideas and structure of this chapter have benefited from discussion with many colleagues, people with dementia, and carers. Special thanks to people who attend Dementia Conversations at Bowdon Vale, to Barbara Stephens, to members of TIDE, and to a weekly seminar group at Wythenshawe Hospital.

References

1. Visit https://carers.org/key-facts-about-carers-and-people-they-care.

2. Visit https://carers.org/news-item/older-carers-putting-their-health-risk-care-spouses-and-partners.

3. Age UK. *Briefing: Health and Care of Older People in England*. London: Age UK, 2017.

4. Cameron, I., Aggar, C., Robinson, A., and Kurrle, S. Assessing and helping carers of older people. *BMJ* 2011, 343. doi: 10.1136/bmj.d5202.

5. Carers Trust. *Caring about Older Carers: Providing Support for People Caring in Later Life*. London: Carers Trust, 2015.

6. Carers Act 2014. www.legislation.gov.uk/ukpga/2014/23/section/10.

7. Carers Act 2014. For the whole act, visit www.legislation.gov.uk/ukpga/2014/23.

8. National Institute for Health and Clinic al Excellence and SCIE. Joint publication: Dementia: Supporting people with dementia and their carers in health and social care. November 2006. www.scie.org.uk/publications/misc/dementia.

9. SCIE. Assessing the mental health needs of older people. April 2006. www.scie.org.uk/publications/guides/guide03.

10. Imison C, Poteliakhoff E and Thompson J. Older people and emergency bed use: exploring variation. The Kings Fund.

Ideas that change health care. London 2012

11. GOV.UK. Make, register or end a lasting power of attorney. www.gov.uk/power-of-attorney.

12. Mental Capacity Act 2005. www.legislation.gov.uk/ukpga/2005/9/contents.

13. Tidy, C. Advance care planning. Patient: Professional Articles, Primary Care (General Practice), 2005. https://patient.info/doctor/advance-care-planning.

14. Scott, I., Vaughan, L., and Bell, D. Effectiveness of acute medical units in hospitals: A systematic review. *International Journal of Quality in Health Care* 2009, 21(6): 39–407.

15. Clissett, P., Porock, D., Harwood, R., and Gladman, J. Experiences of family carers of older people with mental health problems in the acute general hospital: A qualitative study. *Journal of Advanced Nursing* 2013, 69(12): 2707–16.

16. Jurgens, F., Clissett, P., Gladman, J., and Harwood, R. Why are family carers of people with dementia dissatisfied with general hospital care? A qualitative study. *BMC Geriatrics* 2012, 12: 57.

17. NHS Choices: About dementia. www.nhs.uk/conditions/dementia/about.

18. Guy's and St Thomas' NHS Foundation Trust. Delirium: Information for relatives, carers and patients. https://static1.squarespace.com/static/620644a7f9b6c87ecd6dcc99/t/64527268874dc6336a705c91/1683124840834/Delirium.pdf.

19. National Institute on Aging. Depression and older adults. www.nia.nih.gov/health/depression-and-older-adults.

20. The Mental Capacity (Deprivation of Liberty Standard Authorisation) Regulations 2008. www.legislation.gov.uk/ukdsi/2008/9780110814773/contents.

21. Law Commission. Mental capacity and deprivation of liberty: Current project status. 2017. www.lawcom.gov.uk/project/mental-capacity-and-deprivation-of-liberty.

22. John's Campaign. www.johnscampaign.org.uk.

23. The Butterfly Scheme. www.butterflyscheme.org.uk.

24. Parliamentary and Health Service Ombudsman. Care and Compassion, 14 February, 2011. www.ombudsman.org.uk/publications/care-and-compassion.

25. Care Quality Commission. Dignity and nutrition for older people. 18 March 2013. www.cqc.org.uk/publications/themed-inspection/dignity-and-nutrition-older-people.

26. Francis, R., QR (chair). *Independent Inquiry into Care Provided by Mid Staffordshire NHS Foundation Trust, January 2005–March 2009*. London: Stationery Office, 2010. www.gov.uk/government/uploads/system/uploads/attachment_data/file/279109/0375_i.pdf.

27. Alzheimer's Society. This is me. www.alzheimers.org.uk/info/20113/publications_about_living_with_dementia/415/this_is_me.

28. Giebel, C. et al. South Asian older adults with memory impairment: improving assessment and access to dementia care. *International Journal of Geriatric Psychiatry* 2015, 30(4): 345–56.

29. Willoughby, J. Dementia Friendly Hospitals Charter. https://www.dementiaaction.org.uk/news/28149_dementia_friendly_hospitals_charter_interview_julie_willoughby.

30. What's important to me: A review of choice in end of life care. The Choice in End of Life Care Programme Board, 2015. https://assets.publishing.service.gov.uk/government/uploads/system/uploads/attachment_data/file/407244/CHOICE_REVIEW_FINAL_for_web.pdf.

31. Office for National Statistics. Deaths of care home residents, England and Wales: 2021. https://www.ons.gov.uk/peoplepopulationandcommunity/birthsdeathsandmarriages/deaths/bulletins/deathsinthecaresectorenglandandwales/2021.

32. Dewing, J., and Dijk, S. What is the current state of care for older people with dementia in general hospitals? A literature review. *Dementia* 2016, 15(1): 106–24.

33. La Fontaine, J., Juttla, K., Read, K., Brooker, D., and Evans, S. *The Experiences, Needs and Outcomes for Carers of People with Dementia: A Literature Review*. University of Worcester: Association of Dementia Studies, 2016.

34. Goldberg, S., and Harwood, R. Experiences of general hospital care in older patients with cognitive impairment: Are we measuring the most vulnerable patients' experiences? *BMJ Qual Saf* 2013, 977–80.

35. ILC-UK. The emotional well-being of older carers. ILC-UK London, 2015. https://ilcuk.org.uk/wp-content/uploads/2018/10/The-emotional-well-being-of-older-carers.pdf.

36. Dementia UK, n.d. www.dementiauk.org.

37. TIDE: Together in Dementia Everyday, n. d. http://tide.uk.net.

38. Parker, D., Mills, R., and Abbey, J. Effectiveness of interventions that assist caregivers to support people with dementia living in the community: A systematic review. *International Journal of Evidence-Based Healthcare* 2008, 6(2): 137–72.

39. Selwood, J., Johnston, K., Katona, C., Lyketsos, G., and Livingston, G. Systematic review of the effect of psychosocial interventions on family care-givers of people with dementia. *Journal of Affective Disorders* 2007, 1–3: 75–89.

40. Pickard, L. The effectiveness and cost effectiveness of support and services to informal carers of older people: A review of the literature prepared for the Audit Commission. Discussion Paper. Personal Social Services Research Unit. London School of Economics, 2014.

41. Brodaty, H. Family care-givers of people with dementia. *Dialogues in Clinical Neuroscience* 2009, 11(2): 217–28.

42. Moniz-Cook, E., Vernooj-Dassen, M., Woods, R. et al. A European consensus on outcome measures for psychosocial intervention research in dementia care. *Journal of Aging and Mental Health* 2008, 12(1): 14–29.

43. Prince, M., Comas-Herrera, A., Knapp, M., Guerchet, M., and Karagiannidou, M. *World Alzheimer Report 2016: Improving Healthcare for People Living with Dementia: Coverage, Quality and Costs Now and in the Future*. London: Alzheimer's Disease International (ADI), 2016.

44. Banerjee, S., and Wittenberg, R. Clinical and cost effectiveness of services for early diagnosis and intervention in dementia. *International Journal of Geriatric Psychiatry* 2009, 24(7): 748–54.

45. National Audit of Dementia. Impact of the COVID-19 pandemic on hospital care for people with dementia. RC-PSYCH, n. d. impact-of-covid-19-on-dementia-care-report.pdf (rcpsych.ac.uk).

46. N. Greenwood, STSFT. Visiting during the COVID-19 pandemic. NHS England, n.d.

47. Social care cuts mean thousands with dementia taken to A&E, charity says. *The Guardian*, 17 May 2021.

48. Downar, J., and Kekewich, M. Improving family access to dying patients during the COVID-19 pandemic. *Lancet Respir Med* 4, 2021: 335–7.

49. BBC News. Coronavirus: Family visit plea over dementia patients. 10 June 2020, BBC News. www.bbc.co.uk/news/uk-wales-52984465.

Dementia and Related Disorders

Ayesha Bangash and Farooq Khan

Introduction

Raising the awareness of acute hospital healthcare professionals (HCPs) about dementia and the common symptoms that people with dementia experience can maximise the rate of detection of these symptoms and empower patients and their carers to report them. Improving dementia awareness is a global priority, as stated by the World Health Organization (WHO). In the United Kingdom, the national dementia strategy and a policy paper titled 'Prime Minister's Challenge on Dementia 2020' aim to improve dementia care; specific policy has been created with the aim of improving the care for people with dementia in a hospital setting. The national strategy is supported by non-government organisations such as the Kings Fund, which in 2014 issued a programme titled 'Enhancing the Healing Environment', and the Royal College of Nursing, which in 2013 articulated its five principles in a statement titled 'Commitment to the Care of People with Dementia in General Hospitals'. Both of these initiatives aim to improve the hospital environment by promoting dementia-friendly wards and HCPs' awareness of dementia and of the challenges it presents.

Dementia describes a group of brain disorders that cause gradual cognitive impairment, which becomes serious enough to affect a person's daily functioning (1). Cognition encompasses knowledge, memory, judgement, attention, solving problems and making decisions. Dementia produces a decline both in intellectual functioning and in the ability to undertake personal activities of daily living such as washing, dressing, eating, personal hygiene, and toilet activities (2). How such a decline manifests itself will depend largely on the social and cultural setting in which the patient lives. A person's consciousness is usually not affected. There are currently around 850,000 people with dementia in the United Kingdom (3).

Epidemiology

Estimates of the prevalence of dementia in hospitals vary across published studies but range between 5 per cent and 45 per cent (4–7). Patients with dementia have high rates of hospital admissions: around 6 per cent of people with dementia are in-patients in general hospitals at a given time point, by comparison with approximately 0.6 per cent of over-65s without dementia (8). Although dementia prevalence is high, the proportion of those undiagnosed or unrecognized by healthcare staff in general hospitals is approximately 56 per cent (9). Patients who receive a dementia diagnosis in the community will have this diagnosis recorded by the hospital in 75 per cent cases. This is due to the lack of a formal system of communicating information between healthcare providers (10).

Subtypes of Dementia

Knowing the various types of dementia is vital, since each form of this disease can have a different course and responds differently to treatment. These types are listed in Table 9.1.

The commonest subtypes of dementia are described next.

Alzheimer's Disease

This condition represents an estimated 50 per cent of dementias. The most common early symptom is short-term memory loss. As the disease advances, symptoms can include problems with language, disorientation, inability to manage self-care, and behavioural issues. The disease process is associated with plaques and tangles in the brain and reduction in the activity of the cholinergic neurons. A computerised tomography (CT) or a magnetic resonance imaging (MRI) scan of the brain can show disproportionate atrophy of the medial temporal lobe, particularly of the volume of the hippocampal formations (13).

Vascular Dementia

This condition represents around 25 per cent of dementias (13). This form of dementia occurs in the context of cerebral ischemia (usually caused by poorly controlled cardiovascular disease), which often leads to transient ischemic attacks (TIAs) or strokes. The

Table 9.1 Dementia subtypes

Possible causes of cognitive impairment	
Reversible causes (11)	Hypothyroidism Folate/B12 deficiency Benign CNS tumours Hydrocephalus Chronic subdural haematoma
Irreversible causes (12)	*Degenerative dementias* Alzheimer's disease Dementia with Lewy bodies Frontotemporal dementia Progressive supranuclear palsy Corticobasal degeneration *Vascular dementia* Multi-infarct Subcortical
Infective (11)	Creutzfeldt-Jakob disease HIV
Immunologically mediated (11)	Multiple sclerosis Systemic lupus erythematosus Hashimoto's encephalopathy
Inherited (12)	Huntington's disease Wilson's disease
Psychiatric (12)	Depression (pseudodementia)

temporal relationship between a cerebrovascular event and cognitive deficits is required to make the diagnosis. People present with progressive cognitive impairment, frequently stepwise, after multiple cerebrovascular events. Features are typically the same as in other dementias. However, the presence of cerebrovascular disease on brain imaging and focal neurological signs such as dysarthria and hemiparesis differentiate vascular dementia from other dementias (14). Mixed dementia (i.e. Alzheimer's disease and vascular dementia) represents 5 per cent of dementia cases (13).

Dementia with Lewy Bodies

Dementia with Lewy bodies (DLB) represents an estimated 15 per cent of dementias (13). In contrast to other forms, it typically presents with a more rapid onset and with fluctuating degrees of cognitive impairment, visual hallucinations, and paranoid delusions. Motor features of Parkinsonism are present. The underlying mechanism involves the build-up of Lewy bodies, clumps of alpha-synuclein protein in neurons. Dementia with Lewy bodies is distinguished from dementia in Parkinson's disease by the time frame in which dementia symptoms appear in relation to Parkinson symptoms. In Parkinson's disease with dementia, the onset of dementia occurs more than a year after the onset of Parkinsonian symptoms. Dementia with Lewy bodies is diagnosed when cognitive symptoms begin at the same time as, or within a year of, Parkinsonian symptoms (15). If DLB is suspected when Parkinsonism and dementia are the only presenting features, positron emission tomography (PET) or single photon emission computed tomography (SPECT) imaging may show reduced dopamine transporter activity (16). A DLB diagnosis can also be supported using a dopamine transporter (DaT) scan (17).

Risk Factors for Dementia

The aetiology of dementia is usually multifactorial and poorly understood. Identified modifiable and non-modifiable risk factors for developing the syndrome are described below.

Age

Out of all the people with dementia in the United Kingdom, 5.2 per cent will be under the age of 65 (18). The risk of dementia increases significantly with advancing age. One in fourteen people over the age of 65 (7 per cent) and one in six people over the age of 80 have dementia (17 per cent) (19).

Genetics

Early-onset Alzheimer's disease has a very strong family pattern of inheritance. Studies of families affected by Alzheimer's demonstrate a higher prevalence in the presence of one of the following three genes mutations. These three genes are the amyloid precursor protein (APP) gene and two presenilin genes (PSEN-1 and PSEN-2). Mutations in such genes can cause early onset dementias; however, they are quite rare. Some families probably have a different and unknown mutation (20).

Most people do not develop dementia as a result of a single gene mutation. More than 20 gene variants have been associated with Alzheimer's type of dementia. The variants affect the risk of a person's developing this type of dementia, but do not directly cause it.

They tend to interact with one another and with other factors such as age and lifestyle, to influence the overall risk of getting a late-onset dementia. One gene, Apolipoprotein E, has been associated with an increased risk of late-onset Alzheimer's disease. There are three variants of it, namely APOE e2, APOE e3, and APOE e4 (20).

Gender

Women are more likely than men to develop Alzheimer's type of dementia. In the case of other dementias, men and women have much the same risk. For vascular dementia, men are at slightly higher risk than women, as a result of being at increased risk of atherosclerotic vascular disease and strokes (21).

Ethnicity

South Asian, African, and Afro-Caribbean people are more likely to develop vascular dementia than other ethnic communities. This could be due to their higher risk of stroke, cardiovascular disease, and diabetes (21).

Head Injury

Researchers have reported a link between traumatic head injury and dementia; however, the relationship between the two is not clear (21).

Alcohol

Alcohol use disorders are a major risk factor for all types of dementia (22).

Smoking

People who smoke have a higher risk of atherosclerosis and other types of vascular disease, which may be the underlying causes of the increased dementia risk (22).

Depression

Studies suggest that people who experience depressive episodes are at an increased risk of developing dementia when they are older (21).

Common Presentations of Dementia in a Hospital Setting

Most people with dementia are admitted to hospital for reasons other than dementia. The most common reasons for admissions are falls, broken or fractured hips or hip replacement, urinary tract infections, chest infections, poor nutrition, dehydration, or stroke (9). People living with dementia who are in hospital also have a high prevalence of experiencing delirium at some point during the admission (up to 66 per cent) (9). Behavioural and psychological symptoms of dementia (BPSD) are also common in the hospital, indeed more so than in the community: depression (34 per cent), anxiety (35 per cent), delusions (11 per cent) and hallucinations (15 per cent). The topic of is covered specifically in Chapter 10. Behavioural and psychological symptoms of dementia can occur in the absence of a delirium or can complicate it. The presence of psychological symptoms is associated with an increased incidence of falls and agitation (9, 10).

Approximately 61 per cent of community patients with dementia in the United Kingdom receive a dementia diagnosis, although figures can differ between geographical area (10). When a patient with a dementia diagnosis is admitted to hospital, there is no official system to communicate this information between healthcare providers. If the dementia diagnosis and the symptoms frequently associated with it are not identified and managed, patients can experience negative outcomes regarding morbidity, mortality, and length of stay. Dementia affects roughly half the patients in geriatric medicine departments; it also affects in-patient care, discharge, and the time when a person can live at home. Therefore it is vital for people to receive a timely diagnosis of dementia, both in the community and in hospital settings (10, 23).

Clinical Management

All elderly patients admitted urgently to hospital should be assessed for confusion and memory problems. This can be challenging in acutely unwell people. Delirium is common and virtually always causes deficits in cognitive tests. Medications, particularly those with anticholinergic effects, can affect cognition. Poorly controlled comorbid disease such as diabetes, a depressed conscious level, and sensory impairment can also impact on cognitive testing (23, 24).

Patient Report and Informant History

To make a dementia diagnosis, there should be evidence of significant cognitive decline from a previous level of performance in one or more cognitive domains:

- learning and memory (e.g. inability to learn new information or having forgotten previously recalled information)
- language (e.g. word-finding difficulty)
- executive function (e.g. problems with planning and organization)
- complex attention (e.g. problems with sustained attention)
- visuospatial impairment (problems with interpreting spatial relationships)
- agnosia (e.g. difficulty in recognising faces or objects)
- apraxia (inability to perform a motor task such as buttoning a shirt)

Such cognitive deficits should interfere with one's independence in everyday activities and do not occur in the context of a delirium. Symptoms must be present for at least six months to support a diagnosis (25).

In contrast to dementia, mild cognitive impairment (MCI) involves subjective symptoms (mostly of memory loss) and appreciable cognitive impairment, but there is no obvious impairment in activities of everyday life (11).

Objective Cognitive Assessment Tools

The Mini-Mental State Examination (MMSE) can be used. A score of under 24 out of 30 is suggestive of dementia. The Abbreviated Mental Test Score (AMTS) is also used. The conciseness of this tool is advantageous in busy acute wards, where undertaking longer cognitive tests may not be practical. It is relatively easier for patients with hearing or vision difficulties who do not need a motor response. The Montreal Cognitive Assessment (MoCA) is a 10-minute 30-point cognitive test with executive functioning and attention tasks designed for those who score 24–30 on MMSE. The suggested cut-off is 26 (26, 27). The Addenbrookes Cognitive Examination (ACE-III) has more frontal-executive and visuospatial items than the MMSE. Its diagnostic accuracy is considered to be somewhat superior to that of the MMSE and, despite the longer administration time of 16-20 minutes, ACE-III is recommended in most patient settings, including general hospitals. The cut-off score for dementia is 82-88/100 (28). Further information on psychometric scales in older people can be found in Chapter 21.

Investigations

In order to contribute to supporting dementia subtyping and rule out reversible causes of cognitive impairment, the following investigations are advised (13).

Blood Tests (14)

Full blood count (FBC), CRP Urea and electrolyte (U&E), liver function tests (LFTs), calcium, glucose and lipid profile Thyroid function, vitamin B12 and folate

Neuroimaging

Computerized tomography or MRI of the brain (14); PET, SPECT, and DaT scans of the brain can be considered for DLB (16, 17).

Clinical features generating suspicion of a less common (or atypical) cause of dementia include (12):

- early onset (under the age of 65)
- rapid progression
- family history
- systemic or neurological features other than those associated with the commonly seen dementias

Where less common causes of cognitive impairment are suspected, consider the following investigations:

- formal neuropsychometric assessments, which can help to differentiate normal aging from MCI and neurodegenerative disorders from reversible causes of impaired cognition (e.g. depression) and can also help in the differential diagnosis of dementias that are due to different aetiologies (e.g. Alzheimer's disease versus vascular dementia) (12, 29);
- genetic testing for various conditions such as Huntington's disease, familial Alzheimer's disease, familial prion dementia, and so on (12);
- HIV tests to exclude HIV-associated dementia (12, 30);
- connective tissue serology in suspected central nervous system (CNS) inflammation, for example erythrocyte sedimentation rate (ESR), anti-nuclear factor (ANF), anti-cardiolipin antibodies, anti-neutrophil cytoplasmic antibodies (ANCA), rheumatoid factor, anti-thyroid antibodies, caeruloplasmin level (12);
- electroencephalogram (EEG), which in patients in whom dementia is suspected is useful mainly to rule out delirium, depression, atypical complex partial seizures, and prion disease (12, 31);

- cerebrospinal fluid (CSF) examination can help to identify non-neurodegenerative diseases associated with cognitive or motor decline (or both), for example paraneoplastic syndromes and viral encephalitis (12, 32).

Pharmacological Interventions

There are currently no available medications that can reverse or halt the neurodegenerative processes observed in dementia. However, there are medications that in some people have been shown to help to maintain function – including cognition and behaviours – for longer periods after neuronal damage (22, 33).

Medications for Cognitive Impairment

Two classes of drugs are currently recommended:

- **Acetylcholinesterase (AChE) inhibitors:** donepezil, galantamine, and rivastigmine
- These are recommended in mild to moderate Alzheimer's disease. AChE inhibitors delay the breakdown of acetylcholine released into synaptic clefts and so enhance cholinergic neurotransmission. They help to improve cognition, mood disturbances, and activities of daily living (34). Donepezil or rivastigmine can be given to people with mild to moderate DLB as well as with severe DLB. Galantamine should be given in mild to moderate DLB patients if donepezil and rivastigmine are not tolerated (33).
- Donepezil should be given initially at 5 mg, once daily, at bedtime. After one month the treatment should be assessed, and the dose can be increased to a maximum of 10 mg administered once daily, if necessary (33).
- Galantamine should be given initially at 8 mg, once daily, for four weeks, and then increased to 16 mg, once daily, for at least four weeks. Maintenance treatment is 16–24 mg, once daily, depending on the assessment of clinical benefit and tolerability (33).
- Rivastigmine is given initially at a dose of 1.5 mg, twice daily, and may be increased in steps of 1.5 mg, twice daily, at intervals of at least two weeks, according to tolerance, up to a maximum dose of 6 mg administered twice daily. Alternatively rivastigmine patches are available; initially one should use a 4.6-mg patch per day. This can be increased to a 9.5-mg patch per day for, at least four weeks. Following discharge from hospital, GPs should be requested to seek advice from the memory service for queries regarding AChE inhibitors (33).
- Common side effects include nausea, vomiting, diarrhoea, muscle cramps, loss of appetite, tiredness, headaches, and abnormal dreams (33). Pulse rate should be checked at baseline and at follow-up, as AChE inhibitors are associated with rare incidences of heart block and sinus bradycardia (35).

- **N-methyl-D-aspartic acid receptor antagonists: memantine**
- Memantine blocks the effects of pathologically elevated levels of glutamate that may lead to neuronal dysfunction. It helps to improve cognition, mood disturbances, and activities of daily living (36). Memantine monotherapy is recommended as an option for managing people with moderate Alzheimer's disease who are intolerant of, or have a contraindication to, AChE inhibitors, or people with severe Alzheimer's disease. Consider memantine for people with DLB if AChE inhibitors are not tolerated or are contraindicated. But consider AChE inhibitors or memantine for

people with vascular dementia only if they have a suspected comorbid Alzheimer's disease or DLB (33).

- Memantine is initially given as 5 mg, once daily, and then increased at weekly intervals, in steps of 5 mg, up to a maximum of 20 mg daily. After discharge from hospital, GPs should be advised on the titration regime, and also to seek advice from the memory service for queries. Common undesirable effects are dizziness, headache, constipation, somnolence, and hypertension (33). Memantine undergoes renal elimination; thus eGFR should be checked prior to starting it (37).

Non-Pharmacological Interventions

Most general hospitals are not designed to provide dementia care. Patients tend to be admitted for reasons other than the dementia itself. Therefore the dementia is seldom the treatment priority. Staff training and knowledge around dementia management can be limited. This can result in unmet needs and an increase in behavioural and psychological symptoms of dementia on wards (38, 39).

Dementia care requires appropriate environmental adjustments that have to be arranged by hospital staff. Being in hospital can be disorientating and frightening for a person with dementia. Familiar people and familiar things can provide comfort and reassurance. Family members or close friends should be encouraged to be present. Medications do not always help with behavioural and psychological symptoms of dementia; the staff should recognise that all behaviour communicates a need or a feeling, for example wandering can be due to boredom or to being in pain. Relatives and friends can provide information on what actions or responses are likely to make a person more distressed, as well as insight into behaviours that might seem puzzling. Agitation and aggression can be minimised by allowing patients access to outside areas such as gardens (40).

Aromatherapy, music, massage, or spiritual support are used, but to a lesser extent than in long-term care settings. Research from long-term settings suggests that these interventions can be effective in reducing the behavioural and psychological symptoms of dementia. But they are difficult to implement in a hospital ward when staff members are busy managing the acute ailment, lack knowledge or time, and frequently change over (38).

Discharge to Place of Residence and Community Support

The unfamiliarity of the hospital environment can cause stress for patients with dementia. They should be discharged to their place of residence as soon as possible. Delays in initiating discharge planning can cause delayed admissions (41). Patients who experience physical health problems (such as a fall) to the extent that they would struggle to undertake independent living may require care once they return home. Hospital social services, occupational therapists, and the discharge liaison team, after assessing a patient's needs, can ensure that a suitable care package is arranged to enable living at home; or they may decide that long-term care (assisted living facilities or nursing homes) are a more practical option. Engaging with families can ensure a quick discharge to a place of residence (38).

Patients with suspected dementia or with a dementia diagnosis received in the general hospital should be referred to community specialist mental health services after discharge. This can ensure confirmation of dementia subtype; it also makes sure that the patient is given access to evidence-based non-pharmacological interventions, the dementia adviser service, and support services. Support or psychoeducation groups for family carers can be arranged (14).

Dementia Care and Staff Satisfaction

It is hoped that the HCPs' skill and motivation to provide quality dementia care can be improved and maintained through awareness raising and leadership. HCPs are generally motivated by either extrinsic or intrinsic factors (43). In the instance of dementia care, intrinsic motivation relates to an HCP's enjoyment at helping a person with dementia. The HCP gains extrinsic motivation from being as competent in their professional role as possible, from receiving positive feedback from patients and colleagues, and from the avoidance of punishment. In a busy ward environment, caring for someone with dementia, particularly in the absence of risk to the patient and his ot her immediate environment, can be a poor motivating task (44). There is rarely emotional reward or thanks from patient or family, and there are few negative incentives in the form of punishments that may be administered if the patient is not prioritised; patients with dementia often lack the capacity to complain about poor care and may not have strong advocates acting on their behalf (45). Furthermore, staff in the United Kingdom often feel unsupported and demotivated by a system that often fails to prioritise older people, by organisations that promote task-based care over person centeredness, and by a lack of emphasis on dementia care and training (46). To improve motivation, hospitals are being encouraged to adopt dementia leadership initiatives, such as appointing hospital dementia champions and establishing dementia working groups (47). Progress is slow, however, and recommendations for improving care are often not realised (46).

Patients and their carers are also encouraged to contribute to, and influence, their own care by raising the awareness of HCPs to their individual care needs and through diagnostic information at the time of admission (48, 49). National 'patient passport' schemes provide patients with an information pack that they complete at home and take with them to hospital each time they are admitted. These documents help to inform the staff of an individual's diagnosis, usual needs, likes and dislikes.

Dementia Knowledge and Interpersonal Skills

Knowledge of how to care for people with dementia can be acquired through formal teaching or practical experience. In the United Kingdom, dementia care is usually provided by psychiatrists and psychiatric nurses (50); however, when patients with dementia come into hospital, they are most commonly admitted to elderly medicine, trauma and orthopaedics, and medical wards (51). It might be assumed that, with increased exposure, staff on these wards become more adept at caring for people with dementia; however, in the United Kingdom they do not have formal psychiatric training as a rule and, although psychiatric liaison teams are usually available on a case by case basis, they are not part of the ward's multidisciplinary team (52).

Qualitative data from sixty-four doctors, nurses, and allied health assistants in a UK teaching hospital revealed that members of staff felt that education, induction, and in-service training left them underprepared and not confident to care for confused people. Participants admitted to inadequate knowledge of dealing with mental health problems, a state of affairs that leads to frustration, stress, and avoidance (53). Ninety per cent of nurses describe working with people with dementia challenging or very challenging (54), and several observation studies have shown that, although nurses strive to provide optimum care, that is not always achievable (55, 56).

Similar concerns are formulated by the carers and families of people with dementia, when they come to visit hospital wards. As part of a Royal College of Nursing report (57), 1,481 community carers of people with dementia were surveyed on the theme of barriers to dementia care in a general hospital setting. Seventy-nine per cent of carers felt that the staff had a poor understanding of caring for people with dementia and 75 per cent felt that staffing levels were too low. As part of the same report, 718 HCPs were also surveyed. They cited the pressures of existing workloads (77 per cent of respondents) and insufficient staffing levels (75 per cent) as barriers to care.

Conclusion

Poor dementia care, including untreated psychological symptoms, pain, and delirium, are associated with worse patient outcomes and satisfaction with care (58–62). If the dementia diagnosis or the symptoms commonly associated with dementia are not accounted for, patients are likely to experience adverse outcomes, principally mortality, falls, and delirium (9). Studies generally suggest a mortality rate of 31 per cent at six months and 40 per cent at twelve months (42). Despite challenges, the proactive recognition of dementia and delirium in hospitals is likely to improve patient outcomes, thanks to a growing awareness of the impact of cognitive impairment on long-term outcomes. There is growing evidence of the effectiveness of interventions such as environmental adaptations, staff education, and multi-professional working. Offering effective care to people with dementia in general hospitals can reduce the trauma of a hospital admission, the length of in-patient stay, and other healthcare-related complications and enhance health, well-being, and quality of life for individuals and their families (39, 41).

References

1. Alzheimer's Society. What is dementia? London, Alzheimer's Society, 2017. www.alzheimers.org.uk/download/downloads/id/3416/what_is_dementia.pdf.

2. World Health Organization. *The ICD-10 Classification of Mental and Behavioural Disorders*. Geneva: World Health Organization, 1992. http://www.who.int/classifications/icd/en/bluebook.pdf.

3. Alzheimer's Society. Facts for the media. London, Alzheimer's Society, 2017. www.alzheimers.org.uk/about-us/news-and-media/facts-media.

4. Sampson, E.L., Blanchard, M.R., Jones, L., Tookman, A., and King, M. Dementia in the acute hospital: Prospective cohort study of prevalence and mortality. *Br J Psychiatry* 2009, 195(1): 61–6.

5. Ames, D., Tuckwell, V. Psychiatric disorders among elderly patients in a general hospital. *Med J Aust* 1994, 160 (11): 671–5.

6. Laurila, J.V., Pitkala, K.H., Strandberg, T.E., and Tilvis, R.S. Detection and documentation of dementia and delirium in acute geriatric wards. *Gen Hosp Psychiatry* 2004, 26(1): 31–5.

7. Goldberg, S.E., Whittamore, K.H., Harwood, R.H., Bradshaw, L.E., Gladman, J.R.F., and Jones, R.G. The prevalence of mental health problems among older adults admitted as an emergency to a general hospital. *Age Ageing* 2012, 41(1): 80–6.

8. Russ, T.C., Shenkin, S.D., Reynish, E., et al. Dementia in acute hospital inpatients: The role of the geriatrician. *Age and Ageing* 2012, 41(3): 282–4.

9. Jackson, T.A., Gladman, T.R.F., Harwood, R.H., MacLullich, A.M.J., Sampson, E.L., et al. Challenges and opportunities in understanding dementia and delirium in the acute hospital. *PLoS Medicine* 2017, 14(3), e1002247.

10. Crowther, G.J.E., and Bennett, M.I. How well are the diagnosis and symptoms of dementia recorded in older patients admitted to hospital? *Age and Ageing* 2017, 46: 112–18.

11. Budson, A.E., and Solomon, P.R. *Memory Loss, Alzheimer's Disease and Dementia* (2nd ed.). Elsevier, 2016. See esp. Section II, Differential diagnosis of memory loss and dementia, pp. 47–145.

12. Carson, A., Zeman, A., Myles, L., and Sharpe, M. *Handbook of Liaison Psychiatry*. Cambridge: Cambridge University Press, 2007. See esp. Chapter 14, Neurological disorders, pp. 305–64.

13. Burns, A., and Iliffe, S. Dementia. *BMJ* 2009, 338: b75.

14. Robinson, L., Tang, E., and Taylor, J.-P. Dementia: Timely diagnosis and early intervention. *BMJ* 2015, 350: h3029.

15. Husain, M., and Schott, J.M. *Oxford Textbook of Cognitive Neurology and Dementia*. Oxford: Oxford University Press, 2016. See esp. Chapter 36, Dementia with Lewy bodies and Parkinson's disease dementia, pp. 399–413.

16. McKeith, I.G., Boeve, B.F., Dickson, D.W., et al. Diagnosis and management of dementia with Lewy bodies: Fourth consensus report of the DLB Consortium. *Neurology* 2017, 89(1): 88–100.

17. Yousaf, T., Dervenoulas, G., Valkimadi, P.-E., et al. Neuroimaging in Lewy body dementia. *J Neurol* 2019, 266(1): 1–26. doi: 10.1007/s00415-018-8892-x.

18. Alzheimer's Society. Facts for the media. London, Alzheimer's Society, 2017. www.alzheimers.org.uk/about-us/news-and-media/facts-media. Also Alzheimer's Research UK. Dementia statistics hub. London: Alzheimer's Society, 2018. www.dementiastatistics.org/statistics/prevalence-by-age-in-the-uk/#:~:text=A%20person%27s%20risk%20of%20developing,over%20the%20age%20of%2080.&text=people%20under%2065%20have%20dementia,%2C%205.2%25%20of%20the%20total.

19. Age UK. Later life in the United Kingdom, 2019. London, Age UK, 2019. www.ageuk.org.uk/globalassets/age-uk/documents/reports-and-publications/later_life_uk_factsheet.pdf.

20. Alzheimer's Society. Can genes cause dementia? London, Alzheimer's Society, 2020. www.alzheimers.org.uk/about-dementia/risk-factors-and-prevention/alzheimers-disease-and-genes#content-start.

21. Alzheimer's Society. Dementia risk factors and prevention. London, Alzheimer's Society, 2020. www.alzheimers.org.uk/about-dementia/dementia-risk-factors-and-prevention.

22. Cunningham, E.L., McGuiness, B., Herron, B., and Passmore, A.P. Dementia. *Ulster Med J* 2015, 84(2): 79–87.

23. Russ, T.C., Shenkin, S.C., Reynish, E., et al. Dementia in acute hospital inpatients: The role of the geriatrician. *Age Ageing* 2012, 41(3): 282–4.

24. Leonard, M., McInerney, S., McFarland, J., Condon, C., Awan, F., O'Connor, M., et al. Comparison of cognitive and neuropsychiatric profiles in hospitalized elderly medical patients with delirium, dementia and comorbid delirium–dementia. *BMJ Open* 2016, 6: e009212.

25. American Psychiatric Association. *Diagnostic and Statistical Manual of Mental Disorders* (5th ed.). Arlington, VA: American Psychiatric Association, 2013. See esp. Neurocognitive disorders, pp. 591–643.

26. Pendlebury, S.T., Klaus, S.P., Mather, M., de Brito., and Wharton, R.M. Routine cognitive screening in older patients

admitted to acute medicine: Abbreviated Mental Test Score (AMTS) and Subjective Memory cCmplaint versus Montreal Cognitive Assessment and IQCODE. *Age Ageing* 2015, 44(6): 1000–5.

27. Velayudhan, L., Ryu, S.-H., Raczek, M., Philpot, M., Lindesay, J., Critchfield, M., and Livingston, G. Review of brief cognitive tests for patients with suspected dementia. *Int Psychogeriatr* 2014, 26(8): 1247–62.

28. Noone, P. Questionnaire review: Addenbrooke's Cognitive Examination, III. *Occupational Medicine* 2015, 65: 418–20.

29. Rascovsky, K. A primer in neuropsychological assessment for dementia. Practical Neurology, The Neurology Hub, July–August 2016. https://docs.google.com/viewerng/viewer?url=http://v2.practicalneurology.com/pdfs/pn0716_CF_Neuropsych.pdf.

30. Nightingale, S., Michael, B.D., Defres, S., et al. Test them all: An easily diagnosed and readily treatable cause of dementia with life-threatening consequences if missed. *Pract Neurol* 2013, 13(6): 354–6.

31. Smailovic, U., and Jelic, V. Neurophysiological markers of Alzheimer's Disease: Quantitative EEG approach. *Neurol Ther* 2019, 8: 37–55.

32. Kansal, K., and Irwin, D.J. The use of cerebrospinal fluid and neuropathological studies in neuropsychiatry practice and research. *Psychiatr Clin North Am* 2015, 38(2): 309–22.

33. National Institute for Health and Care Excellence (NICE). *Donepezil, Galantamine, Rivastigmine and Memantine for the Treatment of Alzheimer's Disease.* London: NICE, 2011. donepezil-galantamine-rivastigmine-and-memantine-for-the-treatment-of-alzheimers-disease-pdf-82600254699973 (nice.org.uk).

34. Cochrane. Rivastigmine for people with Alzheimer's disease [internet]. London: Cochrane; 2015 [cited 2020 Dec 19]. Available from: www.cochrane.org/CD001191/DEMENTIA_rivastigmine-people-alzheimers-disease.

35. Rowland, J.P., Rigby, J., Harper, A.C., et al. Cardiovascular monitoring with acetylcholinesterase inhibitors: a clinical protocol. *Adv Psychiatr Treat* 2018; 13(3), 178–84.

36. Cochrane. Memantine as a treatment for dementia. London, Cochrane, 2019. www.cochrane.org/CD003154/DEMENTIA_memantine-treatment-dementia.

37. Lefevre, G., Callegari, F., Gsteiger, S., et al. Effects of renal impairment on steady-state plasma concentrations of rivastigmine: A population pharmacokinetic analysis of capsule and patch formulations in patients with Alzheimer's disease. *Drugs Ageing* 2016, 33(10): 725–36.

38. Ames, D., O'Brien, J.T., and Burns, A. (eds). *Dementia* (5th ed.). Boca Raton, FL: CRC Press, 2017. See esp. Chapter 16, Managing people with dementia in the general hospital, pp. 172–83.

39. Royal College of Psychiatrists. *Who Cares Wins: Improving the Outcome for Older People Admitted to the General Hospital: Guidelines for the Development of Liaison Mental Health Services for Older People.* London: RCPsych, 2005. www.bgs.org.uk/sites/default/files/content/resources/files/2018-05-18/WhoCaresWins.pdf.

40. White, N., Leurent, B., Lord, K., Scott, S., Jones, L., et al. The management of behavioural and psychological symptoms of dementia in the acute general medical hospital: A longitudinal cohort study. *Int J Geriatr Psychiatry* 2015, 32(3): 297–305.

41. Royal College of Psychiatrists. *National Audit of Dementia Care in General Hospitals, 2016–2017: Third Round of Audit Report.* London: RCPsych, 2017. www.rcpsych.ac.uk/docs/default-source/improving-care/ccqi/national-clinical-audits/national-audit-of-dementia/round-3/nad-care-in-general-hospitals-2016-17-third-round-of-audit-report.pdf?sfvrsn=5dffeef8_4.

42. Sheehan, B., Lall, R., Gage, H., Holland, C., Katz, J., and Mitchell, K. A 12-month follow-up study of people with dementia referred to general hospital liaison

psychiatry services. *Age Ageing* 2013, 42, 786–90.

43. Deci, E. and Ryan, R. 2002. *Handbook of Self-Determination Research*. Rochester, NY: University of Rochester Press.

44. Hynninen, N., Saarnio, R. and Isola, A. The care of older people with dementia in surgical wards from the point of view of the nursing staff and physicians. *Journal of Clinical Nursing* 2015, 24(1–2): 192–201.

45. Bradshaw, L.E., Goldberg, S.E., Schneider, J.M., and Harwood, R.H. Carers for older people with co-morbid cognitive impairment in general hospital: Characteristics and psychological well-being. *International Journal of Geriatric Psychiatry* 2013, 28(7): 681–90.

46. Tadd, W. Hillman, A. Calnan, S. Calnan, M. Bayer, T. and Read, S. *Dignity in Practice: An Exploration of the Care of Older Adults in Acute NHS Trusts*. PANICOA, 2011. http://www.bgs.org.uk/ pdf_cms/reference/Tadd_Dignity_in_ Practice.pdf.

47. Banks, P., Waugh, A., Henderson, J., Sharp, B., Brown, M., Oliver, J. and Marland, G. Enriching the care of patients with dementia in acute settings? The Dementia Champions Programme in Scotland. *Dementia (London)* 2014, 13(6): 717–36.

48. The Butterfly Scheme. Home page, November 2014. http://butterflyscheme .org.uk/november-2014.

49. Alzheimer's Society. This is me: A support tool to enable person- centred care. Alzheimer's Society, 2010. www .alzheimers.org.uk/thisisme.

50. Jolley, D., Benbow, S.M., and Grizzell, M. Memory clinics. *Postgraduate Medical Journal* 2006, 82(965): 199–206.

51. Goldberg, S., Whittamore, K., Harwood, R., Bradshaw, L., Gladman, J., and Jones, R. The prevalence of mental health problems among older adults admitted as an emergency to a general hospital. *Age and Ageing* 2012, 41(1): 80–6.

52. Royal College of Psychiatrists. *National Audit of Dementia Care in General Hospitals, 2012–13: Second round audit and update*. Royal Collage of Psychiatrists, 2013. www.rcpsych.ac.uk/ docs/default-source/improving-care/ccqi/ national-clinical-audits/national-audit-of- dementia/round-2/nad-round-2-national- report-2013.pdf?sfvrsn=ed5a6094_2.

53. Griffiths, A., Knight, A., Harwood, R. and Gladman, J.R. Preparation to care for confused older patients in general hospitals: a study of UK health professionals. *Age and Ageing* 2014, 43(4): 521–7.

54. The Alzheimer's Society. 2009. *Counting the Cost: Caring for People with Dementia on Hospital Wards*. Alzheimer's Society. www.alzheimers.org.uk.

55. Nolan, L. Caring for people with dementia in the acute setting: A study of nurses' views. *British Journal of Nursing* 2007, 16(7): 419–22.

56. Cowdell, F. The care of older people with dementia in acute hospitals. *International Journal of Older People Nursing* 2010, 5 (2): 83–92.

57. Royal College of Nursing. *Dignity in Dementia: Transforming General Hospital Care*. Royal College of Nursing, 2011. www.rcn.org.uk/__data/assets/pdf_file/ 0019/405109/RCN_Dementia_project_ professional_survey_findings_.pdf.

58. Sampson, E., White, N., Leurent, B., Scott, S., Lord, K., Round, J. and Jones, L. Behavioural and psychiatric symptoms in people with dementia admitted to the acute hospital: prospective cohort study. *British Journal of Psychiatry* 2014, 205(3): 189–96.

59. Sampson, E., White, N., Lord, K., Leurent, B., Vickerstaff, V., Scott, S. and Jones, L. Pain, agitation, and behavioural problems in people with dementia admitted to general hospital wards: A longitudinal cohort study. *Pain* 2015, 156(4): 675–83.

60. Wancata, J., Windhaber, J., Krautgartner, M. and Alexandrowicz, R. The consequences of non-cognitive symptoms of dementia in medical hospital departments. *International Journal of*

Psychiatry in Medicine, 2003, 33(3): 257–71.

61. Husebo, B.S., Ballard, C., Sandvik, R., Nilsen, O.B., and Aarsland, D. Efficacy of treating pain to reduce behavioural disturbances in residents of nursing homes with dementia: cluster randomised clinical trial. *British Medical Journal* 2011, 343. doi: 10.1136/bmj.d4065.

62. Holmes, J., and House, A. 2000. Psychiatric illness predicts poor outcome after surgery for hip fracture: A prospective cohort study. *Psychological Medicine* 2000, 30: 921–9.

Chapter 1

Behavioural and Psychological Symptoms of Dementia in Hospital Settings

Ravinder Kaur Hayer and George Tadros

Introduction

The term 'behavioural and psychological symptoms of dementia' (BPSD) is a descriptive label for a diverse collection of non-cognitive phenomena that arise as part of the dementia syndrome (1). It encompasses the wide variety of disturbances of mood, thought, perception, personality, and motor activity many people with dementia experience throughout the course of their illness (2). A few examples of neuropsychiatric symptoms and behaviours that are considered under this umbrella term are agitation, depression, aggression, wandering, insomnia, hallucinations, and delusions; all of them have the potential to impact on quality of life and complicate the care of those who live with dementia (3).

The recognition that BPSD are part of the dementia syndrome is by no means novel. As far back as the early twentieth century, Alois Alzheimer described a 51-year-old female patient who presented with jealousy towards her husband, paranoid delusions, auditory hallucinations, and protracted episodes of screaming in addition to the classical cognitive features of the disorder (4). The term itself, however, was not coined until 1996; it was developed by the International Psychogeriatric Consensus Conference of the International Psychogeriatric Association (IPA) Task Force on Behavioural Disturbances of Dementia, in order to effectively capture many of the common challenges that people living with dementia face – along with those charged with their care (5). Although terms such as 'challenging behaviour', 'non-cognitive symptoms', and 'unmet needs' are all used interchangeably to describe this constellation of symptoms and behaviours, there is international acceptance of BPSD as a clinical term (6).

It is important to appreciate that, unlike cognitive and functional deficits – which progress over time, owing to the neurodegenerative nature of the condition – BPSD can occur across all the stages of dementia and have a tendency to fluctuate (7). Furthermore, BPSD are almost universally present during the course of the syndrome, with a 97 per cent five-year prevalence of at least one behavioral and psychological symptom of dementia in individuals with the condition (8). Interestingly, despite being an inherent part of the disorder, BPSD are not deemed in any of the current classification systems as being an essential criterion for a dementia diagnosis (2). They are nonetheless an incredibly important facet of the syndrome, not only having a significant impact in terms of reduction in quality of life for the individuals who experience them, but also contributing to considerable carer burden, increased direct and indirect healthcare costs, and premature institutionalisation (9–11).

The Challenges BPSD Present to Acute Settings

BPSD commonly occur within acute hospitals, affecting 75 per cent of in-patients with dementia at some point during their admission (12). Aggression and activity disturbance are the most frequent behaviours displayed; they are followed by sleep disturbance, depression, phobia, or anxiety, which more than a third of individuals also experience during their hospital stay (12). By contrast, in community populations depression, apathy, and anxiety have been identified as the most prevalent BPSD symptoms (8).

The BPSD displayed in general hospitals have a complex and multifaceted aetiology. Those living with dementia often have their symptoms exacerbated by the disorienting ward environment, and this is further compounded by their acute physical illness, delirium, and pain (13, 14). Medications initiated for physical complaints during an admission may also contribute to BPSD symptoms. For instance, drugs with anticholinergic properties (which are utilised for a variety of indications in clinical medicine) lead to a significant anticholinergic burden, and this can both exacerbate BPSD and worsen cognition (15, 16).

The considerable consequences that hospital admissions have on people living with dementia are well recognised. Indeed, non-professional caregivers of those with dementia have observed the detrimental effects an acute hospital stay can have on their loved ones; as many as 79 per cent describe the admission as having a negative impact on dementia symptoms, and 54 per cent of these describe the extent of this impact as being 'significant' (17). Furthermore, Hessler et al. identified that BPSD in hospital settings not only get associated with a range of complications during routine care and medical interventions but also result in considerable distress for the nursing staff (18). They demonstrated that there are higher rates of physical restraint, specialist psychiatry, and neurology consultations, as well as of the utilisation of multiple psychotropic drugs for patients with BPSD – all evidencing the challenges that the staff experience in trying to manage these behaviours (18).

In order to treat symptoms, it has been demonstrated that almost 40 per cent of patients with BPSD have a pharmacological intervention and 55 per cent a non-pharmacological intervention during their admission to an acute hospital (13). One kind of pharmacological intervention is the use of antipsychotics. Although indicated in some cases, antipsychotics have been perceived to be inappropriately prescribed for managing BPSD by up to a quarter of nursing staff in general hospital settings; and, when considering the risks they carry, this is significant (17). This said, there is a recognition of the many obstacles to using non-pharmacological strategies in acute hospitals. Healthcare professionals are under immense pressure and have limited time; there is insufficient staffing and a constant movement of patients, reports of a lack of the necessary training or specialist support, and an environment that is not always conducive to meeting the needs of those with dementia (19). Despite these challenges, there are effective ways to manage BPSD in hospital environments, and these will be discussed in greater depth later in this chapter.

Classification of BPSD

There is no universally agreed classification system for BPSD symptoms. The 1996 International Psychogeriatric Consensus Conference of the IPA suggested that it is possible to group symptoms into 'behavioural' and 'psychological' categories, as the term would imply (5) – and this is perhaps the most basic classification system for BPSD. The Consensus Conference proposed that behavioural symptoms are those identified by observing the patient (these include physical and verbal aggression, agitation, wandering, and sexual disinhibition), whereas psychological symptoms are predominantly elicited by interviewing persons with dementia and obtaining collateral history from their caregivers (such symptoms include anxiety, low mood, hallucinations, and delusions) (5). It has been suggested, however, that this classification system may be oversimplistic, as it does not consider that some psychological phenomena can also be discerned from an individual's behaviours, for example when someone appears visibly anxious or is responding to unseen stimuli (1).

The Consensus Conference acknowledged that there are various other ways in which BPSD can be classified, and it outlined three alternative approaches: by behaviour type (e.g. aggression), by function (e.g. disordered sleep), and by clusters of symptoms treated as 'syndromes' (e.g. depressive syndrome) (5). Several syndromes that consist of associated BPSD symptoms have since been described by factor-analytical studies with the help of BPSD rating tools. This indicates that BPSD are not solitary phenomena and that some symptoms have a tendency to occur simultaneously (20). In one such study, which was conducted by the European Alzheimer's Disease Consortium, four groups or 'factors' were identified using the Neuropsychiatric Inventory (NPI): a psychosis factor (irritability, agitation, hallucinations, and anxiety), a psychomotor factor (aberrant motor behaviour and delusions), a mood liability factor (disinhibition, elation, and depression), and an instinctual factor (appetite disorders, sleep disorders, and apathy) (20). Interestingly, they could not find an association between mood and apathy, as proposed by Aalten et al., who grouped BPSD into three syndromes: mood/apathy, psychosis, and agitation (20, 21). This highlights that, although attempts have been made to cluster BPSD symptoms in a meaningful way in order to improve the recognition of syndromes and guide their subsequent management, there remains a lack of agreement on how this should be done.

Causes and Contributors

The aetiopathogenesis of BPSD is multifactorial and isolating the various contributing factors is challenging because of the overlapping symptomatology (22, 23). Identical behaviours may arise from different causes and non-identical behaviours may respond to the same management strategy – which highlights the complexities involved in establishing their aetiology (22, 23). A helpful way to consider the causes of BPSD is to explore the factors directly related to the person with dementia and those that are due to external influences.

Patient (Internal) Factors

Dementia-related structural and functional changes have been correlated with specific BPSD symptoms (24). In their systematic review of neuroimaging findings related to BPSD in dementia of the Alzheimer's type, Alves et al. concluded that apathy and psychotic symptoms in dementia are linked with volume reductions or hypo-metabolism in the prefrontal cortex, anterior cingulate, insula, and temporal lobes, whereas white matter lacunes correlate with progression of Alzheimer's disease and are associated with depressive symptoms (24). There are also changes in neurotransmission and neuromodulation, with dopaminergic, serotonergic, noradrenergic dysfunction and altered amino acid levels, all playing a role in BPSD symptomatology (25). The impact this has on the individual may further be influenced by other biological factors, such as the underlying genetic make-up or existing comorbidities (26).

In a review of the available evidence, Cipriani et al. reported that premorbid personality could be a factor in the development of BPSD on account of the potential for personality traits to become exaggerated as dementia advances (27). Psychiatric disorders such as severe depression, anxiety, bipolar affective disorder, schizophrenia – and the psychotropic drugs used to manage them – may also contribute to non-cognitive symptoms (7). For example, it is important to be aware of the potential for benzodiazepines, which are often used in the management of BPSD in the acute hospital setting, to cause, paradoxically, behavioural disinhibition (28). Medications prescribed for physical health symptoms such as bladder antispasmodics, histamine antagonists, Digoxin, Levetiracetam, muscle relaxants, and some antibiotics have also been demonstrated to contribute to both agitation and apathy (29). However, it is not only the introduction of medication that can be problematic. Hospital staff should be vigilant about BPSD that are a direct result of medication withdrawal, particularly from antidepressants, benzodiazepines, or strong analgesics such as opioids (29).

Ballard et al. have highlighted the need for an early detection of urinary tract, chest, and dental infections, as these can frequently lead to BPSD in those with dementia (30). Treatment of these infections, and indeed any other underlying physical health issues such as constipation or dehydration, may resolve BPSD without the need to medicate the symptoms or the behaviours themselves (for more details, see Chapter 11 on the management of delirium) (30). The authors also highlight that sensory deficits, particularly visual and auditory impairment, can precipitate BPSD (30). Therefore all patients with dementia should have their hearing and vision assessed as part of the routine upon admission to hospital, and then corrected where possible; this may involve an intervention as simple as regularly prompting individuals with dementia to wear their spectacles or hearing aids, if they tend to forget about it (30).

Pain is common in people with dementia admitted to acute hospitals and is strongly associated with BPSD symptoms, particularly aggression and anxiety (31). However, as a result of a reduction in the ability to subjectively report it as their cognition declines, pain can often be overlooked and undertreated (32). Pain related to internal organs, the head, and the skin is particularly challenging to assess, as compared to pain originating from the musculoskeletal system (e.g. pain due to arthritis), as the latter can be identified through passive movements (33). Indeed, there should be a high index of suspicion for musculoskeletal pain if there is resistance or aggression displayed by the individual with dementia during interventions that involve moving the limbs, as this movement may well have triggered discomfort. Finally, it is important to recognise the potential for central neuropathic pain. This is caused by white matter lesions that lead to multiple disconnections between areas of the brain, in a process termed 'deafferentiation' (32). Central neuropathic pain is considered to be underdiagnosed in dementia, particularly in those with a vascular aetiology, but also in dementias of the Alzheimer's and frontotemporal type, where it, too, plays a part (32, 34).

BPSD symptoms can arise if a person has needs that are not satisfied. This concept has been explored by Cohen-Mansfield, who proposed the 'unmet needs model of agitated behaviour' (35). The model details three categories of behaviours that can arise from an individual's needs: behaviours to obtain or meet a need (e.g. pacing to provide stimulation); behaviours to communicate a need (e.g. repetitive requests signalling a cry for help); and behaviours that result from an unmet need (e.g. fidgeting due to discomfort) (35). An example of where this model can be usefully applied is in the consideration of inappropriate sexual behaviour (ISB). As a result of the changes in cognition and judgement that individuals with dementia experience, their unfulfilled need for intimacy may express themselves in behaviours that are challenging for those around them. Such behaviours include unwelcome advances, public displays of sexualised behaviour, and, in some instances, physical aggression if their sexual desires are not met (36).

Non-Patient (External) Factors

The hospital setting is often not conducive to meeting the needs of people who live with dementia. A cluttered environment, extremes of noise, and the lack of familiar objects can exacerbate existing non-cognitive symptoms or lead to new ones; and such symptoms are consequently targets for intervention (37). The absence of a routine and the reduced character of opportunities for activity (which causes understimulation) can also contribute to BPSD (37).

A caregiver approach is certainly implicated in the aetiology of BPSD, as the evidence suggests that agitation in those with dementia can be exacerbated by caregivers who display impatience, irritation, or even anger (38). By contrast, when caregivers adopt a supportive attitude and are accepting of individuals' reduced level of functioning, this appears to minimise the risk of the occurrence of hyperactive behaviours (38). In the acute hospital setting, the utilisation of this calm and collected approach by staff may cancel the need for pharmacological interventions and restrictive practices, the latter being more commonly resorted to than one might expect. Indeed, it has been demonstrated that almost a quarter of patients with dementia are subject to restrictive practices (e.g. bed rails or mittens) during their admission. Such treatment can not only worsen BPSD counterproductively, but also have the potential to cause significant physical health complications (13).

Assessment of BPSD

The thorough assessment of BPSD is the cornerstone to being able to devise an individualised, person-centred management plan, where the focus for intervention is well defined and clear. Cloak et al. advise that the aim of the assessment process is essentially to characterise the symptoms, identify reversible causes, ascertain the type and urgency of the management strategies required, and create a baseline for measuring the response to any interventions utilised (29). Central to this process is the careful observation of patients by ward staff members, who are then able to determine with precision the specific behaviours displayed; for example, using a statement such as 'the patient is agitated' (when agitation is an umbrella term that covers a myriad of presentations) is far less helpful than a detailed account of what is *actually* being witnessed (29). Furthermore, the staff should have the necessary systems in place to be able to report symptoms and have them acted upon. The limited evidence base in this area suggests that, while hospital staff members are able to recognise distress in individuals with dementia, they struggle to know how to act upon their observations (39).

The use of antecedent behaviour consequence (ABC) charts can support the task of establishing any chronological links between symptoms and potential causative factors by encouraging the staff to reflect on what happens before, during, and after any incident of BPSD (40). By using a simple table to document the above, patterns may begin to emerge that help with the prediction, prevention, and management of behaviours. For example, does the behaviour always follow a certain intervention? Or does the behaviour occur only during family visits? Or is it that the behaviour is displayed throughout the day without any obvious triggers, but has been noted to respond well to simple verbal reassurance or redirection by staff?

A detailed collateral history further consolidates the information-gathering process, as the patient's usual caregivers can offer valuable insights into the types of BPSD symptoms that the individual habitually displays and into what is already recognised to exacerbate and relieve them in the community. Finally, a thorough physical examination and appropriate investigations complete the assessment. This not only helps to identify any possible underlying causes for the BPSD phenomena but also serves as a baseline measure of physical health before any interventions are introduced.

There is, of course, a subjective element to the assessment of BPSD, and there are challenges with quantifying the symptoms observed. Validated instruments exist to standardise the assessment process, and multiple tools are available to assess depression, anxiety, psychosis, and observed behaviour. Examples include the Behavioural Pathology in Alzheimer's Disease Rating Scale (Behave-AD) and the Neuropsychiatric Inventory (NPI), which are both based on structured interviews and can be used to support the detection and quantification of BPSD (41, 42). That said, these assessment tools do have their weaknesses, not least that they are time-consuming if accurately administered, which limits their usefulness within busy hospital settings (29). The NPI-Q was devised by Kaufer et al. with this feature in mind: it is a relatively succinct, two-page self-administered questionnaire – as opposed to being an interview – and, as such, is more suitable for general clinical practice (43). Whichever (or, indeed, if any) of the many tools available are used, one must be mindful of the fact that they are helpful only if applied consistently and if the results are acted upon. Therefore rating scales should not be a substitute for a thorough assessment based on detailed history and careful observation; rather they should be used to consolidate the information-gathering process and to provide a baseline for the efficacy of interventions to be measured against. These rating scales will be discussed further in Chapter 21.

The clinical significance of pain is exemplified by its being described as the 'fifth vital sign', while healthcare professionals are actively encouraged to assess this symptom regularly, alongside other routine physical observations (and hence with the same frequency) (44). As mentioned earlier, pain is often an underreported contributor to BPSD, and this further reinforces the need to be particularly vigilant about it in people with dementia. The Visual Analogue Scale, the Verbal Rating Scale, and the Numerical Rating Scale are all self-report tools that have been deemed to be valid, reliable, and suitable for use in clinical practice to support the detection of pain (44). However, self-reporting scales have obvious limitations when considering those who, because of their degree of cognitive impairment, struggle to communicate their experience of pain; and it is for this group of individuals that observational pain tools are indicated (45). One such example is the MOBID-2 Pain Scale. This instrument not only enables the assessment of pain on the basis of a response to standardised, guided movements of parts of the body (and therefore of pain related to the musculoskeletal system); it also allows the observation of pain behaviours related to internal organs, head, and skin in those with advanced dementia (46). Another tool commonly used in clinical practice for those with end or late-stage dementia (who are thus unable to articulate their symptoms) is the Abbey Pain Scale (47). This simple tool assesses changes in body language, behaviour, physiology, physical status, vocalisations, and facial expressions as a means of more objectively measuring pain (47). Regardless of the pain scale selected, these instruments need to be regularly repeated after any pain management intervention in order to gauge whether there has been a subsequent improvement in the individual's symptoms.

Management

A guiding principle in the management of BPSD is that prevention is better than cure. Hence strategies based on the information gleaned from the assessment process related to the individual (and in particular what typically triggers and relieves his or her non-cognitive symptoms) should be implemented early on during admission to hospital. An example is simply to ensure that a patient with dementia is placed in a quieter area of the ward, if his or her usual caregivers advise that noise causes this patient distress. If BPSD do arise despite preventative measures, it is vital to treat in the first place any potential underlying causes of the symptoms, such as pain, constipation, or infection. It is also important to consider the severity and the consequences of the neuropsychiatric symptoms in question (30). Given that BPSD are often self-limiting (they resolve or improve in 4–6 weeks), symptoms that are infrequent, are not distressing, and do not pose a risk to the individual or others usually lend themselves to watchful waiting or to a non-pharmacological approach (30). However, it is recognised that this is not always a viable option in the hospital setting, where behaviours may prevent the staff from carrying out essential daily care and medical treatment, or may negatively impact the recovery of other unwell patients. This being said, even in those situations where managing BPSD requires pharmacological strategies, non-pharmacological strategies should continue to be used alongside. Some examples of non-pharmacological strategies that may be helpful will now be considered.

Non-Pharmacological Strategies

In their systematic review of the non-pharmacological approaches used in the management of BPSD, Livingston et al. summarised that behavioural techniques – strategies based on the analysis of ABC charts – are not only effective in reducing neuropsychiatric symptoms: their positive effects can last for some months beyond the interventions themselves (48). They also concluded that psycho-education for caregivers, and possibly cognitive stimulation therapy for those living with dementia, can confer some benefit in reducing BPSD (48). Interventions such as music therapy and Snoezelen (a specially designed room, which combines relaxation with the exploration of sensory stimuli) were limited in their utility by the fact that improvements identified during the session were not sustained in the longer term (48). Livingston et al. made a qualifying statement that the lack of evidence to support other therapies is due to the dearth of robust research in this area and does not necessarily mean that they are ineffective (48).

A non-pharmacological intervention that is certainly gathering interest is aromatherapy. Ballard et al. propose that aromatherapy with lavender and Melissa oil is a generally well-tolerated alternative to psychotropic drugs for the management of BPSD in non-crisis situations (30, 40). Furthermore, there are several ways in which the oils can be used, enabling a personalised sensory experience to be offered on the basis of the individual's presentation; Ballard et al. give the example that inhalation may be more effective than massage in someone who displays motor restlessness (40).

Lyketsos et al. have explored non-pharmacological management strategies and helpfully considered them as falling under four broad categories; 'cognitive interventions' (which include reorientation, providing prompts, and sequencing tasks), 'environmental modifications' (which involve adjusting the noise levels, reducing the visual clutter, or using objects and pictures to provide cues), 'changes in activity demand' (which encourage focusing on routines and scheduled activities and reducing their complexity), and 'interpersonal approaches' (which very much depend on the likes and dislikes of the individual and tailor the communication process to that person's cognitive abilities) (37). In reality, an individual may require a combination of these techniques, some being adopted simultaneously or particular strategies being used in particular situations.

There are other, more specific, non-pharmacological strategies that can be used to manage particular neuropsychiatric symptoms. For example, in sleep disorders, increasing sunlight exposure and encouraging physical activity during the day, while simultaneously ensuring that there is a structured bedtime routine, free from disturbances at night, can all be helpful means of regulating the sleep–wake cycle (49). When considering inappropriate sexual behaviour, the non-pharmacological management includes ensuring that the individual with dementia has opportunities to satisfy his or her natural sexual desires more acceptably and, if behaviours persist, minimising triggers such as suggestive television programmes (50). For those patients who expose themselves in public areas, trousers without front openings can be trialled (after carefully weighing up the risks, benefits, and ethical aspects of these measures) in order to maintain the individuals' dignity and avoid distress to the patients around them (50).

Pharmacological Strategies

For individuals with dementia and BPSD, if non-pharmacological strategies are unsuccessful or if there are significant risks that require urgent intervention, medications can be considered. We must be mindful that this cohort of patients is particularly susceptible to the unwanted effects of drug treatments and therefore a detailed medication history, baseline physical health investigations, and an electrocardiogram should precede the initiation of any psychotropic agents wherever practically possible (26). Once initiated, drugs should be regularly reviewed and withdrawn as soon as it is feasible to do so safely (26). Furthermore, if the patient lacks capacity, decisions around the use of medication should be made in his or her best interest, in line with Mental Capacity Act legal frameworks and good practice, ideally taking into account the person's known wishes and involving his or here carers where the situation allows. In what follows we consider some of the most common BPSD symptoms and the psychotropic drugs that may have a role in managing them.

Aggression and Agitation

The term 'agitation' is non-specific and has been used to describe an array of presentations such as irritability, restlessness, purposeless activity, inappropriate vocalisations – and many more. Acetylcholinesterase inhibitors and Memantine can be used for this indication; the Maudsley guidelines conclude that, while these medications do confer some benefit in reducing behavioural disturbances with dementia, the effect is modest (51). Interestingly, there is evidence to suggest that the combination of Memantine and Donepezil has greater efficacy in the management of BPSD than Donepezil alone (52). Other research has questioned the efficacy of Memantine for this indication; nevertheless, Memantine is still widely used in clinical practice (53). This said, its usefulness in acute hospital settings may be limited by the fact that it requires titration and takes some time to take effect.

Where agitation is severe or aggressive behaviours are associated with significant risk, an atypical antipsychotic may be indicated and is preferable to a first-generation alternative (3). Risperidone is the only licensed antipsychotic for the use of BPSD (1 mg a day has been demonstrated to be the optimum dose), but other antipsychotics may be used off label if risperidone is contraindicated or not tolerated (51,54). In clinical practice, Quetiapine is often used for Lewy body or Parkinson's disease dementia, as it is thought to have a lower risk of worsening the motor features of the condition – a risk associated with all the antipsychotics when used in these types of dementia (51). But caution is to be exercised, as evidence would suggest that Quetiapine is not efficacious for agitation in dementia and can even worsen cognition (55).

For any antipsychotic used in dementia, particular care is needed when balancing the risks against the potential benefits, especially in view of the fact that patients in hospital settings are already susceptible to the side effects, which include hypotension, falls, and QTc prolongation (56). Furthermore, meta-analysed research provides strong evidence for increased risk of strokes with this group of drugs when used in dementia; Banerjee summarises that treating 1,000 people with BPSD with an atypical antipsychotic for around twelve weeks would result in an additional eighteen strokes (3). He found that there is also evidence for the risk of adverse events to increase over time, and therefore he advised that any antipsychotic should be used at the lowest effective dose and for the shortest possible duration (preferably under twelve weeks) (3). It follows that, once such use is initiated, regular reviews should be undertaken and concerted efforts made to reduce or stop the antipsychotic (3). If there is a subsequent relapse of aggression upon withdrawing the antipsychotic, Ballard et al. recommend that an alternative psychotropic be considered, for example an antidepressant (30).

In extremis, rapid tranquilisation, which uses intramuscular medication, may have to be considered. As well as bearing in mind the legal framework for intramuscular drug administration, it is important to consult local trust policy, as this can vary. Where possible, the choice of a drug for rapid tranquilisation should take into account the patient's comorbidities, other prescribed medications, previous response to the medication (if used before), the total daily dosages of psychotropic drugs already administered, and, of course, their preferences, if they are known (57). Although not always feasible during the acute situations in which rapid tranquilisation is required, discussion with the patient's next of kin and family should take place as soon as is practical.

Mood Disorders and Anxiety Symptoms

Meta-analysis data would suggest that the overall evidence of effectiveness for anti-depressants in people with Alzheimer's type of dementia is small, only a few randomised controlled trials having been conducted to date (58). Selective serotonin re-uptake inhibitors (SSRIs) are the most common choice for the first-line management of depression in dementia, but if there are concerns around poor sleep mirtazapine may be more appropriately selected, given its sedative properties (59, 60). Tricyclic antidepressants have become less popular in recent times, being superseded by the newer antidepressants available, which have far better safety profiles and tolerability (61). Another drawback of tricyclic antidepressants is their significant anticholinergic effects, which can cause dry mouth, constipation, ocular complaints, and urinary retention (61). These side effects counter-productively have the potential to aggravate BPSD symptoms, and a meta-analysis by Thompson et al. concluded that they can also further impair cognition in people with dementia (62). With regard to anxiety in dementia, the SSRIs sertraline, fluoxetine, and citalopram have all been demonstrated to be effective, but citalopram has the additional benefit of appearing to reduce the behavioural symptoms associated with anxiety (and can be considered if the QTc interval is within normal limits) (63). These are preferable to benzodiazepines, which not only run the well-established risks of tolerance, dependence, and unpleasant withdrawal symptoms but can also exacerbate cognitive impairment or paradoxically worsen behavioural disturbances (63). That said, benzodiazepines may have a role in the management of anxiety symptoms if used judiciously for short periods (63). Other options include tricyclic antidepressants, venlafaxine, mirtazapine, pregabalin, and buspirone; anticonvulsants and antipsychotics are reserved for exceptional circumstances, given the significant risks they carry (63). Acetylcholinesterase inhibitors may also have a role in both depression and anxiety, as well as in the treatment of the commonly reported symptom of apathy (63, 64).

Sleep Disturbance

Melatonin is a naturally occurring hormone secreted by the pineal gland and is key to the regulation of circadian rhythms. Several studies have investigated the value of exogenous melatonin in improving the sleep–wake cycle in those with dementia and produced mixed results. A meta-analysis of randomised controlled trials concluded that it is well tolerated and may improve sleep efficiency and total sleep time in dementia; however, for Alzheimer's type of dementia more specifically, the evidence for the latter was lacking (65). Sedative hypnotics and atypical antipsychotics have also been demonstrated to ameliorate sleep disturbance in dementia (66). This appears to be due their tranquilising effect and impact on BPSD rather than to an effect on sleep per se, and, given the risk profile of these drugs, justification for their long-term use is limited (66).

Psychotic Symptoms

At times, caregivers will state that an individual with dementia is 'psychotic', but this report needs to be carefully scrutinised. For example, patients with dementia frequently describe confabulated events, such as seeing relatives who have passed away; neverthe-less, unlike true psychosis, they do not hold these beliefs with delusional intensity and in consequence respond poorly to antipsychotics (59). Once psychotic phenomena are confirmed, antipsychotics can be considered, but only if those phenomena are deemed to be distressing to the individuals with dementia or to place them or others at risk. Again, risperidone is the only antipsychotic licensed for psychosis in dementia and the same considerations are required when managing these symptoms on a background of Parkinson's disease dementia and Lewy body dementia, as mentioned earlier (51). When considering those with Parkinson's disease, clozapine has been shown to be an effective treatment of psychotic symptoms; it does not worsen motor function and may in fact improve tremor (67). However, the need for regular blood monitoring and the potential for significant side effects with this drug limit its use in clinical practice.

Toolkit

In response to the concerns around inappropriate prescribing of antipsychotic medication in dementia, the Alzheimer's Society – in conjunction with the Department of Health, Dementia Action Alliance, the College of Mental Health Pharmacy, and the Royal Colleges of Psychiatrists and General Practitioners – developed a paper-based toolkit to guide health and social care professionals in the management of BPSD (68). This toolkit follows a simple, stepped care, 'traffic-light' system in which green represents no symptoms where simple preventative strategies are required, amber is for mild or moderate symptoms that need low-intensity general measures, and red is for severe symptoms that necessitate specific interventions (68). This system encourages the use of two simple flow diagrams, one to use if the person with dementia is already prescribed antipsychotics and the other if he or she is not (68). It is important to note that this toolkit focuses on the needs of people in care home settings and explicitly excludes inpatients within acute hospitals. But it could certainly be adapted for this use and is readily available from the Alzheimer's Society website.

Conclusion

BPSD is a term used to describe a heterogeneous collection of neuropsychiatric behaviours and symptoms, which arise as part of the dementia syndrome. They have been demonstrated to cause distress to the individual with dementia and also to affect adversely those around them. Significantly, BPSD are common in individuals with dementia in hospital settings and have been proven to lead to poorer outcomes and increased healthcare costs. It is therefore clear that the prevention and management of BPSD should be a priority to hospital-based healthcare professionals and an important focus for intervention. For all patients with dementia, the aim is to ultimately develop an individualised plan on admission that pre-emptively addresses any potential causes for BPSD and, in the event that they occur, uses non-pharmacological management strategies as first-line treatment. If these conservative strategies are not feasible or effective, the judicious use of drug treatments can be considered.

References

1. Lawlor, B. Managing behavioural and psychological symptoms in dementia. *British Journal of Psychiatry* 2002, 181(6): 463–5. www.cambridge.org/core/services/aop-cambridge-core/content/view/A8632B904987EE3F2D6132423300182D/S0007125000269286a.pdf/div-class-title-managing-behavioural-and-

psychological-symptoms-in-dementia-div
.pdf.

2. Cerejeira, J., Lagarto, L., and Mukaetova-
Ladinska, E. Behavioral and psychological
symptoms of dementia. *Frontiers in
Neurology* 2012, 3: 73. https://doi.org/10
.3389/fneur.2012.00073.

3. Banerjee, S. *The Use of Antipsychotic
Medication for People with Dementia:
Time for Action*. Department of Health,
2009. http://psychrights.org/research/
digest/nlps/banerjeereportongeriatric
neurolepticuse.pdf.

4. Stelzmann, R.A., Schnitzlein, H.N., and
Murtagh, F.R. An English translation of
Alzheimer's 1907 paper, 'Über eine
eigenartige Erkankung der Hirnrinde'.
Clinical Anatomy 1995, 8: 429–43. https://
doi.org/10.1002/ca.980080612.

5. Finkel, S.I., e Silva, J.C., Cohen, G., Miller,
S., and Sartorius, N. Behavioral and
psychological signs and symptoms of
dementia: A consensus statement on
current knowledge and implications for
research and treatment. *International
Psychogeriatrics* 1997, 8(3): 497–500.
www.researchgate.net/profile/Norman-
Sartorius/publication/313059339_
Behavioral_and_Psychological_Signs_
and_Symptoms_of_Dementia_A_
Consensus_Statement_on_Current_
Knowledge_and_Implications_for_
Research_and_Treatment/links/
5892f43da6fdcc1b4146d7bb/Behavioral-
and-Psychological-Signs-and-Symptoms-
of-Dementia-A-Consensus-Statement-
on-Current-Knowledge-and-
Implications-for-Research-and-
Treatment.pdf.

6. Ireland, N., and Moniz-Cook, E. Getting
our terminology right: The power of
language. *Journal of Dementia Care* 2021,
29(2): 24–27. https://hull-repository
.worktribe.com/preview/3738359/2021%
207%20James%20et%20al%20JDC%20%
20Power%20of%20Langauge.pdf.

7. Kales, H.C., Gitlin, L.N., and Lyketsos,
C.G. Assessment and management of
behavioral and psychological symptoms
of dementia. *British Medical Journal* 2015,
350: 369. https://doi.org/10.1136/bmj
.h369.

8. Steinberg, M., Shao, H., Zandi, P.,
Lyketsos, C.G., Welsh-Bohmer, K.A.,
Norton, M.C. et al. Point and 5-year
period prevalence of neuropsychiatric
symptoms in dementia: The Cache
County Study. *International Journal of
Geriatric Psychiatry* 2008, 23(2): 170–7.
https://doi.org/10.1002/gps.1858.

9. Hurt, C., Bhattacharyya, S., Burns, A.,
Camus, V., Liperoti, R., Marriott, A. et al.
Patient and caregiver perspectives of
quality of life in dementia. *Dementia and
Geriatric Cognitive Disorders* 2008, 26(2):
138–46. https://doi.org/10.1159/
000149584.

10. Ballard, C., Lowery, K., Powell, I.,
O'Brien, J., and James, I. Impact of
behavioral and psychological symptoms
of dementia on caregivers. *International
Psychogeriatrics* 2000, 12(S1): 93–105.

11. Herrmann, N., Lanctôt, K.L., Sambrook,
R., Lesnikova, N., Hébert, R., McCracken,
P. et al. The contribution of
neuropsychiatric symptoms to the cost
of dementia care. *International Journal of
Geriatric Psychiatry* 2006, 21(10): 972–6.

12. Sampson, E.L., White, N., Leurent, B.,
Scott, S., Lord, K., Round, J. et al.
Behavioural and psychiatric symptoms in
people with dementia admitted to the
acute hospital: Prospective cohort study.
British Journal of Psychiatry 2014, 205(3):
189–96. https://doi.org/10.1192/bjp.bp
.113.130948.

13. White, N., Leurent, B., Lord, K., Scott, S.,
Jones, L., and Sampson, E.L. The
management of behavioural and
psychological symptoms of dementia in
the acute general medical hospital:
A longitudinal cohort study. *International
Journal of Geriatric Psychiatry* 2017, 32
(3): 297–305. https://doi.org/10.1002/gps
.4463.

14. Feast, A.R., White, N., Lord, K., Kupeli,
N., Vickerstaff, V., and Sampson, E.L.
Pain and delirium in people with
dementia in the acute general hospital
setting. *Age and Ageing* 2018, 47(6):

841–6. https://doi.org/10.1093/ageing/afy112.

15. Mishriky, R.S., and Reyad, A.A. Pharmacological alternatives to antipsychotics to manage BPSD. *Progress in Neurology and Psychiatry* 2018, 22(1): 30–5. https://wchh.onlinelibrary.wiley.com/doi/pdf/10.1002/pnp.495.

16. López-Álvarez, J., Sevilla-Llewellyn-Jones, J., and Agüera-Ortiz, L. Anticholinergic drugs in geriatric psychopharmacology. *Frontiers in Neuroscience* 2019, 13: 1309. https://doi.org/10.3389/fnins.2019.01309.

17. Alzheimer's Society. *Counting the Cost: Caring for People with Dementia on Hospital Wards*. London: Alzheimer's Society, 2009. www.alzheimers.org.uk/sites/default/files/2018-05/Counting_the_cost_report.pdf.

18. Hessler, J.B., Schäufele, M., Hendlmeier, I., Junge, M.N., Leonhardt, S., Weber, J. et al. Behavioural and psychological symptoms in general hospital patients with dementia, distress for nursing staff and complications in care: Results of the General Hospital Study. *Epidemiology and Psychiatric Sciences* 2018, 27(3): 278–87. https://doi.org/10.1017/S2045796016001098.

19. Pike, G., and Beveridge, K. *Dignity in Dementia: Transforming General Hospital Care*. Hove: Employment Research, 2011. www.rcn.org.uk/clinical-topics/dementia/-/media/bc3abc35d1294ab486fb2f3263808320.ashx.

20. Petrovic, M., Hurt, C., Collins, D., Burns, A., Camus, V., Liperoti, R. et al. Clustering of behavioural and psychological symptoms in dementia (BPSD): A European Alzheimer's disease consortium (EADC) study. *Acta Clinica Belgica* 2007, 62(6): 426–32. www.researchgate.net/profile/Magdalini-Tsolaki/publication/5501629_Clustering_of_behavioural_and_psychological_symptoms_in_dementia_BPSD_A_European_Alzheimer's_disease_consortium_EADC_study/links/0fcfd5110c8d9cb86e000000/Clustering-of-behavioural-and-psychological-

symptoms-in-dementia-BPSD-A-European-Alzheimers-disease-consortium-EADC-study.pdf.

21. Aalten, P., de Vugt, M.E., Lousberg, R., Korten, E., Jaspers, N., Senden, B. et al. Behavioral problems in dementia: A factor analysis of the neuropsychiatric inventory. *Dementia and Geriatric Cognitive Disorders* 2003, 15(2): 99–105. https://doi.org/10.1159/000067972.

22. Ballard, C., Smith, J., Corbett, A., Husebo, B., and Aarsland, D. The role of pain treatment in managing the behavioural and psychological symptoms of dementia (BPSD). *International Journal of Palliative Nursing* 2011, 17(9): 420–4. www.researchgate.net/profile/Bettina-Husebo/publication/51783696_The_role_of_pain_treatment_in_managing_the_behavioural_and_psychological_symptoms_of_dementia_BPSD/links/549303840cf22d7925d5b153/The-role-of-pain-treatment-in-managing-the-behavioural-and-psychological-symptoms-of-dementia-BPSD.pdf.

23. Bird, M., Jones, R.H., Korten, A., and Smithers, H. A controlled trial of a predominantly psychosocial approach to BPSD: treating causality. *International Psychogeriatrics* 2007, 19(5): 874–91. https://doi.org/10.1017/S1041610206004790.

24. Alves, G.S., Carvalho, A.F., de Amorim de Carvalho, L., Sudo, F.K., Siqueira-Neto, J.I., Oertel-Knochel, V. et al. Neuroimaging findings related to behavioral disturbances in Alzheimer's disease: A systematic review. *Current Alzheimer Research* 2017, 14(1): 61–75. https://doi.org/10.2174/1567205013666160603010203.

25. Vermeiren, Y., Le Bastard, N., Van Hemelrijck, A., Drinkenburg, W.H., Engelborghs, S., and De Deyn, P.P. Behavioral correlates of cerebrospinal fluid amino acid and biogenic amine neurotransmitter alterations in dementia. *Alzheimer's & Dementia* 2013, 9(5): 488–98. http://doi.org/10.1016/j.jalz.2012.06.010.

26. Tible, O.P., Riese, F., Savaskan, E., and von Gunten, A. Best practice in the

management of behavioural and psychological symptoms of dementia. *Therapeutic Advances in Neurological Disorders* 2017, 10(8): 297–309. https://doi.org/10.1177/1756285617712979.

27. Cipriani, G., Borin, G., Del Debbio, A., and Di Fiorino, M. Personality and dementia. *Journal of Nervous and Mental Disease* 2015, 203(3): 210–4. http://doi.org/10.1097/NMD.0000000000000264.

28. Paton, C. Benzodiazepines and disinhibition: A review. *Psychiatric Bulletin* 2002, 26(12): 460–2. www.cambridge.org/core/services/aop-cambridge-core/content/view/421AF197362B55EDF004700452BF3BC6/S0955603600001240a.pdf/benzodiazepines_and_disinhibition_a_review.pdf.

29. Cloak, N., and Al Khalili, Y. *Behavioral and Psychological Symptoms in Dementia.* Treasure Island, FL: StatPearls Publishing, 2020. www.ncbi.nlm.nih.gov/books/NBK551552.

30. Ballard, C.G., Gauthier, S., Cummings, J.L., Brodaty, H., Grossberg, G.T., Robert, P. et al. Management of agitation and aggression associated with Alzheimer disease. *Nature Reviews Neurology* 2009, 5 (5): 245–55. https://doi.org/10.1038/nrneurol.2009.39.

31. Sampson, E.L., White, N., Lord, K., Leurent, B., Vickerstaff, V., Scott, S. et al. Pain, agitation, and behavioural problems in people with dementia admitted to general hospital wards: A longitudinal cohort study. *Pain* 2015, 156(4): 675–83. https://doi.org/10.1097/j.pain.0000000000000095.

32. Achterberg, W.P., Pieper, M.J., van Dalen-Kok, A.H., De Waal, M.W., Husebo, B.S., Lautenbacher, S. et al. Pain management in patients with dementia. *Clinical Interventions in Aging* 2013, 8: 1471–82. https://doi.org/10.2147/CIA.S36739.

33. Husebo, B.S., Strand, L.I., Moe-Nilssen, R., Husebo, S.B., and Ljunggren, A.E. Pain in older persons with severe dementia. Psychometric properties of the Mobilization–Observation–Behaviour–Intensity–Dementia (MOBID-2) Pain Scale in a clinical setting. *Scandinavian Journal of Caring Sciences* 2010, 24(2): 380–91. https://doi.org/10.1111/j.1471-6712.2009.00710.x.

34. Scherder, E.J., and Plooij, B. Assessment and management of pain, with particular emphasis on central neuropathic pain, in moderate to severe dementia. *Drugs & Aging* 2012, 29(9): 701–6. https://doi.org/10.1007/s40266-012-0001-8.

35. Cohen-Mansfield, J. Use of patient characteristics to determine non-pharmacologic interventions for behavioural and psychological symptoms of dementia. *International Psychogeriatrics* 2009, 12(1): 373–80.

36. Cipriani, G., Ulivi, M., Danti, S., Lucetti, C., and Nuti, A. Sexual disinhibition and dementia. *Psychogeriatrics* 2016, 16(2): 145–53. http//doi.org/10.1111/psyg.12143.

37. Lyketsos, C.G., Colenda, C.C., Beck, C., Blank, K., Doraiswamy, M.P., Kalunian, D.A. et al. Position statement of the American Association for Geriatric Psychiatry regarding principles of care for patients with dementia resulting from Alzheimer disease. *American Journal of Geriatric Psychiatry* 2006, 14(7): 561–73. https://baycrest.echoontario.ca/wp-content/uploads/2018/01/Position-Statement-of-the-American-Association-for-Geriatric-Psychiatry-Regarding-Principles-of-Care-for-Patients-With-Dementia-Resulting-From-Alzheimer-Disease.pdf.

38. De Vugt, M.E., Stevens, F., Aalten, P., Lousberg, R., Jaspers, N., Winkens, I. et al. Do caregiver management strategies influence patient behaviour in dementia? *International Journal of Geriatric Psychiatry* 2004, 19(1): 85–92. https://doi.org/10.1002/gps.1044.

39. Crowther, G.J., Brennan, C.A., and Bennett, M.I. The barriers and facilitators for recognising distress in people with severe dementia on general hospital wards. *Age and Ageing* 2018, 47(3): 458–65. https://doi.org/10.1093/ageing/afx198.

40. Douglas, S., James, I., and Ballard, C. Non-pharmacological interventions in dementia. *Advances in Psychiatric Treatment* 2004, 10(3): 171–7. www .cambridge.org/core/services/aop-cambridge-core/content/view/ CB4C6A081FFB24A29106998463D8 D8BC/S1355514600001267a.pdf/ nonpharmacological_interventions_in_ dementia.pdf.

41. Reisberg, B., Borenstein, J., Salob, S.P., Ferris, S.H., Franssen, E., and Georgotas, A. Behavioral symptoms in Alzheimer's disease: Phenomenology and treatment. *Journal of Clinical Psychiatry* 1987, 48(5): 9–15.

42. Cummings, J.L. The Neuropsychiatric Inventory: Assessing psychopathology in dementia patients. *Neurology* 1997, 48 (suppl 6): 10–16.

43. Kaufer, D.I., Cummings, J.L., Ketchel, P., Smith, V., MacMillan, A., Shelley, T. et al. Validation of the NPI-Q, a brief clinical form of the Neuropsychiatric Inventory. *Journal of Neuropsychiatry and Clinical Neurosciences* 2000, 12(2): 233–9. https:// neuro.psychiatryonline.org/doi/full/10 .1176/jnp.12.2.233.

44. Williamson, A., and Hoggart, B. Pain: a review of three commonly used pain rating scales. Journal of Clinical Nursing 2005, 14(7): 798–804. https://doi.org/10 .1111/j.1365-2702.2005.01121.x.

45. Corbett, A., Husebo, B.S., Achterberg, W.P., Aarsland, D., Erdal, A., and Flo, E. The importance of pain management in older people with dementia. *British Medical Bulletin* 2014, 111(1): 139–49. https://doi.org/10.1093/bmb/ldu023.

46. Husebo, B.S., Strand, L.I., Moe-Nilssen, R., Husebo, S.B., and Ljunggren, A.E. Pain in older persons with severe dementia: Psychometric properties of the Mobilization–Observation–Behaviour–Intensity–Dementia (MOBID-2) Pain Scale in a clinical setting. *Scandinavian Journal of Caring Sciences* 2010, 24(2): 380–91. https://doi.org/10.1111/j.1471-6712.2009.00710.x.

47. Abbey, J., Piller, N., Bellis, A.D., Esterman, A., Parker, D., Giles, L. et al. The Abbey pain scale: a 1-minute numerical indicator for people with end-stage dementia. *International Journal of Palliative Nursing* 2004, 10(1): 6–13.

48. Livingston, G., Johnston, K., Katona, C., Paton, J., Lyketsos, C.G., and Old Age Task Force of the World Federation of Biological Psychiatry. Systematic review of psychological approaches to the management of neuropsychiatric symptoms of dementia. *American Journal of Psychiatry* 2005, 162(11): 1996–2021. https://doi.org/10.1176/appi.ajp.162.11 .1996.

49. Salami, O., Lyketsos, C., and Rao, V. Treatment of sleep disturbance in Alzheimer's dementia. *International Journal of Geriatric Psychiatry* 2011, 26 (8): 771–82. https://doi.org/10.1002/gps .2609.

50. Black, B., Muralee, S., and Tampi, R.R. Inappropriate sexual behaviors in dementia. *Journal of Geriatric Psychiatry and Neurology* 2005, 18(3): 155–62. https://doi.org/10.1177/ 0891988705277541.

51. Taylor, D.M., Barnes, T.R., and Young, A.H. *The Maudsley Prescribing Guidelines in Psychiatry* (13th ed.). Hoboken, NJ: John Wiley & Sons, Inc., 2018.

52. Chen, R., Chan, P.-T., Chu, H., Lin, Y.-C., Chang, P.-C., Chen, C.-Y. et al. Treatment effects between monotherapy of donepezil versus combination with memantine for Alzheimer disease: A meta-analysis. *PLoS ONE* 2017, 12(8): e0183586. https://doi.org/10.1371/journal .pone.0183586.

53. Maidment, I.D., Fox, C.G., Boustani, M., Rodriguez, J., Brown, R.C., and Katona, C.L. Efficacy of memantine on behavioral and psychological symptoms related to dementia: A systematic meta-analysis. *Annals of Pharmacotherapy* 2008, 42(1): 32–8. https://doi.org/10.1345%2Faph .1K372.

54. Katz, I.R., Jeste, D.V., Mintzer, J.E., Clyde, C., Napolitano, J., and Brecher, M. Comparison of risperidone and placebo for psychosis and behavioral disturbances associated with dementia: A randomized,

double-blind trial. *Journal of Clinical Psychiatry* 1999, 60(2): 107–15.

55. Ballard, C., Margallo-Lana, M., Juszczak, E., Douglas, S., Swann, A., Thomas, A. et al. Quetiapine and rivastigmine and cognitive decline in Alzheimer's disease: Randomised double blind placebo controlled trial. *British Medical Journal* 2005, 330(7496): 874. https://doi.org/10.1136/bmj.38369.459988.8F.

56. Joint Formulary Committee. *Risperidone: British National Formulary.* London: BMJ Group and Pharmaceutical Press. https://bnf.nice.org.uk/drug/risperidone.html.

57. National Institute for Health and Care Excellence (NICE). *Violence and Aggression: Short-Term Management in Mental Health, Health and Community Settings: NICE Guideline* [NG10]. 2015. www.nice.org.uk/guidance/ng10/resources/violence-and-aggression-shortterm-management-in-mental-health-health-and-community-settings-pdf-1837264712389.

58. Orgeta, V., Tabet, N., Nilforooshan, R., and Howard, R. Efficacy of antidepressants for depression in Alzheimer's disease: Systematic review and meta-analysis. *Journal of Alzheimer's Disease* 2017, 58(3): 725–33. http://dx.doi.org/10.3233/JAD-161247.

59. Rosenblatt, A. The art of managing dementia in the elderly. *Cleveland Clinic Journal of Medicine* 2005, 72: S3–13.

60. Kitching, D. Depression in dementia. *Australian Prescriber* 2015, 38(6): 209. https://doi.org/10.18773/austprescr.2015.071.

61. Khawam, E.A., Laurencic, G., and Malone, D.A. Side effects of antidepressants: An overview. *Cleveland Clinical Journal of Medicine* 2006, 73(4): 351–61. http://www.ccjm.org/content/ccjom/73/4/351.full.pdf.

62. Thompson, S., Herrmann, N., Rapoport, M.J., and Lanctôt, K.L. Efficacy and safety of antidepressants for treatment of depression in Alzheimer's disease:

A meta-analysis. *Canadian Journal of Psychiatry* 2007, 52(4): 248–55. https://journals.sagepub.com/doi/pdf/10.1177/070674370705200407.

63. Badrakalimuthu, V.R., and Tarbuck, A.F. Anxiety: a hidden element in dementia. *Advances in Psychiatric Treatment* 2012, 18(2): 119–28. www.cambridge.org/core/services/aop-cambridge-core/content/view/9F1F60CBDAB9ECA1FE74C14715BC642F/S1355514600016345a.pdf/anxiety_a_hidden_element_in_dementia.pdf.

64. Berman, K., Brodaty, H., Withall, A., and Seeher, K. Pharmacologic treatment of apathy in dementia. *American Journal of Geriatric Psychiatry* 2012, 20(2): 104–22. https://doi.org/10.1097/JGP.0b013e31822001a6.

65. Xu, J., Wang, L.L., Dammer, E.B., Li, C.B., Xu, G., Chen, S.D. et al. Melatonin for sleep disorders and cognition in dementia: A meta-analysis of randomized controlled trials. *American Journal of Alzheimer's Disease & Other Dementias* 2015, 30(5): 439–47. https://doi.org/10.1177/1533317514568005.

66. Salami, O., Lyketsos, C., and Rao, V. Treatment of sleep disturbance in Alzheimer's dementia. *International Journal of Geriatric Psychiatry* 2011, 26(8): 771–82. https://doi.org/10.1002/gps.2609.

67. The Parkinson Study Group. Low-dose clozapine for the treatment of drug-induced psychosis in Parkinson's disease. *New England Journal of Medicine* 1999, 340(10): 757–63. https://doi.org/10.1056/NEJM199903113401003.

68. Alzheimer's Society. *Optimising Treatment and Care for Older People with Behavioural and Psychological Symptoms of Dementia: A Best Practice Guide for Health and Social Care Professionals.* Alzheimer's Society, 2011. https://www.alzheimers.org.uk/sites/default/files/2018-08/Optimising%20treatment%20and%20care%20-%20best%20practice%20guide.pdf?downloadID=609.

11

Liaison Old Age Psychiatry Management of Delirium in Acute Hospitals

Mani Santhana Krishnan, Josie Jenkinson, and Rashi Negi

Delirium and Liaison Psychiatry

Delirium is an acute change in mental state causing difficulties in attention, awareness, and arousal, and also fluctuating cognition. There are often multiple underlying causes. Delirium is much more common in older people and affects approximately one in three elderly patients in acute hospitals (1). The presentation is often under-recognised throughout the patient's journey, despite being associated with poor outcomes, higher costs of care, and higher mortality (2, 3). Delirium can be hyperactive (predominantly agitated), hypoactive (predominantly withdrawn and drowsy), or mixed.

The risk of developing delirium increases with increasing physical and biological insults (triggers) on the body. Individuals with a higher degree of frailty are more vulnerable to delirium even when they have less severe insults. After a fractured neck of femur and subsequent surgery, up to 60 per cent of patients will develop delirium (4), and if the person requires admission to an intensive care unit (ICU) the incidence increases to 80 per cent (5). Early detection and intervention improve patient outcomes, but there should also be a focus on prevention, particularly in very high-risk groups such as older people who undergo elective major surgery (6).

Delirium can be very distressing for individuals and their loved ones, who may recall their experiences for the rest of their lives. It can also be very distressing for staff members, who may lack confidence and expertise in the recognition and treatment of delirium.

Given its prevalence in the general hospital setting and its effect on mortality, more work and training are needed to increase awareness of and attention to this condition; compared to other serious conditions, delirium is still very much under-recognised and under-researched. General hospitals vary in the support they provide to people with delirium, which may come in the form of specialist dementia and delirium teams or frailty in-reach services, or may rely on liaison psychiatry services (particularly old age psychiatry services, be they separate or integrated into general liaison services). Unless proven otherwise, any sudden change in mental state should be treated as delirium, and it is important that liaison clinicians are aware of how services work in their individual hospitals and are willing to support them according to need.

The Role of Psychiatric Liaison Services in Delirium Care

Clinicians may hold varied opinions as to who should support people with delirium in the general hospital, and these views can be difficult to reconcile, particularly when resources are scarce. It may come as no surprise that the authors all believe strongly that liaison psychiatrists have an important role to play when it comes to the management of delirium and see it as their core business. Even if services are not resourced to provide direct clinical care to all patients with delirium (which, given the prevalence of the condition, is always likely to be the case), to protect our patients we should, at a minimum, advocate best practice and foster education and training in the general hospitals that we support.

Detection and Screening

As already discussed, delirium is common but underdetected (7, 8). It is well known that lack of detection results in poor patient outcomes (9, 10), and there is much work to be done to improve detection rates both in the emergency department (ED) and on the wards. Liaison services can greatly influence this by providing education, support, and leadership by embedding delirium detection at the front door. There are many ways to do this, for example by embedding screening tools into ED documentation and into ward admissions documentation, by including screening guidance into hospital policies, and by making screening part of the teaching programmes.

There are various screening tools available for delirium, for example the 4AT (11), SQID (Single Question in Delirium) (12), and the CAM (Confusion Assessment Method) (13). A good summary of these, which lists their various advantages and disadvantages, is contained in the SIGN guidelines on delirium (14). The SIGN guideline ultimately recommends the 4AT as the most appropriate screening tool for use in general hospitals. It is brief, free, and easy to use; and it requires no formal training.

Additional resource

A blog by Alasdair MacLullich describes the issues on screening and how to navigate through various screening tools:

    www.deliriumwords.com/delirium-words-1/delirium-detection-in-routine-clinical-care-two-basic-processes

Complex Case Management

Often the management and support of patients with delirium are relatively straightforward operations and people will respond very well to the treatment of the underlying causes. However, some patients may have complex presentations and their management and support will greatly benefit from specialist input. Examples are instances where the person has a severe comorbid mental illness and there are complex prescribing or medico-legal issues, where symptoms are very severe or the diagnosis is not completely clear. Psychiatrists are experts in the assessment and diagnosis of mental disorder, so they are often needed to help to distinguish between delirium and other conditions; and they and can support a holistic management when physical and mental illness coexist.

Hypoactive delirium may be misdiagnosed as depression or dementia, and hyperactive delirium can be confused with mania or psychosis. Key diagnostic features of delirium are the acuity of onset, issues of attention and orientation, fluctuating symptoms, and resolution with the treatment of underlying causes (although this can take weeks, or even months). In delirium, delusions and hallucinations are less likely to be well formed and are often inconsistent, lacking in detail, and not always easily recalled. The longitudinal history and the collateral history are very important in this regard, particularly when trying to ascertain whether there is a possible underlying dementia diagnosis.

Medico-legal frameworks can be difficult to navigate in delirium, and liaison psychiatry services can offer valuable support. Most cases of delirium are likely to be managed using the principles outlined in the Mental Capacity Act and include applications for urgent Deprivation of Liberty and Safeguards (DOLS) authorisations or for forthcoming Liberty Protection Safeguards authorisations; under certain circumstances, however, recourse to the Mental Health Act can be considered, for example if repeated use of restraint and intramuscular medication occurs, or if there is a comorbid mental health condition that impacts on a patient's symptoms.

Patient and Carer Engagement and Support

The experience of having delirium can be very frightening for patients and their loved ones. Involving patients and their families and carers in management wherever possible is an essential part of delirium care. Family and friends are a vital resource in the management of delirium in the hospital setting, and this element of care was impacted greatly as a result of visiting restrictions during the SARS-CoV-2 pandemic. Family and friends may be able to provide reassurance, reorientation, and support around mealtimes or stressful procedures; they also bring in any sensory aids that are needed, as well as familiar items from home. They can provide invaluable feedback on whether the person is different from his or her usual self, or on how the person would behave if he or she were fully recovered. It is important that people are given clear explanations about their condition and are provided with supporting information, including about how they can prevent future recurrence and monitor cognitive functions after the delirium has had time to resolve. Some hospitals have developed their own support leaflets for people with delirium, and it is important that these are given to those who need them.

Additional resource

For hospitals that don't have their own leaflets, generic information leaflets are available, including one developed by SIGN (www.sign.ac.uk/media/1144/pat157.pdf).

Education and Peer Supervision

Liaison services have a key role to play when it comes to the education and training of hospital staff in matters of delirium care, but their capacity to do so may vary extensively, depending on how well developed they are. Ideally, teaching on the topic of delirium should take place across disciplines and professions, at regular intervals. Examples are teaching weekly to EDs, teaching at junior doctors' inductions, and involvement in departmental teaching. Along with structured teaching, ad hoc case-based explanation and informal peer support of hospital colleagues should form part of the input provided by liaison services.

Influencing Local Services

Liaison services are ideally placed to understand the impact of conditions across the whole care system, given the number of agencies and organisations they interface with.

This knowledge of the wider healthcare system is invaluable when one develops and implements delirium pathways and policies. It is particularly important to understand what role community mental health services, integrated care services, and frailty services play and how this role may need to be developed. Liaison teams, particularly if they have a community-facing role or an outpatient facility, may be able to provide support outside the hospital setting, too. Above all, liaison clinicians can be powerful advocates for the development or advancement of delirium care more generally, as a result of the expertise they develop during their support of the general hospital.

Clinical Management of Delirium

Having discussed what an important role liaison psychiatrists can play in delirium care, we will now focus on the clinical management of delirium.

> **Key Principles of Management**
> 1. Take a good history.
> 2. Use a screening tool.
> 3. Identify and treat all possible causes.
> 4. Prioritise a non-pharmacological management of symptoms.
> 5. Use pharmacological management as a last resort, and as safely as possible.
> 6. Have a clear follow-up plan.

Take a Good History

As in all conditions, here too good management starts with an excellent and thorough history. It is important to establish a timeline related to the onset of symptoms, to state whether symptoms fluctuate, and to clarify when the person was his or her usual self for the last time.

Always try to get collateral history, if possible; a collateral history from family, friends, or carers is extremely important and every effort should be made to obtain one. A simple question like 'are they different from their usual self?' is very helpful towards identifying change in the patient's mental state. It may be hard to detect when someone has a hypoactive delirium, whereas, particularly in a busy hospital where staff members are stretched, the agitation of someone who has a hyperactive delirium is much more easily noticed (15).

While taking the history, it is helpful to look out for issues that may predispose someone to developing a delirium (e.g. polypharmacy, multiple comorbidities, sensory impairments, dementia, recent surgery or illness, pain, constipation, changes in environment, poor hydration, and nutritional status).

> **Additional information**
> PINCH ME is a very useful mnemonic for remembering some of the main areas of the history to explore: pain, infection, nutrition, constipation, hydration, medication, environment.

Use a Screening Tool

In general, delirium detection is a two-stage process involving initial screening with the help of a brief simple and sensitive instrument, followed by a formal diagnosis that employs the criteria in the tenth edition of the International Classification of Diseases (ICD). Using a screening tool to detect delirium is quick and easy and should form part of the assessment, alongside conducting a history and full mental state examination.

It has been widely claimed that clinicians lack awareness of the symptoms of delirium and its different subtypes – hyperactive, hypoactive, and mixed (16, 17). Furthermore, many do not have confidence in diagnosing or managing delirium. The situation is compounded further still by patient ward transfers and regular changes in the people who provide care; this is due to staff shift patterns. The consequence is that delirium is underdiagnosed, especially the hypoactive type (16, 17). Delayed detection and failure to diagnose delirium are associated with poor outcomes such as readmission, increased risk of admission to residential care, and high mortality. It is important that screening for delirium is a part of routine care during admission to an acute hospital (16, 17).

Delirium screening starts with raising the awareness of all members of staff, through training. Delirium training should focus on less obvious presentations, for example hypoactivity that can easily be mistaken for 'fatigue' or 'frailty' in seriously unwell or post-operative patients. Other less obvious presentations occur in what is described as a 'prodromal phase', a subtle early prelude to acute delirium. During the prodromal phase, early detection may prevent transition to full delirium. The prodromal phase can include symptoms such as anxiety and general malaise, and a variety of non-specific complaints such as deterioration in cognitive function, reduced pain tolerance, and simply not being oneself (18).

Using a screening tool to detect delirium is quick and easy and should form part of the assessment, alongside conducting a full mental state examination. In general, delirium detection is a two-stage process involving an initial screening with the help of a brief, simple, and sensitive instrument and a formal diagnosis according to the criteria for delirium delineated in ICD10, which is of a high specificity in point of identifying this condition (19).

Screening Tools in the Emergency Department

Emergency departments are the face of modern healthcare systems and, for many older people, the point of admission into the hospital. It has been reported that 15 to 30 per cent of older people have symptoms of delirium on admission to hospital and approximately 50 per cent of patients will develop symptoms during their stay. Hence EDs are a useful place to initiate screening for the symptoms of delirium (20).

There are seven different screening tools that have been trialled in the ED setting:

- the Confusion Assessment Method (CAM) (13)
- the modified Confusion Assessment Method for Emergency Departments (mCAM-ED) (21)
- the Confusion Assessment Method – Intensive Care Unit (CAM-ICU) (22)
- the Delirium Triage Screen (DTS) (23)
- the brief Confusion Assessment Method (bCAM) (23)
- the Neelon and Champagne Confusion Scale (NEECHAM) (24)
- the Richmond Agitation Sedating Scale (RASS) (25)

Screening Tools in the General Hospital

Currently the 4AT is the most widely used screening tool. This is due to its simplicity, validity, and ease of use even in difficult presentations. Other simple tests that have high sensitivity and relative specificity for diagnosing delirium are the digital spatial span, serial sevens, and naming months backwards. All of these could be in principle used as initial screening tools (26).

The routine use of delirium detection screening tools in acute hospitals was explored in a recent study. The response rate was very high: 91 per cent of hospitals in the United Kingdom provided data. Of these, 95 per cent used a formal delirium assessment process and 85 per cent had guidelines or pathways in place for managing delirium. The 4AT was the most widely used tool; it was used in 80 per cent of the hospitals surveyed. The confusion assessment method (CAM) was used in 45 per cent of units. Single question to identify delirium (SQID) was used in 36 per cent of units (28).

A 2020 meta-analysis of seventeen studies reviewing the psychometric properties of the 4AT reported a pooled sensitivity of 0.88 and a pooled specificity of 0.88. Furthermore, the tool was shown to be pragmatic and feasible in a clinical setting. The validation studies included were performed in general medical wards, geriatrics wards, EDs, and surgical wards (28).

Together with the accompanying education and training of nursing staff, the incorporation of the 4AT into the routine care of all patients aged 65 and older admitted to two acute medical units resulted in an increase in the use of the 4AT from 40 per cent to 61 per cent and improved the assessment of the causes of delirium in 94 per cent of cases, going up from 73 per cent (29).

Other available screening tools have practical issues with their implementation in the general hospital setting. A systematic review of screening tools (30) included the Confusion Assessment Method (CAM), the Delirium Rating Scale, the Nurses' Delirium Screening Checklist, the Single Question in Delirium, the Memorial Delirium Assessment Scale and the 4As test. The Confusion Assessment Method (CAM) was found to be the instrument most widely used to identify delirium, but specific training is required to ensure optimum performance. The Delirium Rating Scale and its revised version were found to perform best in the psychogeriatric population, but requires psychiatric training. The Nurses' Delirium Screening Checklist appeared best suited to the surgical and recovery room setting. The Single Question in Delirium showed promise in oncology patients. The Memorial Delirium Assessment Scale, while demonstrating good measures of validity in the surgical and palliative care setting, may be better used as a measure of delirium severity. The 4As Test performed well when delirium was superimposed on dementia, but it requires further study (16).

Although screening tools can be very useful, the importance of eliciting a good collateral history cannot be overemphasised, as patients may not be able to give a clear account of their own symptoms. Observing, monitoring, and recording the patient's overall level of arousal throughout the interaction can be considered just as important as baseline vital signs observations.

Identify and Treat All Possible Causes

Apart from undergoing a comprehensive physical examination, patients should be investigated thoroughly and appropriately, and all possible causes of delirium should be addressed. The set of investigations completed is usually termed a 'confusion screen' and may vary by hospital, but would generally include urinalysis, ECG, chest X-ray, neuroimaging, and a blood panel usually consisting of FBC, U+E, LFT, TFT, bone profile, B12 and folate, CRP, ESR and vitamin D, and other testing depending on the history. If the patient is older or frail, then he or she is likely to benefit from a comprehensive geriatric assessment (see Chapter 19). Some hospitals offer in-reach frailty services that provide it and, if they don't, it may be appropriate to ask for admission to an older people's specialist hospital ward (geriatric ward) or frailty ward. Medications should be reviewed and optimised, particular attention being paid to any drugs that may increase the anticholinergic burden, as these can worsen confusion.

Prioritise Non-Pharmacological Management

Non-pharmacological management of the symptoms of delirium should be optimised; alongside the treatment of the underlying causes, this is one of the most important aspects of delirium care. Optimisation is easily said, but much harder to implement in a busy hospital setting. Noise and distractions should be reduced as much as possible, but people's ability to make sense of what is happening to them should be optimised by ensuring that they have any glasses or hearing aids that they usually use and that they have them on or in. People should be regularly reorientated and given access to natural light, as well as to a clock and calendar they can see easily. Any moves between or within wards should be kept to a minimum. For people who have delirium superimposed on dementia, use of the 'This is me' document developed by the Alzheimer's Society (www .alzheimers.org.uk/get-support/publications-factsheets/this-is-me) can be very helpful, as well as any existing positive behavioural support plans.

Figure 11.1 is a useful visual aide-memoire for the recognition and management of delirium, and it can be reproduced and used freely.

Use Pharmacological Management as a Last Resort, as Safely as Possible

There is little evidence of any specific pharmacological treatment for delirium. The common medication classes that are used in the management of delirium are benzodiazepines and antipsychotic medications. There is a limited role for benzodiazepines in the management of delirium, specifically in frail older adults.

When a patient is severely agitated or distressed and presents with significant psychotic features, cautious use of antipsychotic medication may be considered, after a full, comprehensive review of the risks versus benefits of a pharmacological treatment. The latter may become necessary for treating behavioural and psychological symptoms of delirium such as agitation, aggression, disinhibition and so on, which in practice increase risks not only to the patients who suffer with delirium but also to the professionals who care for them and to other patients on the wards.

Antipsychotic medications can increase the risk of cerebrovascular events and can have a range of problematic anticholinergic, extrapyramidal side effects, QT prolongation, sedation, and falls. In a meta-analysis performed in 2019, the results of cohort studies that included the general population indicated a more than double risk of stroke, albeit with substantial heterogeneity (pooled HR 2.31, 95 per cent CI 1.13) (31).

Hence it is critical to use these medications as a last resort, in the short term, in extremely low doses, targeting specific symptoms, and with very close monitoring and review. It has been recommended to review this usage weekly, with a view to stopping it altogether. Furthermore, the trial of medications should be a multidisciplinary team decision that takes into account all pros and cons, has clear documentation, and communicates explicitly with those who receive the medication and with their families. It is also important to discuss how this medication would be given: orally, intra-

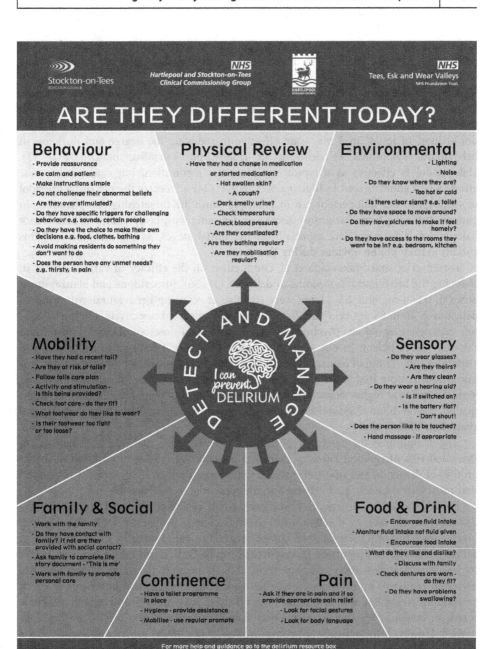

Figure 11.1 Delirium wheel (https://madeinheene.hee.nhs.uk/Portals/0/Faculty%20of%20Patient%20Safety/ Delirium/Delirium%20Wheel.pdf?ver=2020-04-22-143742-007; see also the SIGN guideline risk reduction poster, www.sign.ac.uk/media/1424/sign157_poster.pdf)

muscularly, or (in some cases) covertly, after a clear discussion with the family about risks versus benefits, in line with the principles of the Mental Capacity Act and in line with any local policy.

Much of the early literature describing the pharmacological management of behavioural symptoms advocated haloperidol as the mainstay of treatment. This is reflected in the Cochrane database's systematic review, which has shown that low doses of haloperidol – doses of less than 3 mg – are effective in reducing the degree and duration of behavioural symptoms of delirium in elderly post-operative patients (32, 33). Haloperidol is effective as a typical antipsychotic medication, but causes more side effects when administered in higher doses. NICE (34) advocates the use of haloperidol or olanzapine, but haloperidol can in principle cause life-threatening complications in patients suffering from Parkinson disease or dementia with Lewy bodies (DLB). Hence haloperidol is best avoided, especially in the initial stages, as the symptoms of this condition may not be obvious during this time.

Larsen et al. and Prakantana et al. commented on the efficacy of various agents in reducing the behavioural symptoms of delirium (35, 36). Risperidone and olanzapine at doses of 0.5–4 mg and 2.5–11 mg were effective at reducing behavioural symptoms in delirium in 80 to 85 per cent and 70 to 75 per cent of cases respectively. On the basis of our experience as old age psychiatrists, we estimate that doses substantially lower than this may be sufficient. In our experience, most people will respond to up to 2 mg of risperidone or 7.5 mg of olanzapine without experiencing any major adverse effects. It is important to note that most atypical antipsychotic medications lose their pharmacological benefits at higher doses. It is worth mentioning that there are currently no high-quality double-blind randomised trials available for patients with these behavioural symptoms of delirium.

The Committee on Safety of Medicines (37) issued a warning highlighting an increased risk of cerebral vascular events in patients with delirium who have a background of dementia and who were treated with risperidone or olanzapine. It is believed that most antipsychotic medications have the potential to increase this risk.

Benzodiazepines are usually considered when delirium is associated with withdrawal from alcohol, or if sedation is required such as in cases of DLB. Short-acting lorazepam is usually the preferred choice, as it has a rapid onset, a short duration of action, and sedative properties. In suspected cases of DLB, rivastigmine has been found to be more effective than placebos (38). It is important that benzodiazepines are reviewed regularly by the prescriber; they should be discontinued after one week of continuous treatment, if delirium has been resolved. It is important to note that there is a lack of evidence for their use and that they may well prolong or worsen delirium overall. However, these drugs are commonly used in clinical practice and may play a role in helping people who are terrified of the experience caused by their delirium symptoms.

As a rule, when prescribing in delirium, one must always balance the risk of the prescribed agent against its potential benefits. One should do this by having as clear a view of the clinical scenario as possible, and the treatment should be discussed with all interested parties. The arguments for and against treatment should be clearly set out, while also considering the legal framework for its administration. The paucity of published evidence available to guide our treatment decisions and the existing ambiguity make confident prescribing harder still. Most are agreed, however, that prescribing does have a place, so long as it is done cautiously, thoughtfully, minimally, and in a multidisciplinary team.

Prescribing for acute delirium symptoms is, overall, an under-researched area with many layers of complexities. It is important to note that these patients may be perceived as lacking in capacity because of the presence and severity of the symptoms. As these symptoms invariably increase the risk to patients and their caregivers, the best interest principle of the Mental Capacity Act is often applied in clinical practice. It is highly advised that anyone needing these medications on the grounds of risk should go through an extensive risk versus benefit analysis and that these medications are regularly reviewed to show clear justification for ongoing use.

Here are a few thoughts on antipsychotic medication in the management of delirium.

- It is not a treatment for delirium, but helps to manage severe agitation; you need to weigh risk versus benefit.
- Always consider side effects such as QT prolongation, sedation, falls, and extrapyramidal side effects.

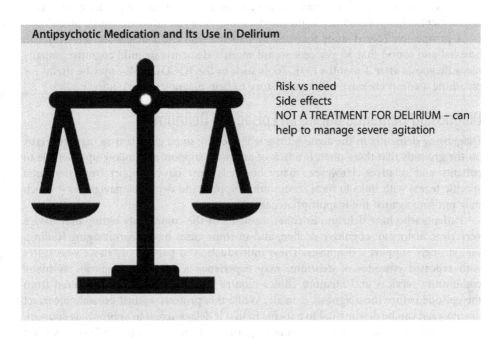

Antipsychotic Medication and Its Use in Delirium

Risk vs need
Side effects
NOT A TREATMENT FOR DELIRIUM – can help to manage severe agitation

Have a Clear Follow-Up Plan on Discharge and Community Care

There are a variety of ways in which patients experiencing delirium may be followed up after hospital discharge – ways that mainly depend on local service arrangements.

For example, these patients may return to an elderly care outpatient clinic or an acute medicine clinic, may be seen by their GPs, or may be referred to local integrated care services or to a memory clinic. It is important that patients are given an opportunity to talk about their experiences, which may have been very distressing, and receive appropriate supportive information about the risk and the prevention of further episodes.

Cognitive function should also be reviewed by someone who is trained in its assessment, and the patient should be referred for further investigations and should receive a more detailed assessment from a specialist, if needed. It can be difficult for organisations other than GP practices to refer to specialist memory clinics, and this needs to be considered carefully from the perspective of delirium discharge pathways. Those who organise services should consider accepting referrals from other secondary care clinics or from integrated care systems, to avoid delays in accessing this input. At Tees, Esk, and Wear Valley NHS Foundation Trust, as part of a quality improvement project, patients who had some cognitive problems at the time of discharge from hospital were followed up in a pilot post-delirium clinic set up by the liaison psychiatry service at twelve weeks after discharge. Of 300 patients followed up by the clinic, around 30 per cent recovered completely, 30 per cent needed referral to a memory clinic, and 30 per cent needed ongoing observation for further deterioration (unpublished data).

Delirium Superimposed on Dementia

Delirium can coexist with dementia. Sometimes we see patients who present to acute hospitals with delirium but have a background history of longer-term cognitive impairment. This poses some diagnostic dilemmas and can affect discharge planning.

A prospective cohort study followed up patients who had a diagnosis of delirium in hospital and found that 38 per cent would merit a dementia or mild cognitive impairment diagnosis after 3 months (39). Tools such as the IQCODE (40) may be useful for obtaining a comprehensive collateral history to help diagnostic work-up.

Diagnosing Dementia during an Episode of Delirium

Diagnosing dementia in the acute setting is viewed by some clinicians as inappropriate, on the grounds that there often is a lack of adequate support and follow-up available to patients and relatives. However, many hospitals now have support from dementia specific teams with links to local community support and dementia navigators – which may mitigate against the inappropriateness view.

Patients who have delirium in either the acute or the community setting may have a very clear history of cognitive decline, and in some cases have neuroimaging findings that strongly support a diagnosis. These individuals, and particularly those who suffer with repeated episodes of delirium, may experience a delay in diagnosis, as many community services and memory clinics require that the person has recovered from the episode before the diagnosis is made. While this protects against possible incorrect diagnoses, it can be detrimental to patients in that it delays access to appropriate support.

It would be good to take a pragmatic approach to such cases and, where there is a means of organising suitable post-diagnostic support, a diagnosis should not be delayed if it is clear. If there is some doubt but the diagnosis is felt to be likely, a working diagnosis could be helpful to the patient: it would support appropriate care planning, and there would be a subsequent review by a specialist to confirm the diagnosis.

Delirium Pathways and Aftercare

Clinical pathways are useful in terms of supporting the consistent management of delirium across various services. Clinical terms should be clear in references to 'delirium pathway' in local services: these pathways should be well described and form part of a coherent policy. Pathways should be common knowledge and should be embedded in practice, clearly shared by liaison services and acute trusts. Pathways may be more to do with assessment, aftercare, or funding arrangements and it is important that old age liaison consultants are well versed in local arrangements.

Examples

Reach Out Project - Cumbria
www.cntw.nhs.uk/services/reach-out-delirium-service/
https://madeinheene.hee.nhs.uk/Portals/0/Faculty%20of%20Patient%20Safety/
Delirium/Delirium%20Marchathon/Reach%20out%20Delirium%20Service%20project
%20-%20CNTW.PDF?ver=2021-03-13-121241-970
Delirium Dementia Outreach Team (DDOT) - Sunderland
www.stsft.nhs.uk/services/dementia-care

Education

The key components of delirium education are awareness, knowledge, and skills. Consistent and regular education, whether formal or informal, will help in identifying at-risk patients; early detection methods, including the screening of patients at risk, will also improve through education.

Awareness

It is well established that the incidence of delirium is high at presentation to hospital and increases in specific populations and settings (older adult wards, post-operative settings, and ICU). Delirium causes significant distress to those who suffer it, their friends and family, and the staff members who care for them.

Delirium has been associated with increase in morbidity and with worsening cognition in older adults. It can result in death (41).

Despite its morbidity, mortality, and long-term consequences, delirium in acute settings is under-detected. Early detection and the treatment of the underlying cause improve chances of recovery.

The management of delirium involves the whole team of care professionals. There is a need to raise awareness across all staff groups, from the front-of-the-house reception staff to everyone in the hospital.

Audits and quality improvement projects have highlighted the importance of delirium education to all care staff (medical, nursing, and allied healthcare professionals). Education is crucial to identifying at-risk patients and to early detection (42).

Skills

Good, compassionate, holistic care is important and delivers high-quality results in cases of delirium. Communicating with patients who are confused, distressed, and frightened is a key skill. Supporting staff to learn about de-escalation and training them in the relevant skills will improve outcomes for patients. Such skills include the capacity to use screening tools like 4AT, CAM and specific tools like the CAM-ICU.

Knowledge

Liaison psychiatry services play a key role in regularly providing formal and informal education to teams and staff groups. Delirium is everybody's business. Once awareness has been raised, the regular provision of teaching is needed to address the knowledge gap:

- risks of untreated delirium;
- delirium superimposed on dementia;
- differential diagnosis of delirium;
- supporting family and carers.

Delirium Is Everybody's Business

Delirium awareness, detection, and management should be embedded in services across acute hospitals. Education is important every step of the way, in order for the staff to engage with all professionals, with patients, and with their carers.

References

1. Fuchs, S., Bode, L., Ernst, J., Marquetand, J., von Känel, R., and Böttger, S. Delirium in elderly patients: Prospective prevalence across hospital services. *Gen Hosp Psychiatry* 2020, 67: 19–25.

2. Leslie, D.L., Marcantonio, E.R., Zhang, Y., Leo-Summers, L., and Inouye, S.K. One-year health care costs associated with delirium in the elderly population. *Arch Intern Med* 2008, 168 (1): 27–32.

3. McCusker, J., Cole, M., Abrahamowicz, M., Primeau, F., and Belzile, E. Delirium Predicts 12-Month Mortality. *Arch Intern Med* 2002, 162(4): 457.

4. Olofsson, B., Lundström, M., Borssén, B., Nyberg, L., and Gustafson, Y. Delirium is associated with poor rehabilitation outcome in elderly patients treated for femoral neck fractures. *Scand J Caring Sci* 2005, 19(2): 119–27.

5. Vasilevskis, E.E., Han, J.H., Hughes, C.G., and Ely, E.W. Epidemiology and risk factors for delirium across hospital settings. *Best Pract Res Clin Anaesthesiol* 2012, 26(3): 277–87.

6. Flinn, D.R., Diehl, K.M., Seyfried, L.S., and Malani, P.N. Prevention, diagnosis, and management of postoperative delirium in older adults. *J Am Coll Surg* 2009, 209(2): 261–8; quiz 294.

7. Barron, E.A., and Holmes, J. Delirium within the emergency care setting, occurrence and detection: a systematic review. *Emergency Medicine Journal* 2013, 30(4).

8. Laurila, J.V., Pitkala, J.H., Strandberg , T.E., and Tilvis, R.S. The impact of different diagnostic criteria on prevalence rates of delirium. *Dementia and Geriatric Cognitive Disorders* 2003, 16(3).

9. La Mantia, M.A., Messina, F.C., Hobgood, C.D., and Miller, D.K. Screening for Delirium in the emergency department: A systematic review. *Annals of Emergency Medicine* 2014, 63(5): 551–60.

10. Neto, A.S., Nassar, A.P., Cardoso, S.O., Manetta, J.A., Pereira, V.G.M., Esposito, D.C., Damasceno, M.C.T., and Slooter, A.J. Delirium screening in critically ill patients: A systematic review and meta-analysis. *Critical Care Medicine* 2012, 40 (5): 1946–51.

11. Bellelli, G., Morandi, A., Davis, D.H.J., Mazzola, M., Turco, R., Gentile, S., Ryan, T., Cash, H., Guerini, F., Torpilliesi, T., Del Santo, F., Trabucchi, M., Annoni, G., and MacLullich, A.M.J. Validation of the

4AT, a new instrument for rapid delirium screening: a study in 234 hospitalised older people. *Age and Ageing* 2014, 43(4): 496–502.

12. Sands, M.B., Dantoc, B.P., Hartshorn, A., Ryan, C.J., and Lujic, S. Single Question in Delirium (SQiD): Testing its efficacy against psychiatrist interview, the Confusion Assessment Method and the Memorial Delirium Assessment Scale. *Palliative Care* 2010, 24(6).

13. Inouye, S.K., van Dyck, C.H., Alessi, C.A., Balkin, S., Siegal, A.P., and Horwitz, R.I. Clarifying confusion: The confusion assessment method. A new method for detection of delirium. *Ann Intern Med* 1990, 113(12): 941–8.

14. The Scottish Intercollegiate Guidelines Network (SIGN) 157: Guidelines on Risk Reduction and Management of Delirium. Scottish Intercollegiate Guidelines Network. *Medicina (Kaunas)* 2019, 55(8): 491. doi: 10.3390/medicina55080491.

15. Crowther, G.J.E., Brennan, C.A., and Bennett, M.I. The barriers and facilitators for recognising distress in people with severe dementia on general hospital wards. *Age Ageing* 2018, 47(3): 458–65.

16. Kakuma, R., du Fort, G.G., Arsenault, L., Perrault, A., Platt, R.W., Monette, J. et al. Delirium in older emergency department patients discharged home: Effect on survival. *J Am Geriatr Soc* 2003, 51(4): 443–50.

17. Siddiqi, N., House, A.O., and Holmes, J.D. Occurrence and outcome of delirium in medical in-patients: A systematic literature review. *Age Ageing* 2006, 35(4): 350–64.

18. De Jonghe, J.F.M., Kalisvaart, K.J., Dijkstra, M., van Dis, H., Vreeswijk, R., Kat, M.G. et al. Early symptoms in the prodromal phase of delirium: A prospective cohort study in elderly patients undergoing hip surgery. *Am J Geriatr Psychiatry* 2007, 15(2): 112–21.

19. Chuen, V.L., Chan, A.C.H., Ma, J., Alibhai, S.M.H., and Chau, V. Assessing the Accuracy of International

Classification of Diseases (ICD) Coding for Delirium. *J Appl Gerontol* 2022, 41(5): 1485–90.

20. Mariz, J., Costa Castanho, T., Teixeira, J., Sousa, N., and Correia Santos, N. Delirium diagnostic and screening instruments in the emergency department: An up-to-date systematic review. *Geriatrics* 2016, 1(3): 22.

21. Grossmann, F.F., Hasemann, W., Graber, A., Bingisser, R., Kressig, R.W., and Nickel, C.H. Screening, detection and management of delirium in the emergency department: A pilot study on the feasibility of a new algorithm for use in older emergency department patients: The modified Confusion Assessment Method for the Emergency Department (mCAM-ED). *Scandinavian Journal of Trauma, Resuscitation and Emergency Medicine* 2014, 22(1): 19.

22. Ely, E.W., Inouye, S.K., Bernard, G.R., Gordon, S., Francis, J., May, L., Truman, B., Speroff, T., Gautam, S., Margolin, R., Hart, R.P., and Dittus, R. Delirium in mechanically ventilated patients: validity and reliability of the confusion assessment method for the intensive care unit (CAM-ICU) *J Am Med Assoc* 2001, 286: 2703–10.

23. Han, J.H., Wilson, A., Vasilevskis, E.E., Shintani, A., Schnelle, J.F., Dittus, R.S., Graves, A.J., Storrow, A.B., Shuster, J., and Ely, E.W. Diagnosing delirium in older emergency department patients: Validity and reliability of the delirium triage screen and the brief confusion assessment method. *Ann Emerg Med* 2013, 62(5): 457–65.

24. Neelon, V.J., Champagne, M.T., Carlson, J.R., and Funk, S.G. The NEECHAM Confusion Scale: Construction, validation, and clinical testing. *Nurs Res* 1996, 45(6): 324–30.

25. Ely, E.W., Truman, B., Shintani, A., Thomason, J.W.W., Wheeler, A.P., Gordon, S., Francis, J., Speroff, T., Gautam, S., Margolin, R. et al. Monitoring sedation status over time in ICU patients: The reliability and validity

of the Richmond Agitation Sedation Scale (RASS). *J Am Med Assoc* 2003, 289: 2983–991.

26. Hall, R.J., Meagher, D.J., and MacLullich, A.M.J. Delirium detection and monitoring outside the ICU. *Best Pract Res Clin Anaesthesiol* 2012, 26(3): 367–83.

27. Tieges, Z., Lowrey, J., and MacLullich, A.M.J. What delirium detection tools are used in routine clinical practice in the United Kingdom? Survey results from 91% of acute healthcare organisations. *Eur Geriatr Med* 2021, 12(6): 1293–8.

28. Tieges, Z., Maclullich, A.M.J., Anand, A., Brookes, C., Cassarino, M., O'Connor, M. et al. Diagnostic accuracy of the 4AT for delirium detection in older adults: Systematic review and meta-analysis. *Age Ageing* 2021, 50(3): 733–43.

29. Bauernfreund, Y., Butler, M., Ragavan, S., and Sampson, E.L. TIME to think about delirium: Improving detection and management on the acute medical unit. *BMJ Open Qual* 2018, 7(3).

30. De, J., and Wand, A.P.F. Delirium screening: A systematic review of delirium screening tools in hospitalized patients. *Gerontologist* 2015, 55(6): 1079–99.

31. Zivkovic, S., Koh, C.H., Kaza, N., and Jackson, C.A. Antipsychotic drug use and risk of stroke and myocardial infarction: A systematic review and meta-analysis. *BMC Psychiatry* 2019, 19 (1): 189.

32. MacSweeney, R., Barber, V., Page, V., Ely, E.W., Perkins, G.D., Young, J.D. et al. A national survey of the management of delirium in UK intensive care units. *QJM* 2010, 103(4): 243–51.

33. Wang, W., Li, H.L., Wang, D.X., Zhu, X., Li, S.L., Yao, G.Q. et al. Haloperidol prophylaxis decreases delirium incidence in elderly patients after noncardiac surgery. *Crit Care Med* 2012, 40(3): 731–9.

34. NICE. Delirium: prevention, diagnosis and management in hospital and long-term care. Clinical guideline [CG103], 28 July 2010.

35. Larsen, K.A., Kelly, S.E., Stern, T.A., Bode, R.H., Price, L.L., Hunter, D.J. et al. Administration of olanzapine to prevent postoperative delirium in elderly joint-replacement patients: A randomized, controlled trial. *Psychosomatics* 2010, 51 (5): 409–18.

36. Prakanrattana, U., and Prapaitrakool, S. Efficacy of risperidone for prevention of postoperative delirium in cardiac surgery. *Anaesth Intensive Care* 2007, 35(5): 714–9.

37. Mowat, D., Fowlie, D., and MacEwan, T. CSM warning on atypical psychotics and stroke may be detrimental for dementia. *BMJ* 2004, 328(7450): 1262.

38. McKeith, I., del Ser, T., Spano, P., Emre, M., Wesnes, K., Anand, R. et al. Efficacy of rivastigmine in dementia with Lewy bodies: A randomised, double-blind, placebo-controlled international study. *The Lancet* 2000, 356(9247): 2031–6.

39. Jackson, T.A., MacLullich, A.M.J., Gladman, J.R.F., Lord, J.M., and Sheehan, B. Undiagnosed long-term cognitive impairment in acutely hospitalised older medical patients with delirium: A prospective cohort study. *Age Ageing* 2016, 45(4): 493–9.

40. Jorm, A.F., and Jacomb, P.A. The Informant Questionnaire on Cognitive Decline in the Elderly (IQCODE): Socio-demographic correlates, reliability, validity and some norms. *Psychol Med* 1989, 19(4): 1015–22.

41. Richardson, S.J., Davis, D.H.J., Stephan, B.C.M., Robinson, L., Brayne, C., Barnes, L.E. et al. Recurrent delirium over 12 months predicts dementia: Results of the Delirium and Cognitive Impact in Dementia (DECIDE) study. *Age Ageing* 2021, 50(3): 914–20.

42. Tauro, R. Delirium awareness: Improving recognition and management through education and use of a care pathway. *BMJ Qual Improv Rep* 2014, 2(2).

Resources

Delirium App

Colleagues in the Midlands have developed an app to support staff (free); two of the authors of the present chapter collaborated in this work. The app has information on screening tools and simple non-pharmacological interventions.

Delirium Videos

Delirium Decision support Tool App, including 4AT calculator:
https://apps.apple.com/gb/app/sign-decision-support/id1525349118

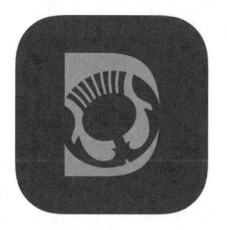

SIGN Decision Support [4+]

Tools based on SIGN Guidelines
SIGN Executive
Designed for iPad

★★★★★ 5.0 • 1 Rating

Free

Other Links

SIGN Guidelines
www.sign.ac.uk/our-guidelines/risk-reduction-and-management-of-delirium/
www.sign.ac.uk/media/1423/sign157.pdf
NICE guidelines
www.nice.org.uk/guidance/cg103
Links to Health Education England North East Delirium Resources
https://madeinheene.hee.nhs.uk/PG-Dean/Faculty-of-Patient-Safety/Delirium-Project/
Delirium-Resources
Toolkits
Scottish Delirium Association - Delirium Pathway
www.signdecisionsupport.uk/risk-reduction-and-management-of-delirium/
iHub Delirium Toolkit from Health Improvement Scotland
https://ihub.scot/project-toolkits/delirium-toolkit/delirium-toolkit/
Toolkit and training resources from Dementia United - Manchester
https://dementia-united.org.uk/delirium-toolkit-training-resources/
Delirium Hub - BGS
www.bgs.org.uk/deliriumhub

Chapter 12

Depression and Associated Disorders

Wendy Burn, George Crowther, and Eimear Devlin

Introduction

The experience of being admitted to hospital can be devastating. The person in hospital is already physically unwell and is placed in an unusual, often hectic, and at times frightening environment. What is more, while in hospital, some patients are given bad news and have to come to terms with changes to their level of premorbid independence and functioning. It is perhaps unsurprising that the prevalence of depression and associated mood disorders among hospitalised older people is more than twice its counterpart in the community (1). Those who are susceptible to depression or have it already may see the emergence of new or more severe symptoms, and even in those with no previous history of a mood disorder symptoms can rapidly develop.

At the opposite end of the spectrum, mood can become elated as well as depressed. This may be associated with an emotional reaction to a stressful situation, new medication, or the relapse of a pre-existing mental illness.

For the clinician, diagnosing mood disorders in hospital can be complex. Neurological disorders, delirium, and fluctuating levels of consciousness can inhibit the patient's verbal communication and subsequent ability to convey his or her experience. Even when symptoms associated with a mood disorder are discovered, the context of that experience needs careful unpicking. Mood can be transiently and catastrophically impacted by organic disorders, medications, ongoing somatic symptoms, bad news about diagnoses, or the hospital environment itself. The clinician has to be careful not to assign potentially stigmatising diagnoses to normal human emotion. This is more easily said than done in a hospital setting; while community psychiatrists have the opportunity to conduct a longitudinal assessment over weeks or months, the liaison psychiatrist's assessment period is usually only as long as the patient's hospital stay.

Further muddying the diagnostic waters are depression associated with dementia and hypoactive delirium. Dementia is common in around 42 per cent of all hospital admission over the age of 75, and of those with dementia around 34 per cent may be expected to experience associated depression (2, 3). It is also estimated that around 20 per cent of older people in hospital will experience delirium at some point during their admission; many of these will have hypoactive symptoms, which have considerable overlap with the symptoms seen in depression – but treatment strategies are very different (1, 4).

Once a diagnosis is established, treatment options require careful thought. Access to psychological therapies can be resource- and time-limited, and prescribing decisions can be complex when you have to bear in mind multiple comorbidities and polypharmacy. On the other hand, a failure to treat can lead to increased length of hospital stay and to risks associated with self-harm, suicide, or self-neglect (5).

These complexities mean that clinicians need a good understanding of the prevalence, risk factors, complex presentations, and differential diagnoses of mood disorders, both low and high, in older people in a hospital setting. This chapter aims to set these out, before going on to discuss the varied treatment options available.

Epidemiology

Older people in a hospital setting can either be admitted with active depressive symptoms or develop new or more severe symptoms as an in-patient. The point prevalence of depression in older people in hospital is around 29 per cent (range 5–58 per cent) (1, 6, 7). In the United Kingdom it is estimated that around 9 per cent of depression diagnoses recorded in hospital are new, the remainder being recorded on admission, depression being a pre-existing condition (8). The diagnostic rate of depression in older people in hospital often doesn't reflect prevalence, however (1, 8); it is estimated that the documented prevalence of depression in this group is only 13 per cent (8). In addition, it must be considered that depression is independently prevalent in people with dementia (9), and in a hospital setting the prevalence of depression in those with comorbid dementia is around 34 per cent (3, 10).

Adjustment disorders in older people in a hospital setting are common, but an exact figure is unclear, which perhaps highlights the challenges of making the diagnosis. In the United Kingdom the prevalence of adjustment disorders among older people in the community is around 2–3 per cent (11). In the United States the prevalence among hospitalised younger people is around 12 per cent (12).

Severe depression with psychotic symptoms is a less common clinical scenario. Psychotic symptoms present in 5.3 per cent of major depressions (13), and the lifetime risk of developing a depression with psychotic features is around 0.35–1 per cent (14). However, due to a symptom profile that often precipitates self-neglect and malnutrition via nihilistic or negative delusions, patients with psychotic depression will often require hospital admission for artificial feeding or hydration, and therefore will be over-represented.

Risk Factors for Developing or Exacerbating Mood Disorders in Hospital

In older people, the biggest predictor of developing a future mood disorder is past history. Those who recover from a first episode of depression have a 50 per cent lifetime chance of developing a subsequent episode, and those with two or more episodes of depression have an 80 per cent chance of recurrence (15). Those with a history of recurrent depression will have between five and nine episodes throughout their lifetime (15, 16). The aetiology of depression is multifactorial – a complex interplay of genetic predisposition, personality structure, early life experience, social environment, and personal circumstance (17). Many of these risk factors are static and, when considering the older person, are therefore largely unmodifiable. However, a knowledge of them allows us to have a better understanding of who is at risk, so that allowances designed to minimise future relapse may be made and appropriate monitoring may take place.

Apart from the impact of receiving a new medical diagnosis, some specific medical conditions and drugs, too, are associated with depression; the most common ones are

Table 12.1 Medical conditions associated with significant depressive symptoms (24).

Endocrine diseases

Addison's disease
Cushing's syndrome
hyperprolactinaemia
thyroid disorders: hypothyroidism, thyrotoxicosis, hyperparathyroidism

Infectious diseases

encephalitis
hepatitis
influenza
mononucleosis

Neurological diseases

Alzheimer's disease
brain tumours
epilepsy
head injury
Huntington's chorea
multiple sclerosis
normal pressure hydrocephalus
Parkinson's disease
stroke

Other diseases

AIDS
folate deficiency
lung cancer
pancreatic cancer
pernicious anemia
systemic lupus erythematosus

listed in Table 12.1. Of particular note are conditions associated with a very high prevalence of a mood disorder:

- Parkinson's disease: 35 per cent clinically significant depressive symptoms, 17 per cent major depression (18).
- Post-stroke: pooled estimate of developing clinically significant depression, 33 per cent (19).
- Post-myocardial infection: 31 per cent of patients develop significant depressive symptoms, 20 per cent develop severe depression (20).
- Alzheimer's-type dementia: in the community, 25 per cent develop symptoms of major depression, 27 per cent minor depression, and the prevalence almost doubles in a hospital setting (3, 21).

One should bear in mind that the relationship between the medical illness and depression is complex and often difficult to establish with clarity, because of the number of variables. For example, some diseases are clearly associated with depression on account of the disability, uncertainty, or functional loss they cause. There is also increasing and intriguing evidence that inflammation can cause depression (22). It has been suggested that the cytokines produced in inflammation transmit an inflammatory signal across the blood–brain barrier. This activates microglia, with resulting collateral damage to nerve cells that in turn leads to depression (23).

Changes to a patient's medications are commonplace in a hospital setting. Drugs are stopped when they are ineffective or thought to be causing intolerable side effects, and new agents are commenced. Side effects from psychotropic medications can be a cause for admission or are sometimes identified when a person is in hospital. Common examples are a selective serotonin re-uptake inhibitor (SSRIs)-induced hyponatremia, postural hypotension induced by mirtazapine, lithium toxicity, or, more rarely, serotonin syndrome. Such events can occur both in people who have recently started an antidepressant or after long-term use. In such cases the drug is either stopped abruptly or reduced, which in turn can precipitate a relapse of the mood disorder. The liaison psychiatry team in this instance needs to be aware of those at risk and of their relapse indicators and consider alternative treatment strategies as necessary. Long-term drugs such as benzodiazepines may also be discontinued abruptly, causing withdrawal or a troubling re-emergence of the very symptoms that these drugs were prescribed to treat.

Less commonly, medications that that can precipitate depressive symptoms are commenced. A list of the more commonly associated agents is displayed in Table 12.2. While not all patients who begin to take these agents need monitoring, where the medications have been recently initiated, they should be considered a potentially reversible cause of a mood disorder.

In people both with and without a predisposition to a mood disorder, the simple event of being admitted to a general hospital can be a distressing factor. Major risk factors for developing depression in older people in the community are disability, a new medical illness, poor health status, poor self-perceived health, bereavement, and sleep disturbance (26). In a hospital setting, these are all common occurrences. Furthermore, the hospital environment can often be noisy, crowded and poorly lit (27), some patients are isolated, and even in multi-bedded bays they may feel lonely and bored.

Table 12.2 Medications associated with significant depressive symptoms as a side effect (25)

Common
levodopa
baclofen
methylphenidate

Uncommon
ciprofloxacin

Rare
chloroquine
mefloquine

Frequency unknown
corticosteroids (e.g. prednisolone, hydrocortisone).
antidepressants of all classes
levothyroxine – if dose too high

Common Presentations of Depression in a Hospital Setting

Diagnosing a mood disorder in a general hospital setting can be challenging; symptoms can overlap with other syndromes, patients often have communication difficulties, and many mood states may be entirely appropriate in the circumstances.

Appropriate Mood Reactions

Sadness and fear are normal and regularly experienced human emotions. Sadness can be experienced for many reasons, but a common causative theme is loss and loneliness. By their very nature, the circumstances that bring people into the hospital often cause loss of independence or functionality and can also cause fear, given the risk they may pose to our health or the suffering they bring about. What is more, patients are constantly exposed to drugs, procedures, and environments that pose a tangible danger to the self, let alone their isolating and confusing character. It would be abnormal for a person not to feel sadness or fear at some point; this does not make them depressed or anxious. It is one of the clinician's roles to establish when these emotions grow more severe or persistent and come to be part of a disorder.

Both DSMV and ICD10 classify acute stress reactions or disorder. They both define this category as a response to exposure to a stressor; this response occurs shortly after the event (ICD10, 1 hour) and persists for two days, but not for more than four (28, 29). The benefit for the patient of classifying this condition is, however, questionable.

Adjustment Disorders

When a person is exposed to a prolonged and stressful change in circumstances, this can have a more easily definable effect on that person's mood. Adjustment disorders arise as a direct consequence of stress or unpleasant circumstances, and the disorder would not have occurred in the absence of that stressor or circumstance. In ICD10 this disorder is divided into three subtypes: depressive, mixed anxiety, and depressive and mixed disturbance of emotions and conduct (28). In DSMV, the subcategories or subtypes are six: with depressed mood, with anxiety, with mixed anxiety and depressed mood, with disturbance in conduct, with mixed emotions and disturbance of conduct, and unspecified (29).

The psychological symptoms of an adjustment disorder include anxiety, worry, irritability, depression and poor concentration. They are often associated with somatic symptoms such as palpitations, tremor, and autonomic arousal (17). Symptoms must have started within one (ICD10) or three months (DSMV) of the stressful change in circumstances and be understandably related to it (28, 29). The majority of adjustment disorders are short-lived, typically lasting only a few months, but some can persist for years and can be associated with aberrant behaviour such as repeated self-harm and aggression (17).

Depressive Disorder

Depressive disorders are categorised as mild, moderate, and severe in both ICD10 and DSMV. The common symptoms and classification criteria are described in Table 12.3. For a diagnosis to be made, symptoms should have been present for a minimum of two

Table 12.3 The symptoms needed to meet the criteria for a depressive episode, according to ICD10 and DSMV (28, 29)

ICD 10		DSMV
Core symptoms • depressed mood • loss of interest and enjoyment • reduced energy and decreased enjoyment Typical symptoms • disturbed sleep[*] • diminished appetite[*] • reduced confidence • reduced self-esteem • ideas of guilt and worthlessness • pessimistic thoughts • ideas of self-harm and suicide		Symptoms • depressed mood for most of the day, almost every day • diminished interest in almost all activities, most of the day • fatigue and loss of energy • insomnia or hypersomnia[*] • change in appetite or significant weight loss (>5% body weight)[*] • psychomotor agitation or retardation • feelings of worthlessness and guilt • diminished ability to concentrate or think • recurrent thoughts of death or suicide
Mild	2 core symptoms and 2 typical symptoms	5 symptoms with minor social or occupational impairment
Moderate	2 core symptoms and 3 typical symptoms	5 symptoms with variable social or occupational impairment
Severe	3 core symptoms and 4 typical symptoms	5 symptoms with major social or occupational impairment

[*] Somatic symptoms.

weeks (28); in practice, however, particularly in a hospital setting, this timeframe can be blurred. For example, if symptoms occur in the context of a change in circumstances and persist for the entire duration of the hospital stay but abate on or nearing discharge, this may not justify a diagnosis. However, if symptoms occur rapidly after the discontinuation of an antidepressant in hospital and match the patient's typical relapse indicators, then a shorter timeframe to diagnosis may be entirely justifiable.

There are, inevitably, cases where differentiating between an adjustment disorder and a depressive disorder causes diagnostic uncertainty. Almost everyone in hospital has experienced a recent stressful circumstance, just by virtue of entering the hospital. In such instances, careful history taking in order to ascertain the trigger of the emotional response can be essential. Past history (including information from collateral sources) helps us to understand symptom severity and chronicity, too.

Some symptoms commonly witnessed in depressive disorders are sleep disturbance (including early morning wakening), anorexia, weight loss, and psychomotor retardation. These are often referred to as biological or somatic symptoms of depression and they have considerable overlap with other syndromes, for example cancer, pain, or hypoactive delirium. Any assessment of an older person in hospital should always consider the aetiology of individual symptoms and whether there are other explanations for them other than a mood disorder.

Depressive Disorder with Psychotic Symptoms

As depression severity worsens, so does the intensity of each symptom. Patients often experience increasingly intense feelings of guilt and worsening psychomotor retardation. This can lead to the development of psychotic symptoms, which are usually negative in their content. Delusional themes are typically mood-congruent, focusing on topics such as poverty, ill health, persecution, or death (nihilistic). Some patients experience negative auditory hallucinations, hearing derogatory comments about them, or olfactory hallucinations, for example that they smell of rotting flesh or waste (30). Psychotic symptoms, where present, always need careful exploration, as they can put the patient at significant risk, in particular for self-neglect, refusal of care, and refusal of food and fluids.

Dementia and Delirium

Delirium is a medical emergency, and is prevalent in around 20 per cent of older people admitted to hospital (1) and 66 per cent of people with dementia in hospital (31). A significant proportion of these patients present with hypoactive symptoms such as lethargy, sedation, psychomotor retardation, and reduced spontaneity (4). These symptoms can mimic symptoms seen in depression and can cause diagnostic confusion in the unsuspecting clinician. When in doubt, one should conduct a thorough examination and rule out delirium before making a diagnosis of depression.

Communication Difficulties

The psychiatrist's key diagnostic tool is communication; however, a hospital environment is not always conducive to good communication. Patients are often in multi-bedded bays, with beds partitioned only by material curtains (32). Ideally interviews should be conducted in a quiet private room, but this may not be possible if the patient is bed-bound or if such a room is not available. The lack of privacy can inhibit answers and cause significant anxiety for patients, especially if they are already fearful of the stigma related to mental health problems.

Even when the conditions of interviewing are maximised, many older people in hospital struggle to understand the information presented to them because they have sensory deficit, have difficulty grasping it because they have cognitive impairment, or have difficulty communicating their responses because they have dysphasia or aphasia. When assessing a patient's mood, every effort should be made to compensate for communication barriers in order to improve the quality of diagnostic information where possible.

Standardised Diagnostic Tools

There are numerous standardised diagnostic tools to assist clinicians in diagnosing depression in a hospital setting. Most of them are self-report questionnaires administered by clinicians (33). Like all diagnostic tools, they do not replace clinical skill, nor are they able to capture the nuances of communication that can be observed in conversation; but they can provide a useful and objective review of symptoms. The most commonly cited tools are the Geriatric Depression Scale (GDS) (34) and the Brief Assessment Schedule Assessment Cards (BASAC) (35). The GDS circulates in several versions of varying length and has the greatest body of evidence to support its use. Pooled results of the evidence show that the GDS 15 has a sensitivity of around 74 and a specificity of 81 for diagnosing depression (33). Multiple other tools exist, for example the Hospital Anxiety and Depression Scale (HADS) (36), the Evans Liverpool Depression Rating (37), the Self-Reported Depression Scale (38), and the Popoff index of Depression, but all these tools have a limited evidence base to support their use (39).

Specifically designed for people with depression in dementia is the Cornell Scale for Depression in Dementia. This is a 19-item tool completed by a clinician after interviewing the patient and nursing staff, and, to repeat, it is specifically oriented at people with dementia (40).

In a busy hospital setting, expecting healthcare professionals to know how to access specific screening tools and how to use them is not always realistic. Unless some specific guidance is in place, choosing which screening tool to use can cause the assessor anxiety; and, even when a tool is selected, it is often time-consuming and complex. It is therefore unsurprising that depression screening tools are rarely seen to be used in clinical practice (41).

Clinical Management and Therapeutic Issues

Prevention

A possible advantage of being in a general hospital setting is the potential for close monitoring for mental health symptoms and the availability of preventative resources set up to minimise the risk of the development of a mental disorder. To use this advantage, all healthcare professionals need to be aware of what a mood disorder is, its prevalence, and how it presents. Nevertheless, a high standard of undergraduate mental health training cannot be assumed (42). Liaison psychiatry teams should therefore strive to offer their general hospital colleagues appropriate training, where possible. This should be done via formal teaching administered to all professionals, via mental health awareness campaigns, and via informal, ward-based education.

Despite this training, many healthcare professionals feel ill equipped to monitor or diagnose mental health problems (41, 43). Subtle or minor symptoms can feel less important than other medical issues, and clinicians often feel less than confident about diagnosing mood disorders, or they feel that symptoms are 'justifiable'. Furthermore, patients can be embarrassed to talk about depressive symptoms (8, 44). To improve the rate of accurate diagnosis of mood disorders, clinicians should have access to up-to-date mental health records, standardised rating scales (as described above), and, where appropriate, guidance on managing mood disorders. These simple measures should be – and are – widely available in most hospitals, yet they constitute much underused resources (8).

Non-Pharmacological Management of Depressive Symptoms

Active monitoring

In people with people with mild depression or sub-therapeutic depressive symptoms, active monitoring of the person's mental state may be warranted (45). In an acute hospital setting, this measure can be particularly pertinent if the patient is awaiting a procedure or a diagnosis that potentially causes anxiety. Specific follow-up of symptoms may not be warranted or practically available from a specialist liaison team – in which case follow-up by the patient's ward team or general practitioner on discharge may be appropriate.

Sleep Hygiene

Ward environments often are busy, noisy, crowded, and uncomfortable. Bedtime routines are usually determined by ward procedure rather than by individual preference, and uncomfortable somatic symptoms can cause discomfort and resulting insomnia. Ensuring that a good sleep hygiene is maintained is recommended in the management of mood disorders (45). But, in the hospital environment, the practical barriers to achieving it can be insurmountable. Even so, it is rarely the case that nothing can be done. Whenever possible, patients should be moved to a side room (after the impact caused by social isolation has been taken into account), familiar bedside items of comfort can be brought in by family and friends, and the staff on the ward should try to maintain a peaceful environment at night as much as possible.

Somatic Symptom Control (Including Control of Pain)

Somatic symptoms such as pain, nausea, shortness of breath, and dizziness are common in older people admitted to the hospital. Severe and persistent symptoms can both cause and perpetuate mood disorders (46); hence removing any potential triggers should be beneficial. Patients believed to be in pain should be assessed appropriately and, if necessary, referred to specialised pain teams for advice on analgesia.

Removing Triggers Where Possible

When the aetiology of a mood disorder is believed to be idiopathic or related to a specific medical condition, the causative agent should be removed, if it is safe to do so. In instances where a drug believed to be causing a mood disorder is necessary to maintain or save life, or where the benefits of the treatment are deemed to outweigh its negative impact on the patient's mental state, both this state and the element of risk should be monitored closely. Any medications should be used in minimal dosage and for the shortest duration, and alternatives to treatment should be sought where possible.

Social Interventions

Social stressors can be a major risk factor for developing a mood disorder (47). Admission to hospital can be socially isolating, people are away from family, carers, and pets, and may in some cases never return to their home, for example if they are discharged to residential care. The impact that this may have on a person's mental state should always be considered and minimised when practically possible.

Reasonable adjustments to allow family and friends to visit should be made where it's possible to facilitate them, and in cases where a person does not have regular visitors hospital voluntary services can be a very useful source of support and company.

If there is concern that a person's holistic and religious needs are not being met, the hospital's chaplaincy services should be summoned to provide a range of support measures, regardless of whether the situation is impacting on that patient's mental state or not.

In a hospital setting it is largely impractical to consider any exercise or sport-based therapies, but intensive physiotherapy – which leads to improved engagement, physical activity, and more confidence in mobilising – may have a similar effect.

Psychological Therapies

In specialties where significant sudden changes to functioning are common or where diagnoses carry poor prognoses, it is recommended that psychologists be available to provide targeted therapies (48). Examples are oncology and major trauma wards. In an in-patient hospital setting, however, the practicalities of providing such a service to the majority of patients is limited.

Cognitive behavioural therapy (CBT) is recommended for treating persistent sub-threshold depressive symptoms or mild to moderate depressive disorder (45). This kind of treatment can take the form of self-guided CBT, computerised CBT, or therapist led CBT, lasting up to twelve sessions.

In patients without significant cognitive decline and with available resources (access to a computer and the ability to use it), self-guided or computerised CBT can be recommended. It is, however, usually impractical to initiate it in a busy hospital ward setting, where patients are acutely unwell. Patients with mild to moderate depression, at or near the point of discharge, could instead be referred for CBT in the community.

Providing therapist-led CBT in an acute hospital setting would rarely be recommended, owing to the unpredictability of patients' length of stay, which limits the number of therapy sessions, the availability of resources, and patients' ability to engage in therapy while acutely unwell. Where psychological therapies are recommended, they can be initiated either by a community mental health team or by a general practitioner on discharge.

Pharmacological Interventions

For people with moderate to severe depression, where non-pharmacological therapies have been ineffective or are impractical, antidepressant therapy should be envisaged – either as a sole treatment or in combination with non-pharmacological therapies (45). In prescribing to older people, one should bear in mind drug administration, absorption, medical comorbidity, polypharmacy or potential interactions, and side effects of the drug. As a general rule, all medications should be stared at the lowest practical dose and titrated to work slowly. While older people in hospital starting on antidepressant medications are arguably monitored more closely than their community counterparts, they often are frail and potentially vulnerable to side effects.

Drug Administration Route

The possible administration routes of antidepressants are oral or intravenous (IV), depending on drug choice. In patients who have an unsafe swallow or are unable to swallow, orodispersible preparations of medications are an alternative to tablets or capsules. For patients who cannot tolerate tablets or capsules or who are being fed via a nasogastric (NG) or percutaneous endoscopic gastrostomy (PEG) route, liquid formulations can be considered. Where an oral, NG, or PEG administration is not possible, an IV administration of antidepressants is possible. Table 12.4 lists commonly available antidepressants and alternative formulations.

Table 12.4 Commonly prescribed antidepressants available in alternative forms (25) (light grey = available, dark grey = unavailable)

Drug	Orodispersible	Liquid	IV
citalopram	unavailable	available	available
fluoxetine	Sublingual liquid	available	unavailable
paroxetine	unavailable	available	unavailable
mirtazapine	available	available	available
trazadone	unavailable	available	unavailable
amitriptyline	unavailable	available	unavailable
escitalopram	unavailable	available	unavailable

Absorption of Antidepressants

Slow gastric mobility, low Ph, and impaired blood flow can all reduce drug absorption in older people; nevertheless, the absorption of most drugs is thought to remain largely unchanged (49). Patients who have undergone significant bowel resection are the exception; in their case, particularly when prescribing modified release preparations of tablets, the active levels of the drug absorbed may be much lower than expected. One could consider administering orodispersible or liquid formulations instead (see Table 12.4).

Choosing an Antidepressant Therapy

Antidepressant choice should be guided by the patient's history (what drugs have and have not worked previously), comorbidity, depressive symptom profile, available route of administration, and potential side effects of the drug.

For antidepressant-naïve patients, it is recommended that the first line treatment should be with a selective serotonin reuptake inhibitor (SSRI). Where a SSRI is ineffective, mirtazapine is usually the second line choice. Where two antidepressants have failed to be effective, a serotonin and noradrenaline reuptake inhibitor (SNRI) such as venlafaxine or duloxetine should be considered (45).

In some instances, an antidepressant may be considered as a first line or as a preferable treatment option, on account of its side effect profile or other properties – for example mirtazapine in patients with coexisting insomnia, poor appetite, and weight loss, or amitriptyline in patients with coexisting neuropathic pain. Table 12.5 displays the most commonly prescribed antidepressant classes and the pros and cons of each, which may aid treatment decisions.

Treatment Adjuvants

Once several antidepressants have been trialled and have failed to benefit the patient, adjuvant therapies may be considered. In the liaison psychiatry setting, this patient group invariably has a history of depression before admission and will likely be known to a community psychiatry team. Information on previous treatments that have been tried and failed should be sought and, where possible, a timeline should be established

Table 12.5 The most commonly prescribed antidepressant classes and the pros and cons of each (25, 50)

Drug	Pros	Cons
SSRI	• Generally well tolerated. • Safer in overdose. • Generally safe in cardiac disease and post-myocardial infarction, and minimal effect on cardiac conduction other than citalopram and escitalopram on QTc interval.	• Increased risk of GI bleeds in those already at risk, compounded if prescribed with NSAIDS, warfarin, and aspirin. • Headaches and GI side effects common. • Sexual dysfunction. • Fluoxetine and fluvoxamine CYP450 enzyme inhibitors – caution with interactions. • Hyponatraemia. • Fluoxetine – long half-life.
Tricyclics	• Sedative. • Chronic pain syndromes.	• Sedative. • Postural hypotension. • Cardiac conduction effects; prolongation of QTc and QRS complex, especially in overdose. • Anticholinergic side effects.
Mirtazapine	• Sedative. • Appetite stimulant. • Less likely to cause hyponatremia than SSRIs. • Second line of treatment after SSRIs.	• Sedative. • Postural hypotension.
SNRI's	• Second line treatment after two previous antidepressants. • Minimal effect on QTc. • Possible adjunctive therapy	• Headaches and GI common side effects. • Sexual dysfunction.

documenting what drugs have been tried, when, and with what effects (positive and negative). This can help to inform future treatment strategies.

The most commonly used treatment adjuvants consist in adding a second antidepressant, adding lithium therapy, or adding an antipsychotic.

The most commonly used and cited antidepressant dual combination is mirtazapine and venlafaxine. Trial data have shown a modest effect in people who failed to responded to monotherapy and the combination is relatively well tolerated, though the potential for serotonin syndrome should be considered (51).

Lithium adjuvant therapy for treatment-resistant depression is recommended by NICE guidelines (45). Its effectiveness is well established; but, given its narrow therapeutic window (plasma levels between 0.4–0.8 mmol/L) and its renal excretion and nephrotoxic effects, it can be difficult to initiate this therapy in older people with existing comorbidity.

The evidence base for using antipsychotics as treatment adjuvants is varied, the most commonly cited drugs being olanzapine, quetiapine, risperidone, and aripiprazole (50).

But, as with any antipsychotics, the side effect profile of this drugs in older people (falls, sedation, stroke) must be considered carefully (52).

Other potential treatment adjuvants are bupropion, buspirone, or T3 (51).

Providing Artificial Feeding and Hydration

In patients with severe depression, self-neglect with refusal of oral food and fluids is a relatively common presentation. Refusal of food and fluid should be thoroughly assessed. In the first instance, this should be done via a full gastrointestinal history and examination, which should cover oral care and hygiene, dental care (assessing for pain or inability to chew), swallow assessment, a full abdominal examination, and, where indicated, abdominal x-rays. A food and fluids chart should be kept, monitoring all intake (including via NG or IV routes), and urine and stool output should be documented. Regular blood tests should be conducted to monitor renal function, albumin, phosphate, and magnesium.

The medical teams caring for the person who refuses food and fluids should carefully liaise with a dietician and establish a refeeding plan, with appropriate monitoring. In some instances, artificial hydration via IV access or artificial feeding via a nasogastric (NG) tube will have to be considered. It is likely that in such instances the person who refuses food and fluids will also refuse the proposed intervention. The decision as to whether to proceed with artificial feeding or hydration against the will of the patient should be taken after careful consideration of the patient's capacity to refuse the treatment and after an assessment of his or her mental state and of the aetiology behind the food and fluids refusal. Under both the Mental Capacity Act and the Mental Health Act, artificial nutrition and hydration must be judged to be in the patient's best interest, and decisions should be made only after pondering the patient's earlier wishes, the views of his or her next-of-kin or power of attorney (where appropriate), and those of the medical team.

Electroconvulsive Therapy

The use of electroconvulsive therapy (ECT) is recommended for severe and treatment-resistant depression (45). In the acute hospital setting, where depression is life-threatening, emergency ECT treatment may be envisaged most commonly after refusal of food and fluids. In patients where food and fluid refusal is significant enough to require NG feeding or IV rehydration, admission to the general hospital is almost certainly indicated. In consequence, the liaison psychiatrist may encounter this scenario relatively frequently.

ECT is a well-established and effective treatment (53). But it necessitates the use of a general anaesthetic, and the treatment is a significant intervention in itself. Coordinating the care of people who need both medical attention and ECT for a severe depressive episode requires careful coordination between the liaison psychiatry team, patients and their family, the ward nursing staff, the medical team, anaesthetic departments, the ECT department, and the local Mental Health Act office (where such patients are detained under a section of the Act). Nursing staff and healthcare professionals in the general hospital are often not used to managing patients before an ECT – for example keeping them nil by mouth or organising medications that prolong or reduce the seizure threshold, as staff members of mental health in-patient units do. If the ECT is performed on a site away from the general hospital, the transport of detained patients and the legal framework for it will also need to be facilitated. Liaison teams should provide written and verbal guidance to members of staff and regularly review their policy and procedure.

Mania

Mood disorders encompass a spectrum of emotions and, although this is less common, mood can become elated as well as depressed. Just like depressive disorders in hospital, mood disorders where elation is a feature can be difficult to diagnose, particularly when they present for the first time. After assessing the symptoms, the clinician must consider all possible aetiologies that may have their roots in physical health care, pharmacology, and psychiatry. In what follows we will consider how elation may present in a hospital setting and what risks it may pose, before describing common differential diagnoses and finally exploring treatment options.

Epidemiology

While psychiatric disorders that are common in somatic patients, such as depression and substance abuse, (54) have received increased scientific attention over the past few years, other psychiatric disorders, such as bipolar disorder or mania, have been less studied (55). As a result, there is a paucity of evidence available to ascertain reliably the prevalence of elated mood or bipolar in acute hospital settings. What is documented shows a marked disparity in the prevalence of bipolar in hospital, which is 5–12 per cent, vis-à-vis the prevalence in the community, which is 0.1 per cent (56). This is an important area for further study, particularly if we bear in mind the morbidity and mortality effects on patients who experience mood disorders, as well as the impacts of elated mood on decision-making and, at times, on the discharge destination, be that 24-hour care or admission to an acute psychiatric hospital.

Presentation

Mania typically presents in hospital as an abnormally elevated or irritable mood, accompanied by challenging symptoms such as distractibility, indiscretions, grandiosity, flight of ideas, hyperactivity, decreased need for sleep, and talkativeness (29).

Episodes of elated mood can cause a number of problems for patients and those tasked with caring for them while they are admitted to hospital. There are a number of risks to be careful about when managing patients who present with elated mood in hospital. These include grandiosity, which prompts risky behaviours caused by feelings of being invincible and impossible to get harmed. Grandiosity can also lead to difficult interactions with staff and other patients; and such interractions, when coupled with irritability, may instigate verbal and or physical aggression. Disinhibition can lead to both inappropriate verbal interactions and physical behaviour. It can take the form of being sexually inappropriate or that of being careless with belongings, finances, and so on. These behaviours can pose a risk to others, but also make the patient vulnerable to exploitation by others. Distractibility can cause problems with eating and drinking that are due to short attention spans and lead to a reduction in nutritional intake. Hyperactivity and a reduced need for sleep are not only disruptive to others in a ward environment, among unwell patients in the hospital, but also detrimental to the patient's physical well-being, as they lead to complications and prolonged hospital stays.

Table 12.6 Symptoms needed to meet the criteria for a manic episode according to ICD10 and DSMV (28, 29).

ICD 10	DSMV
Core symptom	Core symptom
• Predominantly elevated/expansive/ irritable mood	• Distinct period of abnormal and persistent elevated, expansive, or irritable mood. Abnormally and persistent goal-directed behaviour/energy, lasting for at least a week and present throughout most of the day, nearly every day (any duration if hospitalization required).
• Duration of at least a week (unless severe enough to warrant psychiatric hospital admission)	
At least three of the following (four if mood is only irritable) – which leads to severe interference in daily living and functioning:	
• Increased activity or physical restlessness	Three of more of the following should persist and be present to significant degree, representing a noticeable change from usual behaviour
• Increased talkativeness (pressure of speech)	• Inflated self = esteem/grandiosity
• Flight of ideas or subjective feelings of thoughts racing	• Decreased need for sleep
	• More talkative than usual / pressure to keep talking
• Loss of normal social inhibitions, leading to inappropriate behaviour	• Flight of ideas / subjective experience that thoughts are racing
• Decreased need for sleep	• Distractibility as reported or observed
• Inflated self-esteem / grandiosity	• Increase in goal-directed activity (socially, at work, at school; sexually or psychomotor agitation)
• Distractibility or constant changes of activity/plans	
• Reckless behaviour whose risks are not recognised, e.g. overspending, reckless driving	• Excessive involvement in activities that have a high potential for bringing painful consequences (unrestrained buying sprees, sexual indiscretions, etc.)
• Marked sexual energy / sexual indiscretions	

A difference is drawn between manic episodes with and manic episodes without psychotic symptoms. Hypomanic episodes according to both diagnostic manuals: mood elevated/irritable for at least four days, three of the above symptoms present, leading to some interference with personal functioning in daily living.

Table 12.6 gives more details of the diagnostic criteria for manic and hypomanic episodes, according to ICD10 and DSMV.

Aetiology

There are many different reasons why an older adult may present with symptoms of elated mood while admitted to hospital with physical health concerns. The period of elated mood may be due to a psychiatric condition previously diagnosed or presenting for the first time. It may be secondary to a physical health problem, or a side effect of medications that the patient has been taking in the community or has started anew during his or her hospital admission.

Identifying the cause of an older person's presenting with elated mood during an acute hospital admission can be difficult. It requires detailed history taking to be done by those experienced in recognising and diagnosing mood disorders. It also requires appropriate clinical investigations, a mental state examination carried out by the liaison psychiatry team over multiple visits, a collateral history of the patient's premorbid presentation, and a history of mental and physical health problems.

There are a number of differential diagnoses to consider when assessing patients who present with elated mood in the hospital setting.

Delirium

As discussed earlier in relation to depressive presentations in the hospital setting, delirium is found in around a fifth of elderly patients in hospital (1), and this proportion rises to two thirds among patients with dementia (31). The most common type of delirium observed in hospital is that of a mixed picture, where patients experience fluctuations in their activity levels, agitation, mood, and behaviour (4). The hyperactive aspect of the mixed picture can mimic the symptoms of mania. Given the high morbidity and mortality associated with delirium in older people, delirium should always be ruled out in older patients who present with unusual behaviour while in hospital.

Attention Deficit Hyperactivity Disorder

The core features of this neurodevelopmental disorder can be and often are confused with those of a manic or hypomanic presentation, particularly if the attention deficit hyperactivity disorder (ADHD) has gone undiagnosed from childhood.

The core features in question are inattention, hyperactivity, and impulsivity (57). The main differentiation between their manifestation in ADHD and in a manic or hypomanic episode is that in mania these symptoms are of acute onset, and they are abnormal for the individual.

Here collateral history obtained from family, friends, and primary care can be invaluable in determining the timeframe of the symptoms and can support a formal assessment to review the case for a possible diagnosis of ADHD.

Intoxication with Psychoactive Substances: Stimulants, Hallucinogens, Alcohol

Clinically this may be indistinguishable from elated mood as a result of a functional psychiatric disorder. Nevertheless, thorough history obtainment from the patient and, collaterally, from others as well as through longitudinal observation with appropriate testing for common causative agents (urine or blood testing), we can determine whether a patient's presentation is resultant from acute intoxication or from withdrawal from a psychoactive substance rather than from a primary mood disorder.

Anxiety Disorders

Admission into hospital is a stressful and upsetting time for most. Some may experience an increase in pre-existing anxiety; others may develop anxiety in relation to the significant psychosocial stressors associated with a hospital admission.

As a consequence of the cognitive and psychomotor symptoms of anxiety, patients may present with symptoms similar to those of an elated mood. Such symptoms include inattention, poor concentration, irritability, restlessness, sleep disturbance, and pressured or overinclusive speech (28).

Generally people who experience anxiety rather than mania or hypomania display concomitant somatic symptoms of anxiety that are not typically seen in people with elated affective episodes. These symptoms typically include palpitations, sweating, shaking, dry mouth, difficulty breathing, chest pain, abdominal distress, dizziness, muscle tension, and feeling on edge (28).

Schizophrenia Spectrum Disorders

Schizophrenia spectrum disorders are typified in general by distortions of thinking and perception, that is, delusions and hallucinations accompanied by incongruent or blunted affect (28). By comparison, in a manic or hypomanic episode with psychotic symptoms the predominant symptom is mood disturbance (elation); the patient may also experience mood-congruent psychotic symptoms, but these are felt to be directly related to the mood disturbance.

Despite this, there are occasions when patients with marked psychotic symptoms also experience mood disturbance alongside their psychosis. This is when careful professional assessment from those experienced in assessing and diagnosing mental illness is needed.

Patients who are found to experience both affective (mood) and schizophrenic (psychotic) symptoms concurrently and with equal predominance and who not meet the criteria for either a schizophrenia or a mania diagnosis would be diagnosed with schizoaffective disorder of the manic type (28). Differentiating this condition can be a complicated and nuanced process, which may require a longer period of assessment and observation than what can be provided during an acute hospital admission.

Some patients who meet primary diagnostic criteria for schizophrenia can also appear to experience prominent affective changes with fleeting and fragmented hallucinations, bizarre and unpredictable behaviours, and what is general described as a 'fatuous' affect with incoherent speech (28). This may look similar to a manic episode with psychotic symptoms. However, such patients would be diagnosed with a subtype of schizophrenia, namely hebephrenic schizophrenia. This typically presents initially in a younger age group, yet older patients in the hospital may experience a relapse of this disorder during an acute admission.

Personality Disorders

Personality disorder is a diagnosis made when there is an observed deeply ingrained and enduring pattern of behaviour that manifests as inflexible responses to a broad range of personal and social situations. They are considered to be disorders only when there is a significant deviation from the way in which the majority of others in a particular culture perceive, think, feel, and especially relate to people and to themselves. Such patterns tend to be stable and to encompass multiple domains of behaviour and psychological functioning. They also tend to emerge earlier in life, but can be acquired later in life, as a result of constitutional and social experiences (28).

A number of behaviours are shared with mania and responses related to impulsivity, unpredictable and labile emotions, and incapacity to control, as observed in those with emotionally unstable personality disorder (28). Just like patients with emotionally unstable personality disorder, those with histrionic personality disorder can present with behaviours that mimic the ones observed in manic or hypomanic patients – namely labile affect, self-dramatization, theatrical presentation, exaggerated expression of emotions, egocentricity, self-indulgence, lack of considerations for others, excitement or attention seeking (28).

In these situations the core diagnostic criteria of mania or hypomania are not met. It is of particular importance in these cases to gain collateral history for a longitudinal overview of the patient's pervasive pattern of behaviours, both in general and at times of significant psychosocial stress. This will aid the differentiation of an affective disorder from associated behavioural presentations and personality disorders.

Bipolar Affective Disorder

Bipolar disorder is marked by alternating mood elevation (mania or hypomania) and depression. Hypomania is defined as elevated states without significant functional impairment. Bipolar I disorder is characterised by the occurrence of one or more manic episodes or mixed episodes, and bipolar II disorder is characterised by the occurrence of one or more hypomanic episodes (9).

The common symptoms and diagnostic criteria for a manic or hypomanic episode can be found in Table 12.6.

According to ICD10, at least two episodes of affective disturbance must occur for a diagnosis of bipolar affective disorder to be made, and one of them must be of a manic, hypomanic, or mixed polarity (28). By contrast, DSMV permits a single episodes of mania, hypomania, or mixed affective state to diagnose bipolar affective disorder (29).

One cause for the relapse of bipolar and for the fact that patients experience a manic or hypomanic episode during an acute hospital admission related to their physical health is cessation of their psychotropic maintenance medications, for example mood stabiliser or antipsychotic therapy. These medications are usually stopped by the treating team because their impact on the patient's physical health raise concerns (e.g. acute kidney injury and lithium therapy, deranged liver function and sodium valproate, or cardiac arrhythmias and antipsychotics). It is advisable that treating teams that need to stop the maintenance therapy of a patient with a known history of bipolar affective disorder liaise with the liaison psychiatry team for advice and support on how to do it safely.

Risk Factors for Developing or Exacerbating Mood Disorders in Hospital

There is a concept of secondary mania, which is an elated mood directly linked to organic causes such as neurological, endocrine, and pharmacological problems. The limited research available, which describes older patients who present with new-onset elated mood or mania, has shown that this mood abnormality is more likely to be secondary, in other words to result from an underlying cause rather than from a primary mental health diagnosis – by comparison with the situation among younger adults (58).

There is debate as to whether mania as a secondary syndrome is a different entity from the primary affective disorder. The diagnosis is made clinically and is based upon good history taking, which should include collateral, appropriate physical investigations,

Table 12.7 Medical conditions associated with significant manic symptoms (66)

Endocrine diseases

Thyroid: hypo/hyperthryroidsm
Cushing's syndrome

Infectious diseasesesencephalitis

encephalitis
hepatitis
influenza
mononucleosis

Neurological diseases

Alzheimer's disease
brain tumours
epilepsy
head injury
Huntington's chorea
multiple sclerosis
Parkinson's disease
stroke
neurosyphillis
pseudbulbar palsy

Other diseases

AIDS
systemic lupus erythematosus
Fahr's disease
Wilson's disease

mental state examinations, and behavioural observations. Regardless of whether secondary mania is a distinct process in itself, the literature agrees that the management of elated or manic mood in those with concurrent medical illnesses should be focused on the underlying medical illness and on controlling the acute symptoms of mania, in order to alleviate the patient's distress and minimise risks (59).

Psychiatric morbidity is common in neurology patients (60). Table 12.7 lists common neurological conditions associated with elated mood. Neuroimaging studies have demonstrated more severe atrophy and cerebral vascular lesions in older bipolar patients than in age-matched depressed patients and in control cases (61–63). There is a risk that, after a cerebrovascular event (or stroke), patients may develop elated mood (64, 65), although this is much rarer than depressive disorders.

Affective psychiatric comorbidity is seen not only in patients with primary neurological disorders; commonly it can be a symptom in other diseases than affect the central nervous system. Table 12.7 lists the common endocrine, infectious, and other diseases that can cause elated mood.

Medications can also cause elated mood. Table 12.8 lists a number of the medications with elated mood or mania cited as a side effect of their use.

Table 12.8 Medications associated with manic symptoms as a side effect (67)

Common
corticosteroids

Uncommon
antidepressants of all classes
pramipexole

Rare
antipsychotics
anticonvulsants

Frequency unknown
aminophylline
disulfiram
ifosfamide
co-careldopa
co-beneldopa

Treatment

By comparison with what can be actioned in the community, admission to hospital provides an opportunity for close monitoring and timely intervention. It is important to have good links between liaison services and general medical colleagues in order to ensure prompt recognition and referral of any affective disorders. Unlike patients with depressed mood, those with elated mood are likely to be recognised more frequently, on account of their incongruity in a hospital setting; managing their behaviours creates challenging scenarios for the treating teams.

When considering the management of elated mood, is it essential to look at it in stages. These stages are acute, intermediate, and longer-term management. We will now look that management options available for these stages.

The Acute Stage

This stage may require a number of different non-pharmacological interventions as well as consideration of pharmacological intervention, depending on the risk–benefit evaluation of the level of distress that the patient is experiencing and of the risks to oneself and others.

Non-Pharmacological Interventions

Active Monitoring

Active monitoring is especially important in patients admitted to hospital who have a previous diagnosis of bipolar affective disorder, as the stresses associated with an acute admission may cause a manic or hypomanic relapse. This risk of relapse will be made all the higher if, as discussed earlier, such patients have their maintenance psychotropic (mood stabilizer or antipsychotic) therapy stopped. In these cases it is important for the treating teams to involve the liaison psychiatric team in supporting safe cessation and giving advice for it. The input from the liaison psychiatric team may take the form of a pragmatic 'watch and see' approach of monitoring for signs of relapse, and it may be that the patient is discharged home before a detailed assessment of his or her mental state can be carried out or before his or her maintenance therapy is restarted. In such instances, the liaison psychiatry team should consult with its community mental health colleagues or to the intensive home-based treatment teams, for ongoing assessment and monitoring upon discharge.

Sleep Hygiene

Poor sleep or decreased need for sleep is not only a symptom of manic or hypomanic episodes, it can be a precipitant for developing mania or hypomania. Given their acute 24-hour character, ward environments are not always conducive to patients' getting a full, restful night's sleep. This, however, does not preclude attempts to make environmental changes, for example by moving a patient to a quieter side room or bay, by reducing the stimulus around a patient as much as possible at night, in order to prompt sleep, and by minimising the number of night-time interventions.

Somatic Symptom Control (Including of Pain)

Patients presenting with elated mood can also be experiencing common somatic symptoms associated with their physical ill health, but because of their altered mental state they may be unable to communicate these symptoms as effectively or as articulately as they otherwise might. In view of this, teams should monitor and treat as appropriate any symptoms that cause discomfort, for example pain, nausea, vomiting, or shortness of breath. Management of these potential triggers can reduce either patients' risk of developing a disordered mood or, if the latter is already present, possible points of added distress that can lead to agitation or aggression.

Removing Triggers Where Possible

Where the elated mood is thought to be a direct result of medications or physical health problems, the causative medication should be stopped, if possible, or reduced to the lowest possible dose if the treatment is life-saving or no appropriate alternative is available.

If the elated mood is resultant from an underlying physical health problem, treating the physical problem should lead to improvement in the affective symptoms.

Pharmacological Interventions

Pharmacological intervention for management in the acute phase of an episode of elated mood should be used in conjunction with the aforementioned non-pharmacological approaches. Depending on the assessment of the risks to the patient and to others, it may be that initial management with psychotropic medication is required in order for non-pharmacological measures to be implemented safely.

As in all prescribing in old age, careful thought and consideration should be given to how the drug is administered, how it is absorbed, medical comorbidity, polypharmacy, and the side effect profile of the drug. All medications are started at the lowest possible therapeutic dosing and titrated up slowly, while factoring in the level of distress and the risks of the patient's remaining untreated for longer.

Once the decision has been made that pharmacological intervention is warranted, there are three main types of psychotropic medications that are used in the management of acute manic or hypomanic episodes. These are antipsychotics, benzodiazepines, and hypnotics. As mentioned previously, all these medications come with side effects, and the choice of the most appropriate medication depends on the cause of the elated mood as well as on the patient's comorbidities and on other prescribed medications.

Another important aspect to consider in treating those with mania or hypomania is that of capacity and legal frameworks. Is the patient deemed to lack capacity to consent to pharmacological treatment or to remaining in hospital? Does the patient require a legal framework to authorise admission, for example the Mental Capacity Act or the Mental Health Act in the United Kingdom? This is as a vital consideration in every case.

For patients who present with mania and agitation, a rapidly acting oral antipsychotic or benzodiazepine therapy may be required. Each hospital should have a local guideline on the management of agitation or disturbed behaviour within its trust, and that guideline will include the first line medication options and advice on when and how to escalate for further support.

The common first line oral options for mania with agitation are haloperidol, olanzapine, risperidone, quetiapine or lorazepam (67).

It may be that oral administration is not possible, yet on the balance of risk versus benefit it is felt to be in the patient's best interest to be treated. In these instances restraint and administration of intramuscular medications may be required, with drugs such as haloperidol, olanzapine, aripiprazole or lorazepam (67). Advice about the legal framework under which the treatment is needed can be sought from the liaison mental health team or from local mental health legislation teams.

For acute manic and hypomanic patients presenting without agitation, oral treatment can be offered in the form of oral antipsychotics such as haloperidol, olanzapine, risperidone, quetiapine, and aripiprazole (68) or oral benzodiazepines such as lorazepam, diazepam, and clonazepam (67).

If poor sleep is a significant problem and is not addressed through the use of antipsychotics or benzodiazepines, oral hypnotics or sedating antihistamines at night can be commenced – for example zopiclone, zolpidem or promethazine (67). The use of these drugs needs careful attention to the risk they pose of causing reduced coordination and falls.

When acutely agitated presentations are managed effectively and safely, one needs to judge whether the patient's elated mood results from a manic episode indicative of bipolar affective disorder or of some other aetiology, as this will determine whether longer-term therapy with antipsychotics or mood stabilisers is indicated. Again, this decision may not be made during the patient's stay in the general hospital, but it would require follow-up, either through transfer to an acute psychiatric in-patient hospital or by the intensive home-based treatment teams that exist in the community.

If the manic episode occurs in the context of bipolar affective disorder and trials of antipsychotic therapy have been unsuccessful or not tolerated, a mood stabiliser can be added. Lithium can be commenced as a mood stabilizer to treat a manic episode. If lithium is not suitable because of physical comorbidities or because the patient does not wish to engage in regular blood monitoring, sodium valproate can be commenced (69). It is not advised to commence lamotrigine for the management of a manic episode. Regular therapy with an antipsychotic or a mood stabiliser will require ongoing observation and assessment by community mental health or in-patient psychiatry teams on discharge from the general hospital. This is also required for those patients who were previously on maintenance antipsychotic or mood stabiliser therapy, which is stopped or reduced during their admission to the general hospital because of physical comorbidities.

Conclusion

It is the privilege of the liaison psychiatrist to be able to see a vast range of presentations of mood disorders and their consequences. This can often create challenging assessments and can lead to complex treatment decisions. Successfully navigating all this requires careful examination and an understanding of both the physical and mental health conditions and the interplay between the two. Initiating successful treatment plans requires liaison in its truest form: one needs to negotiate a rationale for the assessment and to communicate it to patients, to their community carers, to their clinical team, and to those who continue their care in the community on discharge.

References

1. Anderson, D.A., B. Baldwin, B. Barker, A. Forsyth, D. Guthrie, E. Holmes J. Ratcliffe, and J. Richman, A. *Who Cares Wins: Improving the Outcome for Older People Admitted to the General Hospital.* Royal Collage of Psychiatry, 2005. www.bgs.org.uk/sites/default/files/content/resources/files/2018-05-18/WhoCaresWins.pdf.

2. Sampson, E., Blanchard, M., Jones, L. et al. Dementia in the acute hospital: Prospective cohort study of prevalence and mortality. *British Journal of Psychiatry* 2009, 195(1): 61–6.

3. Sampson, E., White, N., Leurent, B. et al. Behavioural and psychiatric symptoms in people with dementia admitted to the acute hospital: Prospective cohort study. *British Journal of Psychiatry* 2014, 205(3): 189–96.

4. Peterson, J.F., Pun, B.T., Dittus, R.S. et al. Delirium and its motoric subtypes: A study of 614 critically ill patients. *Journal of the American Geriatrics Society* 2006, 54(3): 479–84.

5. Holmes, J., and House, A. Psychiatric illness predicts poor outcome after surgery for hip fracture: A prospective cohort study. *Psychological Medicine* 2000, 30: 921–9.

6. Goldberg, S., Whittamore, K., Harwood, R. et al. The prevalence of mental health problems among older adults admitted as an emergency to a general hospital. *Age and Ageing* 2012, 41(1): 80–6.

7. Cullum, S., Tucker, S., Todd, C. et al. Screening for depression in older medical inpatients. *Int J Geriatr Psychiatry* 2006, 21(5): 469–76.

8. Tooke, B., Aimola, L., Corrado, O., Crawford, M., Hood, C., Plummer, K., and Quirk, A. *Survey of Depression Reporting in Older Adults Admitted to Acute Hospitals.* Royal College of Psychiatrists, 2018. www.rcpsych.ac.uk/docs/default-source/improving-care/ccqi/ccqi-research-and-evaluation/capss/studies/depression-survey-report-older-adults-2018.pdf?sfvrsn=3ed9de11_4.

9. Cerejeira, J., Lagarto, L., and Mukaetova-Ladinska, E.B. Behavioral and psychological symptoms of dementia. *Fronters in Neurology* 2012, 73(3), 1–21.

10. Hessler, J.B., Schäufele, M., Hendlmeier, I. et al. Behavioural and psychological symptoms in general hospital patients with dementia, distress for nursing staff and complications in care: results of the General Hospital Study. *Epidemiology and Psychiatric Sciences* 2017: 1–10.

11. Maercker, A., Forstmeier, S., Enzler, A. et al. Adjustment disorders, posttraumatic stress disorder, and depressive disorders in old age: Findings

from a community survey. *Comprehensive Psychiatry* 49(2): 113–20.

12. Strain, J.J., Smith, G.C., Hammer, J.S. et al. Adjustment disorder: A multisite study of its utilization and interventions in the consultation-liaison psychiatry setting. *General Hospital Psychiatry* 1998, 20(3): 139–49.

13. Gaudiano, B.A., Dalrymple, K.L., and Zimmerman, M. Prevalence and clinical characteristics of psychotic versus nonpsychotic major depression in a general psychiatric outpatient clinic. *Depression and Anxiety* 2009, 26(1): 54–64.

14. Jaaskelainen, E., Juola, T., Korpela, H. et al. Epidemiology of psychotic depression: Systematic review and meta-analysis. *Psychol Med* 2018, 48(6): 905–18.

15. Kessler, R.C., and Walters, E.E. Epidemiology of DSM-III-R major depression and minor depression among adolescents and young adults in the national comorbidity survey. *Depression and Anxiety* 1998, 7(1): 3–14.

16. Mundt, C., et al. (eds). *Interpersonal Factors in the Origin and Course of Affective Disorders*. London: Gaskell/Royal College of Psychiatrists, 1996.

17. Harrison, P., Cowen, P., Burns, T., and Fazel, M. *Shorter Oxford Textbook of Psychiatry* (7th ed.). Oxford: Oxford University Press, 2018.

18. Reijnders, J.S., Ehrt, U., Weber, W.E. et al. A systematic review of prevalence studies of depression in Parkinson's disease. *Mov Disord* 2008, 23(2): 183–9; quiz 313.

19. Hackett, M.L., Yapa, C., Parag, V. et al. Frequency of depression after stroke. *A Systematic Review of Observational Studies* 2005, 36(6): 1330–40.

20. Thombs, B.D., Bass, E.B., Ford, D.E. et al. Prevalence of depression in survivors of acute myocardial infarction. *Journal of General Internal Medicine* 2006, 21(1): 30–8.

21. Ballard, C., Bannister, C., Solis, M. et al. The prevalence, associations and symptoms of depression amongst dementia sufferers. *Journal of Affective Disorders* 1996, 36(3): 135–44.

22. Bullmore, E. *The Inflamed Mind*. London: Short Books, 2018.

23. Yirmiya, R. Depression in medical illness: The role of the immune system. *West J Med* 2000, 173(5): 333–6.

24. Goodwin, G.M. Depression and associated physical diseases and symptoms. *Dialogues in Clinical Neuroscience* 2006, 8(2): 259–65.

25. *British National Formulary* (69th ed.). London: BMJ Group and Pharmaceutical Press, 2015. https://rudiapt.files.wordpress.com/2017/11/british-national-formulary-69.pdf.

26. Martin, G., and Dendukuri, N. Risk factors for depression among elderly community subjects: A systematic review and meta-analysis. *American Journal of Psychiatry* 2003, 160(6): 1147–56.

27. The Kings Fund. Is your hospital dementia friendly? The Kings Fund, 2014. www.kingsfund.org.uk/sites/default/files/media/ehe-hospitals-dementia-assessment-tool.pdf and www.kingsfund.org.uk/projects/enhancing-healing-environment.

28. World Health Organisation. *The International Statistical Classification of Diseases, 10th Revision: Classification of Mental and Behavioural Disorders: Clinical Descriptions and Diagnostic Guidelines*. Geneva: World Health Organization, 1992.

29. American Psychiatric Association. *Diagnostic and Statistical Manual of Mental Disorders* (5th ed.). Arlington, VA: American Psychiatric Publishing, 2013.

30. Lykouras, E., Malliaras, D., Christodoulou, G.N. et al. Delusional depression: Phenomenology and response to treatment. *Acta Psychiatrica Scandinavica* 1986, 73(3): 324–9.

31. Fick, D.M., Agostini, J.V., and Inouye, S.K. Delirium superimposed on dementia: A systematic review. *Journal of the American Geriatrics Society* 2002, 50 (10): 1723–32.

32. Goldberg, S., Whittamore, K., Pollock, K. et al. Caring for cognitively impaired

older patients in the general hospital: A qualitative analysis of similarities and differences between a specialist medical and mental health unit and standard care wards. *Int J Nurs Stud* 2014, 51(10): 1132–43.

33. Dennis, M., Kadri, A., and Coffey, J. Depression in older people in the general hospital: A systematic review of screening instruments. *Age and Ageing* 2012, 41(2): 148–54.

34. Yesavage, J.A., Brink, T.L., Rose, T.L. et al. Development and validation of a geriatric depression screening scale: A preliminary report. *Journal of Psychiatric Research* 1982, 17(1): 37–49.

35. Adshead, F., Cody, D.D., and Pitt, B. BASDEC: A novel screening instrument for depression in elderly medical inpatients. *BMJ* 1992, 305: 397.

36. Hamilton, M. Development of a rating scale for primary depressive illness. *Br J Soc Clin Psychol* 1967, 6(4): 278–96.

37. Evans, M.E. Development and validation of a brief screening scale for depression in the elderly physically ill. *International Clinical Psychopharmacology* 1993, 8(4): 329–31.

38. Koenig, H.G., Meador, K.G., Cohen, H.J. et al. Self-rated depression scales and screening for major depression in the older hospitalized patient with medical illness. *J Am Geriatr Soc* 1988, 36(8): 699–706.

39. Kitchell, M.A., Barnes, R.F., Veith, R.C. et al. Screening for depression in hospitalized geriatric medical patients. *J Am Geriatr Soc* 1982, 30(3): 174–7.

40. Alexopoulos, G.S., Abrams, R.C., Young, R.C. et al. Cornell Scale for Depression in Dementia. *Biol Psychiatry* 1988, 23(3): 271–84.

41. Crowther, G.J.E., Bennett, M.I., and Holmes, J.D. How well are the diagnosis and symptoms of dementia recorded in older patients admitted to hospital? *Age and Ageing* 2016.

42. National Confidential Enquiry into Patient Outcome and Death. *Treat as One: Bridging the Gap between Mental and Physical Healthcare in General Hospitals*. National Confidential Enquiry into Patient Outcome and Death, 2017. http://www.ncepod.org.uk/2017report1/downloads/TreatAsOne_FullReport.pdf.

43. Cowdell, F. The care of older people with dementia in acute hospitals. *International Journal of Older People Nursing* 2010, 5 (2): 83–92.

44. Burroughs, H., Lovell, K., Morley, M. et al. 'Justifiable depression': How primary care professionals and patients view late-life depression? A qualitative study. *Fam Pract* 2006, 23(3): 369–77.

45. National Institute for Health and Care Excellence. *Depressoin in adults: recognition and management*. 2018 (now updated to 2022). ww.nice.org.uk/guidance/cg90.

46. McWilliams, L.A., Cox, B.J., and Enns, M.W. Mood and anxiety disorders associated with chronic pain: An examination in a nationally representative sample. *Pain* 2003, 106(1): 127–33.

47. Hammen, C. Stress and depression. *Annual Review of Clinical Psychology* 2005, 1(1): 293–319.

48. Ehlers, A., and Clark, D. Early psychological interventions for adult survivors of trauma: A review. *Biol Psychiatry* 2003, 53(9): 817–26.

49. Bowker, L., Price, J., and Smith, S. *Oxford Handbook of Geriatric Medicine* (2nd ed.). Oxford: Oxford University Press, 2012.

50. Taylor, D., Paton, C., and Kapur, S. *Prescribing Guidelines in Psychiatry* (12th ed.). Oxford: Wiley Blackwell, 2015.

51. Warden, D., Rush, A.J., Trivedi, M.H. et al. The STAR*D project results: A comprehensive review of findings. *Current Psychiatry Reports* 2007, 9(6): 449–59.

52. Banerjee, S. *The Use of Antipsychotic Medication for People with Dementia: Time for Action*. Department of Health UK, 2009. https://psychrights.org/research/digest/nlps/banerjeereportongeriatricneurolepticuse.pdf.

53. The UK ECT Review Group. Efficacy and safety of electroconvulsive therapy in depressive disorders: A systematic review and meta-analysis. *Lancet* 2003, 361 (9360): 799–808.

54. Krautgartner, M., Alexandrowicz, R., Benda, N., et al. Need and utilization of psychiatric consultation services among general hospital inpatients. *Soc Psychiatry Psychiatr Epidemiol* 2006 41(4): 294–301.

55. World Health Organization. The world health report 2003: Shaping the future. WHO, 2003. https://apps.who.int/iris/handle/10665/42789.

56. Sampson, E.L., Blanchard, M.R., Jones, L., Tookman, A., and King, M. Dementia in the acute hospital: Prospective cohort study of prevalence and mortality. *British Journal of Psychiatry* 2009, 195(1): 61–6.

57. NICE. Attention deficit hyperactivity disorder. NICE, November 2022. https://cks.nice.org.uk/topics/attention-deficit-hyperactivity-disorder.

58. Depp, C.A., and Jeste, D.V. Bipolar disorder in older adults: A critical review. *Bipolar Disord* 2004, 6(5): 343–67.

59. Torales, J., Gonzalez, I., Barrios, I., Ventriglio, A., and Bhugra, D. Manic episodes due to medical illnesses: A literature review. *J Nerv Ment Dis* 2018, 206(9): 733–8.

60. Lykouras ,L., Vassiliadou, M., and Adrachta, D., et al. Illness behavior in neurological inpatients with psychiatric morbidity. *Eur Psychiatry* 2006, 21(3): 200–03.

61. Fujikawa, T., Yamawaki, S., and Touhouda, Y. *Silent cerebral infarctions in patients with late-onset mania. Stroke* 1995, 26(6): 946–9.

62. Shulman, K.I., and Herrmann, N. The nature and management of mania in old age. *Psychiatr Clin North Am* 1999 22(3): 649–65, ix.

63. Cassidy,, F., and Carrol, l. *Vascular risk factors in late onset mania, BJPsych Med* 2002, 32(2): 359–62.

64. Nagaratnam, N., Wong, K.-K., and Patel, I. Secondary mania of vascular origin in elderly patients: A report of two clinical cases. *Archives of Gerontology and Geriatrics* 2006, 43(2): 223–32.

65. Arai, H., Matsumoto, S., Sekiyama, R., and Fukuoka, T. Secondary mania after cerebral infarction in the recovery phase: Case report. *Progress in Rehabilitation Medicine* 2018, 3: 2018–21.

66. Semple, D., and Smyth, R. Bipolar illness. In *Oxford Handbook of Psychiatry* (4 ed.), Oxford: Oxford Academic, online ed., 1 June 2019). https://doi.org/10.1093/med/9780198795551.003.0007 and https://oxfordmedicine.com/view/10.1093/med/9780198795551.001.0001/med-9780198795551-chapter-7#med-9780198795551-chapter-7-div1–3).

67. NICE. British National Formulary (BNF). NICE, 31 May 2023. https://bnf.nice.org.uk.

68. NICE. Bipolar disorder: Assessment and management. NICE, 24 September 2014. www.nice.org.uk/guidance/cg185.

Chapter 3

Prevention of Suicide and Self-Harm in Older People

Peter Byrne and Cate Bailey

For the individuals concerned, for their families and friends, for the health and other professionals whom they have met or tried to access, and for the wider society, death by suicide is the worst possible outcome. Clinicians and coroners interrogate the final common pathways of suicide, but this chapter looks further back. Recent events (precipitants) combine with pre-existing factors to overwhelm a person's coping skills and resilience (social capital, spirituality, help-seeking behaviours) and orient that person towards an act of self-harm. Risk factors that have consistently been associated with suicidal ideation and attempts in older people are:

- current mental disorders, particularly anxiety with comorbid depression (where hopelessness increases the risk);
- bereavement, especially the death of a spouse;
- physical illnesses (especially cancer, pain, and neurological conditions, especially ones that cause functional disability);
- neurocognitive disorders;
- alcohol misuse and dependence;
- social exclusion and isolation;
- economic stress, for example difficult transitions;
- impaired decision-making and problem solving.

Multidimensional and integrated approaches that consider biological, psychological, and social factors and how the past may influence the present are key in preventing suicide and self-harm in older adults. The nature of the act of self-harm and any changes in intention after the event are important factors, but the outcome (life or death) is frequently determined by chance and by factors beyond the control of the individual:

- access to lethal methods during a crisis;
- method failure, for example ligature breaks;
- physiological response, for example that the person vomited a potentially fatal overdose or did not absorb ingested tablets;
- chance discovery by others.

The 5Ps approach (Box 13.1) is a clear paradigm with which to assess people who present to emergency departments (EDs) and other settings, but in many domains older people are at higher risk of death. The approach also places preventative strategies outside hospital settings.

Before identifying health professionals' points of assessment and intervention, we need to reduce the negative influences of chance. Many people choose a violent means of

Box 13.1 Key areas (the 5 Ps) that determine current and on-going risk of suicide

Factor	Areas to explore with patient and informants	Areas where older people are more vulnerable
Problem: the nature of self-harming event; ask why you are seeing this patient right now, and in this setting. Was there unprompted disclosure of suicidal ideation? Did the patient initiate the consultation?	Perceptions of the lethal nature of self-harm; violent acts linked to future death by suicide; note the role of chance (see text) in the act's not resulting in death; degree of planning; final acts (making a will, putting affairs in order, suicide note etc.); discovery: did the person actively self-report?	Most suicides occur in the home and older people are more likely to live alone: less common discovery; fewer physical reserves (liver, renal, cognitive impairment etc.) to reverse the adverse effects of self-harm; diminished gag reflex / aspiration; medication interactions.
Precipitating: recent events, the 'last straw'; many younger adults have no precipitant and have decided on self-harm in the last hour(s) before they act.	Exit events, transitions, losses: personal (especially spousal bereavement), health, financial, changes in location – key event might be a recent hospital discharge, loss of caring role. Consider the meaning of losses to the person. Exposure to suicide method: direct or mediated experiences	More losses as we live longer; losses that may seem small can reactivate earlier losses, or have a greater significance (death of a distant relative, a pet, or a neighbour), or relate to future activities (moving to residential care, loss of the ability to drive or travel to attend a local club)
Predisposing: male gender; older age; personal/family history; medical and psychiatric history; history of previous self-harm, often unreported; misuse of alcohol and substances; current social context; personality traits: impulsivity, rigidity, neuroticism with low extroversion; narcissism; unique occupation (doctor, farmer) or setting (prisoners, even those about to achieve release; anyone in police custody)	Family history of mental disorders, and (less strongly predictive) family history of suicide; adverse childhood events; history of migration; inequalities / lower income – unemployed; *previous self-harm predicts future self-harm*; **alcohol** as dependence/misuse or as a means of disinhibition (Dutch courage) in the suicide act. Access to lethal methods (access to high lethality medications, e.g. insulin, morphine, tricyclic antidepressants, some cardiac meds).	Over 75 years old (independent risk factor for suicide); living alone (in order of decreasing risk): divorced, separated, widowed and lonely; comorbid physical conditions, ***especially cancer, chronic pain, and neurological diseases*** (any that result in functional disability), including dementia; with cognitive decline, more impulsive, with impaired decision-making and problem solving; poverty; perceived burdensomeness; difficult retirement; undisclosed alcohol misuse more likely in older people

Box 13.1 (cont.)

Perpetuating: (1) mental state exam findings uncover current, *distressing* symptoms; and (2) attitudes to mental disorders and their treatments

(1) current depressive symptoms with negative ruminations or, worse, nihilistic or guilty delusions; unpleasant anxiety symptoms; **hopelessness** = loss of hope with ongoing suicidal ideation and intent, even a plan; auditory hallucinations, especially abusive, or commands, e.g. 'kill yourself'; poor sleep.

(2) negative, self-stigmatising attitudes (shame, guilt) to having depression and suicidality; antipathy to psychiatric interventions; nonadherence to treatments.

(1) depression more common, less frequently diagnosed, and less likely to be treated in older populations; self-blame and negative/guilty cognitions ('I am a burden to my family') may be culturally sanctioned; psychotic features may be understated or untreated – sometimes because of concerns about potential side effects of antipsychotics.

(2) clinicians may have lower expectations about treating depression or may judge symptoms as 'rational suicide'; older adults are less likely to be referred for talking therapies, despite good outcomes (see text).

Protective: resilience, coping skills, sense of community and social capital, health seeking behaviours

Stable finances, safe homes and good domestic relationship(s); supportive contacts with family of origin, own family and extended family; work contacts and other accessible social networks; spirituality and religious beliefs; cultural beliefs about suicide.

Older people may be more likely than others to live alone; may have financial insecurity; may have outlived or be distanced from family of origin; may be estranged from own family; current residence may be a temporary or permanent residential care placement; their children likely to have started their own families; former work colleagues and neighbours may have moved on.

Main sources: 8; 15; 25; 57.

suicide: hanging or strangulation, jumping from a height, falling into water, cuts to major blood vessels or (in the United States and other countries with poor gun control laws or none) gunshot injuries. Clinicians should avoid direct or closed questions about the suicide method, but are encouraged to ask directly about the immediate environment and about access to firearms (1). It is challenging to restrict access to suicide methods (see public health measures), and it is worth stating that, with each violent method attempted, older people have considerably less physical reserves for overcoming the insult. The same is true of deliberate overdosing: organ function declines with age, multiple medications before overdose are the rule, not the exception, and alcohol excess (which occurs in two out of three of deaths by suicide) reduces the excretion of toxins (see Box 13.1).

Every person is different: we change with life experience, but most younger people have moderate and rising levels of autonomy (financial, home, vocational status, networks) and are striving to achieve more. Autonomy may be a key (recent) loss in older people (Box 13.1), and cognitions may be negative about the contrast between how things used to be and perceived current status. Ageing brings us all closer to facing death, potential disability, and reduced independence, whether or not these fears are held consciously in mind. Many of the changes in older age, such as loss of health, vitality, potency, professional role, and social position, may be viewed as a narcissistic wounds from which there is little recovery (2). While many older adults negotiate these shifts with minimal difficulty, others may experience emotions such as shame, fear, anger and disgust. Changes that come with ageing can produce a re-experiencing of early losses or vulnerabilities, which resurface. This tests a person's ability to trust and tolerance of interdependence, which are heavily influenced by the care they received in early life, as well as by the quality of the care offered now (2). These social factors are highly individual. They determine the nature of hope (for the future), and thereby serve as strong predictors of death by suicide.

Van Orden and Deming (1) have hypothesised a link between ageism and suicide in older adults. Previous studies have shown that the internalisation of negative stereotypes of ageing is connected to reduced physical and mental functioning. This reduced functioning could potentially contribute to, or perpetuate, factors such as depression and functional impairment, both of which are also associated with suicide. A sense of being a burden, of disconnection and invisibility within society is also emerging as a factor in suicidal ideation in older adults (1).

Epidemiology

The rates of suicide have been relatively constant in the United Kingdom in recent years, though the economic downturn and austerity led to some rises among middle-aged men thought to be 'left behind' by economic circumstances (3). It should also be noted that the spectrum of suicidal ideation and behaviour in older people may be under-recognised as a result of presentations such as self-starvation or dehydration and coroners' difficulty to reach a verdict of suicide when multimorbidity and polypharmacy are the norm (4). The latest UK figures (see Figure 13.1) show peak suicides in the 45–50-year-olds group, then a 'second peak' for suicide across the age ranges (5).

A large three-centre English study of self-harm in those aged over 60 found rates of 65 per 100,000, which is far lower than the rates in those aged 18–59, namely 380 per

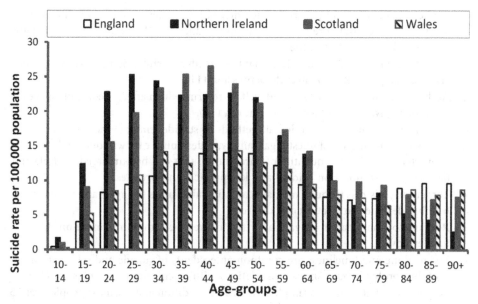

Figure 13.1 Data for 10 years until 2016.
Source: 5.

100,000 (6). Over a 5–8-year follow-up study period, 16.7 per cent of older adults who had presented with self-harm repeated it, and 2 per cent died by suicide. About a half of this 2 per cent took their lives in the first year after the index self-harm, most of them 'switching' from overdose (the initial self-harm episode) to a fatal violent method (6). Numbers were small, and the only predictor of suicide was the use of a violent method in the index episode (6). A recent systematic review identified major risk factors for repeat self-harm among younger older adults – those aged 60–74: such factors are living alone, not being married or partnered, having a current diagnosis of depression, drug and alcohol use, current poor level of functioning, and current psychiatric treatment (7).

Cornell (8) examined the ratio of all acts of self-harm (this includes attempts to end one's life) to deaths by suicide in these age groups. In young people, this ratio varies between 8:1 and 200:1, and in older people it is consistently higher than 4:1. Part but not all of these differences are attributable to the increased vulnerabilities of older people who self-harm (Box 13.1).

Public Health Measures to Reduce Suicide

Primary prevention aims to stop the disorder or the event from happening in the first instance. In this arena, we work primarily to prevent suicide as the outcome, but we use similar multilevel interventions as secondary prevention (early intervention), to engage with someone who has self-harmed, and we treat ongoing morbidity in order to prevent suicide.

Here are a few universal measures that help everyone in the community:

- Reduce alcohol misuse and dependence across all ages: the single best public health measure is minimum alcohol pricing (9).

- Reduce inequalities and poverty, which drive higher rates of self-harm and suicide. Marmot (10) sets out core principles around reducing childhood poverty and giving every child a 'good start in life'.
- Identify and intervene in situations that lead to adverse childhood experiences, which are increasingly linked to later-life depression (11).
- Address the impact of austerity and welfare reform, which affects people of all ages in both their physical and their mental health (12).
- Identify and reduce access to lethal methods of suicide: emulate the great success stories of changing the domestic gas supply, redesigning cars without catalytic converters, limiting the quantity of paracetamol that can be purchased, and placing barriers and warnings on bridges and key public transport sites.
- Target early distress through mental health first aid classes (all ages) and primary care training designed to treat mental disorders.
- Resource primary care to engage and treat depressive symptoms (more on this further down).
- Living alone and loneliness are common antecedents of suicide and self-harm in all ages, but probably have similar associations with suicide across the lifespan (13).
- For everyone with a long-term physical health condition and for most people over 75 years, an appropriate package of care supports them to live as independently as possible. Put another way, functional disability is a modifiable risk factor for suicide (1).
- Collaborate with traditional media (print and broadcast) and with new or social media to improve the quality of suicide reporting (never give details of the method; do not glamorise the deceased or push the line that the person had 'no way out' other than suicide) in order to reduce contagion or imitative suicides.
- In England there are now suicide prevention strategies in every locality. Some of these explore the different challenges of older people.

Selective prevention identifies high-risk groups in order to target evidence-based interventions for them. These are people with a history of self-harm, recent or historical, and older people who have risk factors for death by suicide (Box 13.1), specifically modifiable ones – such as depression, alcohol misuse, isolation, or functional impairment – or pain associated with complex medical comorbidities. In effect this is about providing low-level, acceptable, and accessible psychological interventions, with at least one medical assessment designed to identify later-life depression (14). There is good evidence that antidepressants *as a single intervention* reduce suicide rates in depressed older people, though not in younger adults, and lithium remains a strong protector in all age ranges (15). Also key is redressing discrimination and inequality in the provision of and access to specialist mental health services equipped to treat older adults (16).

Depression: A Powerful Driver of Suicide and Self-Harm, but a Common and Treatable One

The association between suicidal ideation (Box 13.2) and ending one's life is stronger in older people than in other adults and weakest in young people (13). Drivers of these suicidal ideas are a key point for interventions. Among these, the identification and treatment of later-life depression is paramount, and every contact with an older person

---

Box 13.2 Questions to determine the level of suicide risk

The following figure presents a series of sequential questions designed to determine the level of suicide risk.

1. *'In the past couple of weeks, were things ever so bad that you had thoughts that life is not worth living, or that you'd be better off dead?'* [Passive suicide ideation]

If Yes, continue with Question 2

2. *'Have you had any thoughts about hurting yourself or suicide in the past couple of weeks?'* [Active suicide ideation]

If Yes, continue with Questions 2a–2g

2a. *'What have you been thinking of doing?'* [Type of method]

2b. *'How often do you have these thoughts? How long do they stay on your mind?'* [Frequency and persistence]

2c. *'What is going on in your life right now?'* [Life stress (e.g. loss, change in health status)]

2d. *'Do you have a plan for doing this?'* [Specific, detailed suicide plan]

2e. *'Do you intend to harm yourself?'* [Suicide intention]

2f. *'Is anything preventing you from harming yourself? For example, how strong is your desire to live? Do you feel you have a purpose in life? Do you have hope for the future? Do you consider suicide morally wrong or against your religious beliefs? Do you want to avoid causing family and friends pain?'* [Reasons for living]

2g. *'Do you feel you can resist these thoughts? Have you ever done anything to harm yourself? How often do you drink alcohol or use street drugs?'* [Impulse control]

Used with permission from Raue, P.J., Brown, E.L., Meyers, B.S., Schulberg, H.C., and Bruce, M.L. Does every allusion to possible suicide require the same response? *Journal of Family Practice* 2006, 55 (7): 605–12.

---

who struggles with physical health, mental distress, or 'social problems' should include key questions about suicidal ideation. One review found that 45 per cent of persons who died by suicide had seen their primary care provider during the last month of their life; the rate was even higher for older patients than for younger patients. Only 20 per cent had seen a mental health professional (17). A recent systematic review found that 28.9 per cent of older adults who self-harmed had seen their GP within the week, and 62 per cent within the month (7). Only 28.2 per cent were receiving psychiatric care at the time of their self-harm (7). Important settings for identification and intervention are therefore likely to be primary care, general hospital in-patients, and interactions with social care professionals around times of transition in care arrangements, or indeed with any members of the multidisciplinary team (MDT) that works with older people with long-term medical conditions. Comprehensive geriatric assessments led by geriatricians and a specialist MDT have a role in moderating multiple risk factors. Such assessments frequently target multiple interdependent areas such as minimising functional disability and pain, maximising autonomy and connectedness, and planning for the future.

All studies advocate identification of depression by clinical interview, and many recommend structured screening such as the Patient Health Questionnaire (17 18).

The guidelines of the National Institute for Health and Care Excellence (NICE) recommend asking two screening questions of non-cognitively impaired older people on medical wards:

- 'During the past month have you often been bothered by feeling down, depressed, or hopeless?' and
- 'During the past month have you often been bothered by having little interest or pleasure in doing things?'

These questions have been found to be both sensitive and specific and should prompt further inquiry and consideration of referral to specialist services (19). Both the fifteen-item Geriatric Depression Scale (GDS) and a five-item subset also demonstrated sensitivity and specificity for identifying suicidal ideation in elders (14). The five-item subset did not directly inquire about suicidal ideation, asking instead about hopelessness, worthlessness, and life not being worth living. This would suggest that inquiring about these factors opens a helpful way of talking about suicidal ideation. Initial inquiries could then be followed by more specific questions related to plans and intent, in a structured approach (Box 13.2). Scales and screening can act as a useful starting point for further discussion. It is important to note that the phenomenology of depression is different in older adults: agitation is more common than sadness, and somatic complaints are more frequent (20). Comorbid medical conditions, cultural taboos, and low expectations – in patients and clinicians alike – of making a difference mean that depression is often missed or undertreated. Evidence suggests that, despite positive outcomes from talking therapies in older adults, GPs may be reluctant to refer patients for depression, perhaps anticipating onerous and distressing assessment processes (21). A collateral history that identifies recent loss of social function, perhaps minimised by the patient, should prompt further assessment.

Asking about suicide (question 1 in Box 13.2) changes the theme from 'don't ask, don't tell' to a safer interaction. Clinicians need to practice the form of words they intend to use when they start this essential clinical conversation. In older people, physical morbidity is more probable than not, and some of them may see a terminal or severe illness as the means of ending their lives. Thoughts of wanting to hasten death are common: open questions ('what's next? what will happen to you?') are then followed by closed ones ('do you think this illness will kill you? what do you want to happen? what should we do?').

The literature is consistent in describing the utility of depression and suicide awareness training for clinicians (22). This training works for a while, but the effects diminish if the clinician fails to keep asking about suicide as a matter of standard practice, perhaps using a peer learning group to improve the form of words, the timing of conversations, and so on. The best learning is reinforced by good outcomes: treating depression transforms lives.

In keeping with the literature that suggests that poor physical health and mental health are closely related (Box 13.1), integrated approaches or 'chronic care models' are strongly encouraged (23). A large study of thirty-six general practices in the North of England used brief psychological interventions, including behavioural activation and support with the management of drug treatment for patients with depressive symptoms heart disease or diabetes (24). The authors of this study also found that depressive symptoms were reduced and confidence in the self-management of medical conditions increased. Two primary care interventions have used a randomised controlled trial design to explore the effect of a collaborative treatment of depression by comparison with the effect of usual care (25, 26). The IMPACT (25) and PROSPECT (26) interventions both used depression care managers (psychologists, nurses, or social workers in a coordinating role) and options related to education about treatment that included interpersonal or behavioural psychotherapy and follow-up and monitoring of depressive symptoms and medication. The IMPACT treatment arm showed reduced rates of depression and suicidal ideation and a reduction in functional impairment at 6, 12, 18, and 24 months (25).The authors suggested that the most effective components were the personalisation of treatment plans, the fostering of a therapeutic alliance, and the proactive follow-up. At 4, 8, and 24 months, the PROSPECT study demonstrated a significant reduction in suicidal ideation in those with major depression (26).

Indicated Prevention for Four High-Risk Groups

Presenting with New Suicidal Ideas or Actions

Older people who report suicidal ideation, those with a plan to end their lives, or those who have recently attempted to end their lives require intensive support (27). It should also be noted that the spectrum of suicidal ideation and behaviour in older people can manifest as self-starvation, dehydration, or refusal of medical treatment (4). Assessment should be conducted by both medical staff and mental health, in parallel (Box 13.3), with immediate management of the consequences of self-harm and intoxication with substances and potential later withdrawal. A patient declining to engage in any discussion about management or future plans, whether angry or not, is another red flag to increasing risk (4).

It may not be possible for a complete mental health assessment to be conducted if the patient is drowsy or requires treatment for an overdose; however, efforts should be made to continue to assess and formulate a safe immediate management plan. It may include the use of one-to-one nursing while the patient is on a medical ward. Consultation with the patient and the family, as well as the information gleaned from suicide notes, ambulance staff, or other relevant parties, is vital in developing a formulation. General hospital psychiatric teams that treat patients of all ages may not appreciate the complexity and serious intent of these presentations: the recommendation is for a low threshold of admission to hospital. However, after the initial assessment(s), the patient may well be safe to return home, perhaps with the support of a crisis team. Although well established in the care of adults, crisis teams and home treatment teams for older people are not as widely available. There is evidence for such teams in relation to reducing admissions and managing crises at home, but data specifically on suicide rates among older persons while in the care of these teams are not available (28).

Psychiatric In-Patients

Admission to a psychiatric unit is a recognised positive outcome for this first group, but this does not eliminate risks of death by suicide, because most 'in-patient' suicides occur not on the ward, but off the premises, thorough assessment and discussion about voluntary–involuntary status, and any proposed leave is essential. Reassessment as the admission progresses is also vital. Studies specifically focusing on older adult in-patients

Box 13.3 Key approaches after a suicide attempt in older adults

Initial Assessment in A&E and Medical Wards	• Organise a parallel assessment of physical health and mental state with A&E and mental health staff. • Treat the medical consequences of suicide or self-harm attempt. • Gather collateral history from family, friends, ambulance crew, GP, and suicide note (if applicable). • Develop an immediate safety plan after the initial risk assessment; this plan may include the use of one-to-one observation on the medical ward. • Consider appropriate legislation for facilitating mental or physical health treatment, or both (in England, the Mental Health Act; the Mental Capacity Act) • Assessment will guide the need for in-patient treatment or community management. • If it is safe for the patient to return to community, consider using the home treatment team and the community mental health team (CMHT) and provide details for crisis lines to patients, families, and paid carers. • Develop a personalised care plan in order to identify relapse triggers, available supports, and when to seek help. • Communicate with the relevant parties, including the GP and the CMHT.
Psychiatric Inpatient Management	• Avoid out-of-area admissions, if possible. • On admission, provide information regarding ward facilities, the level of observation, and the Mental Health Act. • Develop an immediate plan with observations, leave arrangements (see text), and medication. • Begin discharge planning as soon as patient is admitted, in order to identify factors that may have precipitated admission and may delay discharge. • Carefully consider risk assessment with regard to leave from the ward. • Do repeated and personalised risk assessments during admission, document them, and communicate them to the relevant parties. • Have sufficient staffing levels and make efforts to facilitate a positive engagement. • A multidisciplinary assessment (occupational therapist, physiotherapist, social worker, psychologist, geriatrician, psychiatrist) should develop the biopsychosocial formulation and identify the factors to be targeted by an intervention to reduce suicidal ideation (e.g. functional disability,

Box 13.3 *(cont.)*

	chronic pain, finances, social situation, relationship discord, isolation).
	• Treat mental disorder as appropriate, with pharmacotherapy, and consider referral for psychological therapies.
	• Consider electroconvulsive therapy (ECT) if patient is not eating and drinking or has intense and unrelenting suicidal ideation or psychotic depression.
	• Involve the family where appropriate and acceptable to the patient, bearing in mind safeguarding issues and vulnerability.
	• Begin engagement with the CMHT (or support re-engagement with it).
	• Consider a trial leave before the formal discharge, and liaise with family and community support.
Discharge	• Does the local home treatment or crisis team accept older people?
	• Keep in mind the CMHT support.
	• Arrange discharge meeting with the relevant parties (patient, CMHT staff, family, paid carers, residential care staff).
	• Develop a clear plan for the days after discharge; it should cover the next planned face-to-face contact (guidelines suggest follow-up within 3 days), possible crises (and contacts in case of crisis), quantities of prescribed medication (and their communication to the GP), and ongoing support (which should include psychological interventions).
	• Telephone counselling systems and crisis lines may be considered.

have identified the first week of admission and the first two weeks after discharge as the highest risk period. Both affective disorder and first versus later admission also conferred a higher risk (29). Appleby (30), on the basis of findings from the National Confidential Inquiry into Suicide and Homicide by People with Mental Illness (5), made clear recommendations in this area (see Box 13.4). Bickley (31) reported that short admissions were also associated with an increased risk of suicide. The identification and treatment of mental disorder(s) during admission is paramount. The management of depression is considered elsewhere in this book (Chapter 12), but a large population-based study in patients over the age of 75 demonstrated that the highest risk periods occurred during switching antidepressants and among people who were also prescribed anxiolytics or hypnotics (32). The potential for an emergence or a worsening of suicidal ideation during the initial stages of treatment with selective serotonin reuptake inhibitors (SSRIs) must be considered and managed, but should not deter clinicians from treating depression.

> **Box 13.4** Key elements of a safer care in mental health services (30)
>
> 1. Safer wards
>
> - Removal of ligature points
> - Reduction in absconding
> - Skilled in-patient observation
>
> 2. Care planning and early follow-up after discharge from hospital to community
> 3. No out-of-area admissions for acutely ill patients
> 4. 24-hour crisis resolution and home treatment teams
> 5. Community outreach teams to support patients who may lose contact with conventional services
> 6. Specialised services for alcohol and drug misuse and dual diagnosis
> 7. Multidisciplinary review of patient suicides, with input from family
> 8. Implementation of the National Institute for Health and Clinical Excellence guidance on depression and self-harm
> 9. Personalised risk management, without routine checklists
> 10. Low turnover of non-medical staff

A multidisciplinary approach addresses the various factors that influence an older person's suicidal ideation. The relationship between physical illness, functional disability, and suicidality is complex, but well established (1) (see Box 13.1). Physiotherapy, occupational therapy, and social work have a role in identifying where supports or aids may maximise function and improve quality of life. Chronic pain and suicidality demonstrate a complex relationship, but assertive management, including through referral to specialist pain services, may also have a role in reducing the risk of suicide (33). Regular and repeated risk assessments throughout the period of admission are vital in response to new information and changing circumstances. Ageism covers a multitude of prejudices, so we must not neglect to ask about substance misuse, home environment (debts, hostile neighbours, vulnerability to exploitation), past trauma, or offending history as potential drivers of low mood and suicide. The involvement of family and friends, if available, is important, but we must also take into account the patient's preferences and any safeguarding issues that may have precipitated the suicidal ideation.

For those who demonstrate a profound sense of hopelessness, hypochondriacal delusions, intense suicidality, or refusal to eat and drink, ECT is an evidence-based and frequently life-saving treatment, particularly in an older population. In a study of fifty-three older patients it was found that the odds of suicidal ideation resolution with a course of six sessions was higher for older than for younger patients (34).

A psychological assessment and referral for psychotherapy should be considered, although its timing would depend on the severity of the patient's presentation. Cognitive behavioural therapy (CBT) has an established evidence base for treating depression in older adults (35, 36). More recently, interpersonal therapy (IPT) has been adapted for older adults and showed reduction in suicidal ideation, depressive symptom severity, and increased meaning in life and social adjustment (37). Acceptance and commitment therapy (ACT) may also show promise on account of its transdiagnostic approach and evidence base in comorbid depression and physical health conditions (38). Dialectical behaviour therapy (DBT) has demonstrated utility in the treatment of depression in older patients with comorbid personality disorders (39). Personalised psychosocial treatment is important. It also offers support for developing or repairing relationships and social networks, as these have often deteriorated as a consequence of either depression or some causative factor.

Older Adults with Cognitive Impairment

This is a complex area, where control deficits and rigidity may play a role but exact mechanisms are not clear (40). Recent research also shows that older people who tried to end their lives were more prone to developing dementia at a later stage, independently of medical comorbidities and depression (41). A systematic review of suicidal behaviour in persons with dementia acknowledged that despite methodological limitations there does not appear to be an increased risk in comparison with people who do not have dementia (42). Suicide is rare but associated with comorbidity, particularly with depression, and there is an increased risk in those with young-onset dementia (42). Suicide attempts tend to occur early in the course of the disease. However, Draper (42) has highlighted that early and pre-symptomatic diagnosis (our common current example is Huntington's) may raise further ethical issues and discussions about so-called rational suicide. A 2019 systematic review of rational suicide, where the three authors – Gramaglia, Catali, and Zepegno – could not entirely agree on the conclusions, concedes that this is a real phenomenon in which mental disorder is excluded and capacity is not impaired, but points to 'silent' symptoms of depression and to the slippery slope from the right to die to the social obligation to die, as one perceives oneself as a burden to others (43).

While government targets encourage an early diagnosis of dementia, it is increasingly being realised that a diagnosis given early in the disease process can have significant unintended consequences, some of them harmful (44). The need to inform driving license authorities, the refusal of a travel insurance, and (sometimes) the pressure to hand over one's financial affairs are all potential threats to independence and autonomy. Given the complex relationship between mood, cognition, major life transitions, and suicidal ideation, there is a need to develop psychotherapeutic interventions adapted for older adults with cognitive impairment (45–47). Problem-solving therapy (PST) (45) and problem adaptation therapy (PATH) (46) are evidence-based therapies for late life depression in older adults with cognitive impairment. When compared to supportive therapy, PST has demonstrated the potential to reduce suicidal ideation during and after treatment (45–47).

Of vital importance, too, is acknowledging the high rates of depression, anxiety, and sense of hopelessness among those who act as family carers of people with dementia (48). A cross-sectional study of family carers found that 26 per cent had contemplated suicide more than once in the previous year, and only a half of those had ever told anyone about it (48).Therefore sensitive inquiry into the well-being of carers, mobilisation of supports, and assertive treatment of depression are also a vital aspect of dementia care.

Palliative Care for Older Patients

A desire to die is present in up to a half of terminally ill patients: there is a spectrum that runs from an accepting death to taking action to hasten it, making requests for assisted dying, and having suicidal ideation or plans. Meta-ethnographic studies of the wish to hasten death (WTHD) has identified that such thoughts often emerge as a result of multidimensional suffering, loss of self, fear, and a sense that death is the only way out (49). It has been found that depressive disorder and adjustment disorder are common in patients with a high WTHD. Between 8.5 and 17 per cent of older terminally ill patients have a desire to hasten death (HD), but the treatment of depression reduces HD thoughts (50).

The European Clinical Guidelines for the management of depression in palliative care endorse the evidence-based interventions of good palliative care, facilitating communication between family members, social support, and brief psychological interventions (51).

For patients with more severe depression or at imminent risk of harming themselves, the guidelines advise referral to specialist mental health services. There continues to be a need to integrate mental health and palliative care if one is to provide best practice.

Postvention: What to Do after a Person Takes Their Life

Suicide is a rare event but can define one lost life, and has reverberations way beyond its immediate aftermath. The importance of supporting families bereaved as a result of suicide has been highlighted in an updated national strategy (52). More recently there has been increasing evidence that exposure to suicide increases the risk of subsequent suicide, and a compelling case has been made for interventions for suicide loss survivors (53). The National Suicide Prevention Alliance (NSPA) and Public Health England (PHE) have developed a guide to providing local postvention services (52). Postvention relates to activities developed by or with people who have been bereaved as a result of suicide, in order to prevent adverse outcomes such as more suicide and to support recovery. It is recommend that families and carers be offered prompt and open information and appropriate and effective support.

There are various priorities for clinicians who have cared for patients who have taken their own lives: administrative issues, the well-being of the patient's family, the need for clinical review, training issues, and the well-being of the clinicians themselves (54). Among mental health professionals, some argue that the preparation for a future patient's suicide – which includes advanced clinical training and the development of appropriate procedures and supervision – should be considered an integral aspect of quality services, reflective practice, and meaningful self-care (55). For clinicians left behind by a death by suicide, there are many 'what if?' questions related to the role of chance (as described in our opening paragraph) and to their role in that patient's experience of care. Contact with bereaved families, coroners, and local health providers will be distressing, but these are necessary parts of learning a lesson and moving forward. It should also be noted that reduced rates of suicide have been found in services where there is consistent and stable staffing; and, when deaths by suicide have occurred, they have been reviewed with the patient's family and learning points have been developed (30). Ultimately, as clinicians, we reflect on the complexity of every death by suicide: we respond urgently to the elements we can change, and we work to mitigate every driver, even though many are outside of our control.

Acknowledgements

We thank three fantastic local colleagues in old age psychiatry for their comments on this chapter: Dr. Juliette Brown, Dr. Hugh Grant-Peterkin, and Dr. Rosie Smyth.

References

1. Van Orden, K., and Deming, C. Late-life suicide prevention strategies: Current status and future directions. *Curr Opin Psychol* 2018, 22: 79–83.

2. Garner, J. Psychodynamic work and older adults. *Advances in Psychiatric Treatment* 2002, 8(2): 128–35.

3. ONS. Suicides in the UK: 2018 registrations. Office for National Statistics, 2018. www.ons.gov.uk/peoplepopulationandcommunity/birthsdeathsandmarriages/deaths/bulletins/suicidesintheunitedkingdom/2018registrations.

4. Kiriakidis, S. Elderly suicide: Risk factors and preventative strategies. *Annals of Gerontology and Geriatric Research* 2015, 2(2): 1–6.

5. *The National Confidential Inquiry into Suicide and Safety in Mental Health.* University of Manchester, 2018. https://sites.manchester.ac.uk/ncish.

6. Murphy, E., Kapur, N., Webb, R., Purandare, N., Hawton, K., Bergen, H. et al. Risk factors for repetition and suicide following self-harm in older adults: Multicentre cohort study. *Br J Psychiatry* 2012, 200(5): 399–404.

7. Troya, M.I., Babatunde, O., Polidano, K., Bartlam, B., McCloskey, E., Dikomitis, L. et al. Self-harm in older adults: Systematic review. *Br J Psychiatry* 2019, 214(4): 186–200.

8. Conwell, Y. Suicide in later life: A review and recommendations for prevention. *Suicide and Life-Threatening Behavior* 2001, 31: 32–47.

9. Babor, T., Caetano, R., Casswell, S., Edwards, G., Giesbrecht, N., Graham, K. et al. *Alcohol: No Ordinary Commodity: Research and Public Policy* (2nd ed.). Oxford: Oxford University Press, 2010.

10. Marmot, M., and Bell, R. Fair society, healthy lives. *Public Health* 2012, 126 (Suppl. 1): S4–S10.

11. Cheong, E.V., Sinnott, C., Dahly, D., and Kearney, P.M. Adverse childhood experiences (ACEs) and later-life depression: Perceived social support as a potential protective factor. *BMJ Open* 2017, 7(9): e013228.

12. Cummins, I. The impact of austerity on mental health service provision: A UK perspective. *Int J Environ Res Public Health* 2018, 15(6).

13. Cattell, H. Suicidal behavior. In Copeland, J.R.M., Abou-Saleh, M.T., and Kumar, A. (eds), *Principles and Practice of Geriatric Psychiatry* (2nd ed.). Hobocken, NJ: John Wiley & Sons, Ltd, 2002, pp. 469–72.

14. Heisel, M.J., Duberstein, P.R., Lyness, J.M., and Feldman, M.D. Screening for suicide ideation among older primary care patients. *J Am Board Fam Med* 2010, 23(2): 260–9.

15. Hawton, K., and Pirkis, J. Suicide is a complex problem that requires a range of prevention initiatives and methods of evaluation. *Br J Psychiatry* 2017, 210(6): 381–3.

16. Faculty of Old Age Psychiatry and the Royal College of Psychiatrists. *Suffering in Silence: Age Inequality in Older People's Mental Health Care. College Report 221.* London: Royal College of Psychiarists, 2018.

17. Raue, P.J., Ghesquiere, A.R., and Bruce, M.L. Suicide risk in primary care: Identification and management in older adults. *Curr Psychiatry Rep* 2014, 16(9): 466.

18. Luoma, J.B., Martin, C.E., and Pearson, J.L. Contact with mental health and primary care providers before suicide: A review of the evidence. *Am J Psychiatry* 2002, 159(6): 909–16.

19. Esiwe, C., Baillon, S., Rajkonwar, A., Lindesay, J., Lo, N., Dennis, M. Screening for depression in older adults on an acute medical ward: The validity of NICE guidance in using two questions. *Age Ageing* 2015, 44(5): 771–5.

20. Hegeman, J.M., Kok, R.M., van der Mast, R.C., and Giltay, E.J. Phenomenology of depression in older compared with

younger adults: Meta-analysis. *Br J Psychiatry* 2012, 200(4): 275–81.

21. Collins, N., and Corna, L. General practitioner referral of older patients to improving access to psychological therapies (IAPT): An exploratory qualitative study. *BJPsych Bull* 2018, 42 (3): 115–18.

22. Lapierre, S., Erlangsen, A., Waern, M., De Leo, D., Oyama, H., Scocco, P. et al. A systematic review of elderly suicide prevention programs. *Crisis* 2011, 32(2): 88–98.

23. Conejero, I., Olie, E., Courtet, P., and Calati, R. Suicide in older adults: Current perspectives. *Clin Interv Aging* 2018, 13: 691–9.

24. Coventry, P., Lovell, K., Dickens, C., Bower, P., Chew-Graham, C., McElvenny, D. et al. Integrated primary care for patients with mental and physical multimorbidity: Cluster randomised controlled trial of collaborative care for patients with depression comorbid with diabetes or cardiovascular disease. *BMJ* 2015, 350: h638.

25. Hunkeler, E.M., Katon, W., Tang, L., Williams, J.W., Jr., Kroenke, K., Lin, E.H. et al. Long term outcomes from the IMPACT randomised trial for depressed elderly patients in primary care. *BMJ* 2006, 332(7536): 259–63.

26. Alexopoulos, G.S., Reynolds, C.F., 3rd, Bruce, M.L., Katz, I.R., Raue, P.J., Mulsant, B.H. et al. Reducing suicidal ideation and depression in older primary care patients: 24-month outcomes of the PROSPECT study. *Am J Psychiatry* 2009, 166(8): 882–90.

27. Shah, A., and Zarate-Escudero, S. Elderly suicide and suicide prevention: Mental health and illness of the elderly. *Mental Health and Illness Worldwide* 2017: 575–610.

28. Toot, S., Devine, M., and Orrell, M. The effectiveness of crisis resolution/home treatment teams for older people with mental health problems: A systematic review and scoping exercise. *Int J Geriatr Psychiatry* 2011, 26(12): 1221–30.

29. Erlangsen, A., Zarit, S.H., and Conwell, Y. Hospital-diagnosed dementia and suicide: A longitudinal study using prospective, nationwide register data. *Am J Geriatr Psychiatry* 2008, 16(3): 220–8.

30. Appleby, L., Hunt, I.M., and Kapur, N. New policy and evidence on suicide prevention. *Lancet Psychiatry* 2017, 4(9): 658–60.

31. Bickley, H., Hunt, I.M., Windfuhr, K., Shaw, J., Appleby, L., and Kapur, N. Suicide within two weeks of discharge from psychiatric inpatient care: A case-control study. *Psychiatr Serv* 2013, 64(7): 653–9.

32. Hedna, K., Andersson Sundell, K., Hamidi, A., Skoog, I., Gustavsson, S., and Waern, M. Antidepressants and suicidal behaviour in late life: A prospective population-based study of use patterns in new users aged 75 and above. *Eur J Clin Pharmacol* 2018, 74(2): 201–8.

33. Hooley, J.M., Franklin, J.C., and Nock, M.K. Chronic pain and suicide: Understanding the association. *Curr Pain Headache Rep* 2014, 18(8): 435.

34. Kellner, C.H., Fink, M., Knapp, R., Petrides, G., Husain, M., Rummans, T. et al. Relief of expressed suicidal intent by ECT: A consortium for research in ECT study. *Am J Psychiatry* 2005, 162(5): 977–82.

35. Wasserman, D., Rihmer, Z., Rujescu, D., Sarchiapone, M., Sokolowski, M., Titelman, D. et al. The European Psychiatric Association (EPA) guidance on suicide treatment and prevention. *Eur Psychiatry* 2012, 27(2): 129–41.

36. Allan, C.L., and Ebmeier, K.P. Review of treatment for late-life depression. *Advances in Psychiatric Treatment* 2018, 19(4): 302–9.

37. Heisel, M.J., Talbot, N.L., King, D.A., Tu, X.M., and Duberstein, P.R. Adapting interpersonal psychotherapy for older adults at risk for suicide. *Am J Geriatr Psychiatry* 2015, 23(1): 87–98.

38. Wetherell, J.L., Petkus, A.J., Alonso-Fernandez, M., Bower, E.S., Steiner, A.R., and Afari, N. Age moderates response to

acceptance and commitment therapy vs cognitive behavioral therapy for chronic pain. *Int J Geriatr Psychiatry* 2016, 31(3): 302–8.

39. Lynch, T.R., Cheavens, J.S., Cukrowicz, K.C., Thorp, S.R., Bronner, L., and Beyer, J. Treatment of older adults with co-morbid personality disorder and depression: A dialectical behavior therapy approach. *Int J Geriatr Psychiatry* 2007, 22(2): 131–43.

40. Bredemeier, K., and Miller, I.W. Executive function and suicidality: A systematic qualitative review. *Clin Psychol Rev* 2015, 40: 170–83.

41. Tu, Y.-A., Chen, M.-H., Tsai, C.-F., Su, T.-P., Bai, Y.-M., Li, C.-T. et al. Geriatric suicide attempt and risk of subsequent dementia: A nationwide longitudinal follow-up study in Taiwan. *Am J Geriatr Psychiatry* 2016, 24(12): 1211–8.

42. Draper, B.M. Suicidal behavior and assisted suicide in dementia. *Int Psychogeriatr* 2015, 27(10): 1601–11.

43. Gramaglia, C., Calati, R., and Zeppegno, P. Rational suicide in late life: A systematic review of the literature. *Medicina (Kaunas)* 2019, 55 (10): 656.

44. Brayne, C., and Kelly, S. Against the stream: Early diagnosis of dementia, is it so desirable? *BJPsych Bull* 2019, 43(3): 123–5.

45. Gustavson, K.A., Alexopoulos, G.S., Niu, G.C., McCulloch, C., Meade, T., and Arean, P.A. Problem-solving therapy reduces suicidal ideation in depressed older adults with executive dysfunction. *Am J Geriatr Psychiatry* 2016, 24(1): 11–7.

46. Kiosses, D.N., Ravdin, L.D., Gross, J.J., Raue, P., Kotbi, N., and Alexopoulos, G.S. Problem adaptation therapy for older adults with major depression and cognitive impairment: A randomized clinical trial. *JAMA Psychiatry* 2015, 72 (1): 22–30.

47. Gustavson, K.A., Alexopoulos, G.S., Niu, G.C., McCulloch, C., Meade, T., and

Areán, P.A. Problem-solving therapy reduces suicidal ideation in depressed older adults with executive dysfunction. *Am J of Geriatr Psychiatry* 2016, 24(1): 11–7.

48. O'Dwyer, S.T., Moyle, W., Zimmer-Gembeck, M., and De Leo, D. Suicidal ideation in family carers of people with dementia: A pilot study. *Int J Geriatr Psychiatry* 2013, 28(11): 1182–8.

49. Monforte-Royo, C., Villavicencio-Chavez, C., Tomas-Sabado, J., Mahtani-Chugani, V., and Balaguer, A. What lies behind the wish to hasten death? A systematic review and meta-ethnography from the perspective of patients. *PLoS ONE* 2012, 7(5): e37117.

50. Chochinov, H., and Breitbart, M. *Handbook of Psychiatry in Palliative Medicine* (2nd ed.). New York: Oxford University Press, 2009.

51. Rayner, L., Higginson, I., Price, A., and Hotopf, M. *The Management of Depression in Palliative Care: European Clinical Guidelines.* London: Department of Palliative Care, Policy & Rehabilitation European Palliative Care Collaboration, 2010.

52. PHE and NSPA. *Support after a Suicide: A Guide to Providing Local Services.* London: Public Health England & the National Suicide Prevention Alliance, 2016.

53. Jordan, J.R. Postvention is prevention: The case for suicide postvention. *Death Stud* 2017, 41(10): 614–21.

54. Gibbons, R., Brand, F., Carbonnier, A., Croft, A., Lascelles, K., Wolfart, G. et al. Effects of patient suicide on psychiatrists: Survey of experiences and support required. *BJPsych Bulletin* 2019, 43(05): 236–41.

55. Ellis, T., and Patel, A. Client suicide: What now? *Cognitive and Behavioral Practice* 2012, 19: 277–87.

56. Byrne, P., and Byrne, N. *Clinical Cases Uncovered: Psychiatry.* Oxford: Wiley Blackwell, 2018.

Fear and Anxiety in Acute Settings

Andrew Papadopoulos and Osama Refaat

For many older people, admission to an acute ward is likely to cause a significant degree of anxiety, particularly if they are experiencing confusion, loss, uncertainty surrounding their condition or illness, uncertainty surrounding their future, or if they have a history of struggling with change.

Both the nature and the magnitude of that anxiety is likely to have a significant impact upon a person's response to treatment and capacity to recover and may even pre-empt further physical illness and disability.

While fear and anxiety may prove disabling, they are normal phylogenetic responses to situations, challenges, or expectations that one perceives as threatening or capable of causing harm and in which one feels helpless or hopeless about being able to change one's circumstances for the better.

In acute care settings, anxiety, as well as other mood disorders, can easily go unnoticed in older adults. This may be explained by the complexity of their medical conditions, which in many cases absorb a considerable part of medical attention. Moreover, symptoms of anxiety are commonly subtle in this age group and often go undiagnosed. This contrasts with the significant impact they have on the group's health outcomes. Older people are more likely to minimise psychological distress, or rather convert it into physical symptoms that add to the complexity of the presentation in acute care settings. Somatic symptoms due to general medical conditions and somatic symptoms of anxiety are frequently present together in the same person. They are often difficult to disentangle and require equal attention from the medical team.

Hearing and visual impairment are associated with a higher risk of depression and anxiety in older patients, which adds a significant layer of complexity in acute, poorly lit, and noisy wards (1). The incidence of sensory impairment increases in relation to advancing age. Diminished acuity in vision or hearing (or in both) is frequently associated, in this age group, with difficulty in communicating. In some patients, this may increase the level of anxiety in their day-to-day interactions up to the point of avoidance. Older adults with sensory impairment may also experience a sense of compromised control over the surrounding environment. This may be associated with the fear of leaving the environment that they know and deem safe. Despite being an absolute necessity in most cases, hospital admission, with its sudden upheaval from the familiar home environment and move to a novel hospital environment, can be an anxiety-provoking experience, especially for older adults who suffer variable degrees of sensory impairment.

Patients with dementia may also find the hospital trip and the ward admission to be very stressful experiences (2). Loss of the ability to process new stimuli is an integral part of the lived experience of dementia. Thus, changes in the environment can induce significant confusion and disorientation. Moreover, anxiety can worsen attention, planning, and decision-making capacities, rendering the person with dementia less capable of effective communication with the medical staff in acute settings. Irritability and agitation in hospital wards are often an expression of the underlying physical or psychological discomfort that dementia patients struggle to communicate with any clarity. Providing medical care to dementia patients in acute care settings can be a challenging task. It is the responsibility of the treating staff to preserve patients' dignity while providing the necessary care. It is often useful to create a calm environment for patients, with minimal triggers and distractors. It is also important to provide reassurance and use calming phrases during communication. Sometimes allowing a caregiver to stay with the patient secures a familiar atmosphere and helps the patient to be calmer and less anxious.

Another group of patients that is considered to be generally vulnerable to anxiety and particularly in healthcare settings consists of migrant older adults who are ageing in countries different from their home countries (3). As a result of cultural and language barriers, they may perceive the healthcare services in their host countries as a challenging environment. In acute settings, patients may be anxious about accurately expressing their symptoms to clinicians. Fears may include that the clinician would not be able to help, would give the wrong medications, or would take the wrong decisions if the patient does not express him- or herself correctly. This can put extra pressure on the patient in emergency situations. Patients may also find it difficult to understand the clinician's language but feel embarrassed to ask. Encouraging patients to express themselves while listening and reflecting on what they say will have a good effect, because doing these things helps them feel listened to and enhances their trust in the medical staff. Bilingual healthcare staff and family members can act as interpreters in emergency and unplanned situations; however, where possible, it is always better to arrange for professional interpreters who are not directly involved in the patient's life and have no vested interest. Acknowledging cultural and religious differences whenever they arise can also have a reassuring effect on the patient and his or her caregivers (4).

Older patients with a primary diagnosis of anxiety disorder and with subthreshold anxiety symptoms have equally impaired functioning and increased disability (5). They also use health services more than age-matched controls (6). However, they are less likely to receive appropriate care (6). Comorbid depression and anxiety in older people are associated with higher risk of developing cardiovascular and cerebrovascular diseases (7, 8). Moreover, anxiety disorders that overlap with depression are prevalent after cardiovascular and cerebrovascular events (9). Studies report that anxiety occurs in about one quarter of stroke survivors (10). Additionally, the hospital environment, and especially the acute care experience, are often anxiety-provoking factors; they may trigger a stress response that would, in turn, have its impact on the process of healing and full functional recovery. This highlights the importance of screening for anxiety, assessing its severity, and accordingly integrating an appropriate management for anxiety into the overall care plan.

Normally people's anxiety can be alleviated with regular reassurance, improved social support and relationships, relevant and personalised solutions to their difficulties, or a change in their circumstances that enables them to enjoy a renewed sense of optimism. However, in some cases anxiety can be much more severe, complex, or resistant – enough to affect one's mental health, such that these people will require professional help and treatment by the psychiatry liaison team in order to experience a better quality of life. Factors that account for severe anxiety include:

- an existing mental and physical frailty, illness, and disability particularly in relation to dementia;
- the significance that one's current life circumstances and challenges have for them in relation to their personal welfare and sense of security;
- one's ability to tolerate existing long-term treatments and interventions;
- the availability and quality of social network and material support;
- the opportunity to engage in relevant and meaningful activities and lifestyles;
- Premorbid personality, temperament, and coping styles.

Common Features of Anxiety

1. Related to the autonomic–sympathetic nervous system: elevated heart and respiration rate, sweating, increased production of cortisol and adrenalin, reduction in visceral functioning, divergence of blood flow to major organs, tremor, increased inflammatory reactions
2. Related to emotion and behaviour: agitation, over- or under-compensation, avoidance, sleep disturbance, appetite disturbance (over- or under-eating), irritability, hypervigilance, hypersensitivity reactions, apprehension/fear/worry, reduced attention, concentration, and memory, reduced problem-solving ability

While our bodies are designed to cope with short-term emotional distress, longer-term or more intensive distress is detrimental and can give rise to:

- reduced immunity
- increased risk of mental illness (recurrent depression, psychosis, cognitive impairment)
- increased risk of self-neglect and self-harm
- increased risk of drug and alcohol dependency
- poor recovery from illness
- increased risk of relationship breakdown and social isolation
- loss of self-confidence and self-esteem
- increased risk of physical illness
- lower life expectancy

Types of Anxiety Reactions

Generalised Anxiety Disorder (GAD)

Persistent anxiety over six months, with uncontrollable worry, motor tension, vigilance, and scanning. Not specific to any situation or trigger. May involve persistent ruminative thoughts, concerns, or fears. Increased prevalence in vascular and cortical dementias.

ICD10 Diagnostic Criteria (11)

1. A period of at least six months of prominent tension, worry, and feelings of apprehension about everyday events and problems.
2. At least four symptoms from the following list must be present, of which at least one must be from items (a) to (d).

Autonomic arousal symptoms

    a. palpitations or pounding heart, or accelerated heart rate

    b. sweating

    c. trembling or shaking

    d. dry mouth (not as a result of medication or dehydration)

Symptoms concerning chest and abdomen

    e. difficulty breathing

    f. feeling of choking

    g. chest pain or discomfort

    h. nausea or abdominal distress (e.g. churning in stomach)

Symptoms concerning brain and mind

    i. feeling dizzy, unsteady, faint, or light-headed

    j. feelings that objects are unreal (derealisation), or that one's self is distant or 'not really here' (depersonalisation)

    k. fear of losing control, going crazy, or passing out

    l. fear of dying

General symptoms

    m. hot flushes or cold chills

    n. numbness or tingling sensations

Symptoms of tension

    o. muscle tension or aches and pains

    p. restlessness and inability to relax

    q. feeling keyed up, feeling on edge, or mental tension

    r. sensation of a lump in the throat, or difficulty with swallowing

Other non-specific symptoms

    s. exaggerated response to minor surprises or to being startled

    t. difficulty in concentrating, or mind going blank, because of worrying or anxiety

    u. persistent irritability

    v. difficulty getting to sleep because of worrying

3. The disorder does not meet the criteria for panic disorder (F41.0), phobic anxiety disorders (F40.-), obsessive–compulsive disorder (F42.-), or hypochondriacal disorder (F45.2).

4. Most commonly used exclusion criteria: not sustained by a physical disorder such as hyperthyroidism, an organic mental disorder (F0), or a psychoactive substance-related disorder (F1) such as excess consumption of amphetamine-like substances or withdrawal from benzodiazepines.

Acute Stress Reaction

Short-term anxiety symptoms (over a few days), in response to a stressful life event or challenge.

ICD10 Diagnostic Criteria (11)

A. Exposure to an exceptional mental or physical stressor.
B. Criterion A is followed by an immediate onset of symptoms (within one hour).
C. Two groups of symptoms are given; the acute stress reaction is graded as:

F43.00 mild if only (1) is fulfilled;
F43.01 moderate for (1) plus any two symptoms of (2); and
F43.02 severe for either

- (1) plus any four from (2)
    or
- dissociative stupor.
    1. the criteria B, C, and D for generalised anxiety disorder (F41.1)
    2. any of the following:
        a. withdrawal from expected social interaction;
        b. narrowing of attention;
        c. apparent disorientation;
        d. anger or verbal aggression;
        e. despair or hopelessness;
        f. inappropriate or purposeless overactivity;
        g. uncontrollable and excessive grief (judged by local cultural standards).

D. If the stressor is transient or can be relieved, the symptoms must begin to diminish after not more than eight hours. If the stressor continues, the symptoms must begin to diminish after not more than 48 hours.
E. Most commonly used exclusion criteria: it should occur without the current presence of any other mental or behavioural disorder in ICD10 (except for F41.1 (GAD) and F60 (personality disorders)), and not within three months of the end of an episode of any other mental or behavioural disorder.

Adjustment Reaction

Longer-term anxiety symptoms (1–6 months), in response to a stressful life event or a change in one's circumstances or lifestyle (e.g. loss, relocation, redundancy).

ICD10 Diagnostic Criteria (11)

A. Experience of an identifiable psychosocial stressor not of an unusual or catastrophic type, within one month of the onset of symptoms.
B. Symptoms or behaviour disturbance of the types found in any affective disorders (except delusions and hallucinations), in any disorders in F4 (neurotic, stress-related, and somatoform disorders), and in conduct disorders – so long as the criteria of an individual disorder are not fulfilled. Symptoms may be variable in both form and in severity.

Post-traumatic Stress Disorder (PTSD)

Severe anxiety symptoms, persistent after one month, in response to a life-threatening or catastrophic event. Symptoms would include the following: frequent intrusive thoughts and flashbacks of the trauma, with accompanying nightmares and poor sleep; sensitivity reactions to loud noise, bright light, or sudden social contact (startle response); hypervigilance and apprehension anxiety, reflecting a fear of harm; difficulty with attention, concentration, and memory; general irritability; avoidance behaviour in relation to the cause of the trauma or social situations, particularly crowds; depressed mood, loss of self-confidence; possible feelings of loss or guilt and a sense that harm or death could happen at any moment; loss of trust in the longevity of life (foreshortened future). Symptoms may occur as a recent problem or later on in life, often triggered by some event or experience (latent PTSD).

ICD10 Diagnostic Criteria (11)

A. Exposure to a stressful event or situation (either short- or long-lasting) of exceptionally threatening or catastrophic nature, which is likely to cause pervasive distress in almost anyone.
B. Persistent remembering or 'reliving' the stressor via intrusive flash backs, vivid memories, recurring dreams, or by experiencing distress when exposed to circumstances that resemble or are associated with the stressor.
C. Actual or preferred avoidance of circumstances resembling or associated with the stressor (not present before exposure to the stressor).
D. Either (1) or (2):

1. inability to recall, either partially or completely, some important aspects of the period of exposure to the stressor;
2. persistent symptoms of increased psychological sensitivity and arousal (not present before exposure to the stressor), shown by any two of the following:

   a. difficulty in falling or staying asleep;
   b. irritability or outbursts of anger;
   c. difficulty in concentrating;
   d. hypervigilance;
   e. exaggerated startle response.

E. Criteria B, C, and D all occurred within six months of the stressful event or at the end of a period of stress.

(For some purposes, an onset delayed for more than six months may be included, but this should be clearly specified separately.)

Phobias

Irrational fears leading to anxiety and avoidance. Fear may be learned or innate.

The most common phobias experienced by older people are underpinned by the following fears:

a. a fear of harm perpetrated either by the person who is caring for them or by outsiders;
b. a fear of falling, which may relate to concerns surrounding being left on the ground for long periods of time or experiencing severe pain;
c. a fear of loss, which may reflect loss of independence, loss of cognitive ability, loss of one's home, or loss of a loved one.

While such fears may be completely understandable in that they reflect common experiences in older cohorts, they can be considered phobic when both the likelihood of their occurrence within the person's life is limited and the avoidance response (often triggered by catastrophic thinking) is excessive and debilitating.

ICD10 Diagnostic Criteria (11)

A. Either (1) or (2):

    1. marked fear of a specific object or situation not included in agoraphobia (F40.0) or social phobia (F40.1);

    2. marked avoidance of such objects or situations.

    Among the most frequent objects or situations are animals, birds, insects, heights, thunder, flying, small enclosed spaces, the sight of blood or injury, injections, dentists, and hospitals.

B. Symptoms of anxiety in the feared situation at some time after the onset of the disorder, as defined in criterion B for F40.0 (Agoraphobia).

C. Significant emotional distress due to the symptoms or the avoidance, and a recognition that these are excessive or unreasonable.

D. Symptoms are restricted to the feared situation or to thinking about it.

    If desired, the specific phobias may be subdivided as follows:

- animal type (e.g. insects, dogs)
- nature-force type (e.g. storms, water)
- blood, injection, and injury type
- situational type (e.g. elevators, tunnels)

Dissociative Anxiety

Appearance of physical symptoms and manifestations, but without an identifiable cause (non-epileptic seizures or fugue states: amnesic reactions, hand tremor, paralysis, etc.)

Panic Disorder

Recurrent attacks of severe anxiety, often triggered by a specific thought or situation and accelerated by hyperventilation syndrome (25 per cent of pop). Panic attacks are often underpinned by a specific fear (e.g. fear of being left alone, fear of experiencing pain or suffering, fear of dying, fear of causing harm to others).

ICD10 Diagnostic Criteria (11)

A. Recurrent panic attacks, which are not consistently associated with a specific situation or object and often occur spontaneously (hence the episodes are unpredictable). The panic attacks are not associated with marked exertion or with exposure to dangerous or life-threatening situations.

B. A panic attack is characterised by all of the following:

    a. it is a discrete episode of intense fear or discomfort;

    b. it starts abruptly;

    c. it reaches a crescendo within a few minutes and lasts for at least some minutes;

d. at least four symptoms must be present from the list below, one of which must be from items (1) to (4):

Autonomic arousal symptoms

1. palpitations or pounding heart or accelerated heart rate
2. sweating
3. trembling or shaking
4. dry mouth (not as a result of medication or dehydration)

Symptoms concerning chest and abdomen

5. difficult breathing
6. feeling of choking
7. chest pain or discomfort
8. nausea or abdominal distress (e.g. churning in stomach)

Symptoms concerning brain and mind

9. feeling dizzy, unsteady, faint, or light-headed
10. feelings that objects are unreal (derealisation), or that one's self is distant or 'not really here' (depersonalisation)
11. fear of losing control, going crazy, or passing out fear of dying

General symptoms

12. hot flushes or cold chills
13. numbness or tingling sensations

C. Most commonly used exclusion criteria: the attack is not due to a physical disorder, organic mental disorder (F0), or other mental disorders such as schizophrenia and related disorders (F20–29), affective disorders (F30–39), or somatoform disorders (F45).

Obsessive Compulsive Disorder

May involve regular and intrusive negative thoughts, on their own or accompanied by ritualistic behaviour (or both). Components include an underlying fear of harm to self and others or a fear of disorder and disorganisation, an exaggerated or irrational belief in the immediacy and inevitability of the realisation of the feared scenario, with resultant anxiety in the presence of a specific stimulus or trigger, impaired caudate nucleus that fails to divert or inhibit the intrusive thoughts, and accompanying neutralising activities or rituals (overt and covert), which reduce the anxiety but can themselves become disabling and debilitating for the individual concerned and his or her relationships.

ICD10 Diagnostic Criteria (11)

A. Either obsessions or compulsions (or both), present on most days, for a period of at least two weeks.

B. Obsessions (thoughts, ideas, or images) and compulsions (acts) share the following features, all of which must be present:

1. They are acknowledged as originating in the mind of the patient and are not imposed by outside persons or influences.
2. They are repetitive and unpleasant, and at least one obsession or compulsion must be present that is acknowledged as excessive or unreasonable.
3. The subject tries to resist them (but resistance to some obsessions or compulsions may be minimal if they are very long-standing). At least one obsession or compulsion must be present that is unsuccessfully resisted.
4. Carrying out the obsessive thought or compulsive act is not in itself pleasurable. (This should be distinguished from temporary relief of tension or anxiety).

C. The obsessions or compulsions cause distress or interfere with the subject's social or individual functioning, usually by wasting time.
D. Most commonly used exclusion criteria: the obsession and compulsions are not due to other mental disorders, such as schizophrenia and related disorders (F2), or mood [affective] disorders (F3).

Prevalence in a Hospital Setting

Studies vary considerably; this is a reflection of their geography and of the methodology and assessment tools they deploy. However, as a general rule, they tend to converge on a few basics.

Anxiety disorders show a prevalence of around 10 per cent in the 55+ population, of which 7 per cent are GAD. However, comorbid anxiety with depression is more prevalent than depression or anxiety alone (12). Lenze (2003) (13) suggests that in older people anxiety and depression should be considered to form a continuum.

Fifty per cent of anxiety disorders graduated from adult years, the other 50 per cent are of more recent onset. Comorbid anxiety and depression are predicted by events of loss, ill health, and functional disability. Anxiety alone is predicted by long-standing personality and genetic factors (14–16), for example poor problem-solving ability and negative problem orientation, fear of harm, loneliness, and isolation. Chronic anxiety is predictive of later cognitive impairment (17).

Management

There is no one-size-fits-all approach to the management of anxiety in older people. A comprehensive management plan is required that takes into account the medical, psychological, and social aspects of each individual.

An important part in the management of anxiety in older populations is to revise the patient's current medications and substance history. Older people are generally more sensitive to medication effects, so drug-induced anxiety is not uncommon in this age group. Medications such as corticosteroids, thyroid hormones, oestrogen, antihistamines, Interferon, TNF-alpha, and psychotropics may be associated with anxiety symptoms. Dose adjustment and the replacement or cessation (if possible) of the causative agent will be the treatment of choice, as it avoids burdening the patient with additional medications.

Older people who suffer from anxiety may self-medicate, thus misusing alcohol or benzodiazepines in order to get help with a common problem such as insomnia. It is well established that these substances have a high likelihood of causing dependence and tolerance. People may also self-medicate on over-the-counter medications or medications bought on the Internet. In acute care settings, patients may suffer from anxiety as an integral part of withdrawal from these substances. Hence it is important for clinicians to collect substance history from the patient or from one of the patient's carers who can provide adequate collateral information.

Many treatment approaches are available to clinicians when managing anxiety in older people. Decisions should be based on assessments of the severity and extent of the distress or impairment, as well as on patient preference. An anxiety of mild severity can effectively be alleviated by building a strong therapeutic alliance with the patient. Empathic listening to the patient's fears and illness-related beliefs can considerably improve the clinician's ability to educate the patient about his or her illness and to correct any faulty beliefs that exacerbate anxiety. On the other hand, moderate and severe anxiety often requires psychological treatment, pharmacological treatment, or both combined. Hence it is often useful to assess the severity of anxiety. Rating scales (also covered in Chapter 21) can be a helpful tool to aid this process. Despite the availability of many anxiety rating scales for adults, only a few are suitable for older people: the Short Anxiety Screening Test (SAST), which is a self-report ten-item scale with four-point Likert responses (18), and the Geriatric Anxiety Inventory (GAI), which contains twenty dichotomous items (agree/disagree) (19). GAI also has a shorter five-item version for screening (20).

Psychosocial Treatments

Psychosocial treatments reflect a broad range of non-medical and evidence-based interventions involving activities, discourse, or environmental changes that address a person's needs or treatment goals.

Psychosocial treatments will vary depending on the underlying causes for the person's emotional difficulties, his or her particular preferences for and tolerances of specific interventions, and any contextual influences that can affect the availability and relevance of interventions.

Psychosocial treatments fall into three main types.

Psychological Therapies

Psychological therapies are designed to help the individual and the family change the way in which they appraise and manage their difficulties. They tend to fall into one of three categories: interventions that focus upon cognitive and behavioural processes, known as cognitive–behavioural therapies; interventions that focus upon repressed feelings and drives, known as analytical therapies; and interventions that consider the person as part of a dynamic system, which is in a constant state of flux and transition; these are known as systemic or family therapies.

Such treatments should be undertaken by trained professionals. They include cognitive behaviour therapy (CBT), cognitive analytical therapy (CAT), schema therapy, acceptance and commitment therapy (ACT), mindfulness therapy, counseling, specialist trauma focused cognitive behaviour therapy, eye movement desensitisation and reprocessing (EMDR) therapy, longer-term psychotherapy, psychoanalysis, dialectical behaviour therapy (DBT), and behavioural and systemic family therapy.

Cognitive Behavioural Therapies

Cognitive behavioural approaches seek to identify and change negative, self-limiting, or maladaptive beliefs that people engage with and that tend to limit the extent to which they are capable of exercising control and influence over their fears. Such beliefs can be considered in a number of ways:

➤ *Awfullising*: the individual only engages in the negative aspects of their lives and experiences.
➤ *Exaggerating*: the issue of concern becomes overinflated by comparison with what it should be.
➤ *Catastrophising*: the individual believes that the outcome of a problem, of his or her attempts to cope with it, or indeed of own life will inevitably be negative or catastrophic.
➤ *Magical*: the individual overinvests or is overly optimistic about the ability of an intervention, treatment, or change in circumstances to alleviate his or her problems.

Interventions involve helping people to rethink or reframe the way in which they view their fears and worries and the consequences it has upon their lives. Such interventions may involve offering alternative views, providing education, or setting up behavioural experiments in which a person's actions and achievements in a given task or goal will challenge and change the original negative or self-limiting belief into a positive or self-enabling belief. At times, working psychologically in this way will also require engagement with other, multidisciplinary interventions and practitioners, to assist in meeting the therapeutic goals. For people who have experienced some kind of life-threatening trauma, and particularly if they have post-traumatic stress symptoms, referral to a competent practitioner in trauma-focused CBT or EMDR could be recommended.

Analytical Psychotherapy

Analytical therapy involves a range of approaches drawn from a variety of analytical schools of psychotherapy (Freudian, Jungian, etc.). Each approach will have its own theoretical framework and methods, but will address personality factors that are influential in supporting one's emotional well-being, integrity of personality, and healthy adjustment in response to various challenges – for example the ones that people face in illness, disability, and acute admissions to hospital.

A principal focus of psychoanalytical approaches is on helping the person to identify and manage those psychological *defense* mechanisms that operate to protect one's personality from harm. Common defenses are described in Table 14.1.

Therapy places great emphasis upon the relationship between the therapist and the client; the therapist may become, in the eyes of the client, an object of love, intimacy, parenting, hate, or abandonment. Such *transferences* are encouraged as a way of helping the client work through his or her repressed feelings or emotions. Transferences are based upon the notion that much of what creates anxiety and depression is grounded in the relationships that we have had throughout our lives, and particularly during our childhood.

Table 14.1 Psychological Defenses

Mechanism	Description	Function	Example
Repression	This involves repressing painful or difficult feelings, thoughts, or experiences by pushing them into the unconscious mind.	Protects people from being overwhelmed by their feelings, when such feelings could have the potential of harming or disabling them.	Trying not to think about a distressing thought or feeling; deliberately distracting oneself from a painful conversation.
Denial	This involves stopping painful or unwanted experiences from having to be confronted.	Protects people from the potentially deleterious consequences of having to face their experiences and fears. Denial can be complete or partial	Firmly believing that one's illness is not terminal, or that the doctor is lying about the illness.
Projection	This involves a person's attributing to another person his or her own unacceptable, antisocial, or distasteful feelings, desires, or thoughts about him- or herself.	Protects people from having to accept that they may not be the person that they believe themselves to be but are instead insecure, disloyal, bad, anti-social, selfish, disgraceful, etc.	Blaming the doctors for being diabetic rather than accepting that maybe one has caused the problem through unhealthy living.
Sublimation & Displacement	This involves meeting one's need for gratification, comfort, intimacy, or security from one source or object instead of another.	Ensures that the person remains satisfied or does not have to suffer in any way.	Meeting one's desire for acceptance, warmth, and affirmation, say, from the nursing staff rather than from one's family.
Regression	This involves engaging in a way of being (or responding to a situation) that resembles a way of being (or responding) from an earlier point in the person's life.	The chosen response is one that is likely to have worked successfully in the past and ensures that the person remains safe, stable or in control	Refusing to take medication, or going absent without telling anyone

Systemic Therapies

It is important to recognise that older people's lives are deeply embedded within family, friends, community, and faith. Most older people not only live with, or in close contact with, family but also rely on family for support, connection, love, and purpose. The length of time older people have existed within familial relationships (e.g. with siblings) can vary between 70 and 80 years, and within relationships with children it comes up to possibly 50 years. Understandably, therefore, families and family relationships are key to the well-being of older people (21). Accordingly, families are also challenged by issues arising from a relative's frailty, illness, or disability and consequent admission into acute care. Family members and the wider family, too, are likely to undergo major transitions in their lives if that relative has to experience other and perhaps more permanent transitions, such as into residential care.

The aim of working with families in the context of acute care is to assist the family 'system' to find new ways of coping, relating, and developing, so as to address success-fully the transition and the accompanying challenges that have arisen in their lives as a result of illness or disability and have not been successfully resolved through the use of previously learned coping strategies or resources.

Considering the family as a *system* means recognising that families are more than the sum of the individuals contained in them and that family processes themselves have qualities of their own and exist over and above those of the individuals within the family. As a system, a family is characterised by its norms, rules, expectations, and roles, which are passed down through the generations. Families also exist in a wider systemic context: that of the community and culture they live in – and these in turn have their own norms, expectations, rules, and roles.

In particular, families are characterised by

- ➤ *boundaries*: what is permissible and not permissible in the way individuals relate to one another and to their wider culture and in how they live their lives;
- ➤ *hierarchies*: how status and power are distributed and maintained within the family and how relationships between family members should be defined;
- ➤ *role flexibility*: the capacity that individuals have to adapt to roles in the context of new challenges;
- ➤ *congruent communication*: the ability of family members to communicate effectively, both within the family and outside it, the messages and meanings that they are attempting to communicate;
- ➤ *goodness of fit*: how well the family is able to connect to, be part of, adapt to, and integrate into its community, culture, and lifestyle;
- ➤ *being closed versus being open*: the extent to which families are open to the outside world and are able to accept help, support, and engagement with others. Closed families are characterised by a tendency to remain tightknit and their members have very clear expectations, roles, and ways of behaving with one another;
- ➤ *enmeshment versus differentiation*: the extent to which family members are free to live autonomously and independently within the family while remaining emotionally close and cohesive. Individuals within enmeshed families tend to form interdependent relationships, where boundaries are often lacking or confused;
- ➤ *themes, beliefs, patterns, and scripts*: how the family defines and articulates itself in the wider world in relation to its social and cultural identity, its history and roots, its beliefs and values, its faith and community participation.

Considering families as a system is to view the problems within a family not as 'pathologised', but rather as transitions in which family members have struggled to adapt and in which earlier strategies have not worked. As a result, the system has become stuck, and anxiety was generated. Often the *problems* that families present with can be viewed as their *solutions* to the struggles and challenges they face. As such, families at highest risk of negative outcomes are those that have:

> lack of adequate resources (personal, financial, practical, social, and emotional);
> too many demands;
> poor communication;
> difficulty with role flexibility or adaptive coping styles (rigidity);
> difficulty in accepting help or in engaging with services;
> unresolved anger, conflicts, or ruptures within relationships;
> overly enmeshed or, conversely, overly alienated relationships.

Accordingly, the role of services is to enable and empower families to achieve positive (meaningful, relevant, effective, and stable) transitions by helping them to:

> gain knowledge about and awareness of the changes, conditions, and challenges they face;
> make relevant and meaningful choices regarding the care, services, and interventions they need;
> access and mobilise relevant and adequate resources;
> develop communication;
> develop and maintain new coping styles, skills, or competences;
> resolve conflicts;
> negotiate roles, expectations, and actions;
> grieve their losses;
> identify new meanings and ways for their members to relate to one another;
> identify and access experiences that nurture, support, and enhance quality of life among their members.

The experience of anxiety is likely to reflect family dynamics significantly, and in a number of ways. For example, it may serve to keep family members together; it may help to divert from other problems that the family is facing; or it may be a way of communicating anger or fear about some family members (22).

Movement Desensitisation and Reprocessing

Sometimes hospital-related anxieties and phobias have their roots in the past and are linked to earlier traumatic experiences within a medical setting. These traumatic memories may be too intense for the brain to process, and their unprocessed emotional content can be readily brought up in triggering situations (e.g. when an elderly patient is admitted to a medical care facility). Eye movement desensitisation and reprocessing therapy is rapidly gaining acceptance worldwide as an approved therapeutic approach to deal with past traumatic experiences and their psychological consequences. It desensitises the brain's and the body's responses to traumatic memories. It works with the brain's adaptive information processing (AIP) system to modify the emotional intensity of distressing past experiences. It works well in PTSD, but also in many forms of anxiety, including phobias, panic attacks, and obsessive–compulsive disorder (OCD). The main advantage of EMDR is that it doesn't require full recollection or verbal description of the past traumatic experiences.

Lifestyle Counseling and Coaching

This approach places a focus on exercise, dietary management, social and occupational activities, social relationships, sleep enhancement, and relaxation techniques. Research has recently pointed to the important role that these factors have in both preventing and recovering from anxiety states. Exercise in particular has been shown to be a prophylactic against suffering from both anxiety and depression, and it enhances recovery in those who have experienced depression (37). A variety of professions allied to medicine have important roles to play in this area. These professions are represented by occupational therapists, physiotherapists, dieticians and nutritionists, activity workers, professional coaches, and counsellors.

Building Self-Confidence

While self-esteem has been shown to remain relatively resistant in people over the age of 65, self-confidence can waiver as a result of increasing frailty, loss of abilities, increasing challenges to adopt new ways of functioning or solving problems, or simple attempts to adapt to new and complex environments.

Research undertaken on cognitive ageing suggests that, unlike younger people, older people are more likely to function better using existing well learned skills and abilities rather than attempting to develop new ways of adapting. This is not to say that new skills can't be developed, but rather that they may take longer and may necessitate the person to experience multiple failures before the task is accomplished. Selective optimisation with compensation (SOC) is the name of an approach that seeks to identify a person's existing skills and abilities selectively and to apply them to the challenges that that person faces, while compensating for skills and abilities that are unavailable or may be too problematic to learn. This approach forms the basis of Baltes and Baltes's view of successful aging (23). Here building upon a person's existing strengths while providing that person with compensatory aids and adaptations to his or her environment reflects how this approach is often articulated within rehabilitation programs.

Another approach that has been shown to be highly effective in training people who may have lost some of their abilities in daily living is called 'chaining' (36). In chaining, the task in hand is broken down into small achievable components. Each component is learned, then connected to the next component, until a whole sequence is learned.

A third approach is to change the task demands themselves where possible, so that tasks may be undertaken from within the person's existing repertoire of skills and abilities.

Regardless of approach, care needs to be taken to ensure that the person is able to experience success at the task in hand, so consideration would need to be given to task relevance, timing, available support, and people's capacity to endure what may turn out to be a lengthy and difficult task.

Mindfulness-Based Techniques

A mindfulness approach to managing anxiety is grounded in the teachings of Bhuddism, where self-compassion, focused attention, choiceless awareness, and acceptance are fundamental ways of being that are applied to fear (24). The use of focused relaxation, visual imagery techniques, self-reassurance, ongoing awareness of one's own bodily processes, and engagement with the world around us, together with the exercise of focusing one's attention on the moment, are central to a mindfulness approach. Mindfulness teaching requires both time and practise and should be considered more as a way of living one's life in the context of persistent pain than simply as a set of helpful techniques to control or manage fear and anxiety.

Pharmacological Treatment

Anxiety disorders in older people generally respond well to drug treatment. However, specific phobias respond better to behavioural therapies such as systematic desensitisation. A meta-analysis of clinical trials assessing the efficacy of psychotropic medications in the management of GAD in older population found that medication was superior to the control condition with a pooled odds ratio of 0.32 (95 per cent confidence interval: 0.18–0.54) (25). Effective medications include benzodiazepines, antidepressants, and atypical antipsychotics. In many cases, a comprehensive management plan that includes both psychosocial interventions and psychotropic medications can be applied. Priorities are set according to the patient's preference, as well as according to the clinician's judgement on individualised cases.

Benzodiazepines

Benzodiazepines bind to and allosterically modulate $GABA_A$ receptors, rendering them more sensitive to GABA (γ-aminobutyric acid). The facilitation of the inhibitory GABAergic projections to arousal centres results in sedative, hypnotic, and anxiolytic effects. Tolerance develops rapidly, especially with shorter-half-life benzodiazepines, and this can result in an exacerbation of anxiety symptoms. Hence the key to an appropriate use of benzodiazepines in the management of anxiety is short-term use (2–4 weeks), because long-term use often results in tolerance and more severe withdrawal phenomenon upon discontinuation. Benzodiazepines can also be used while other treatments are initially introduced (such as psychosocial treatment or antidepressants). Side effects associated with the use of benzodiazepines in the elderly include increased risk of falls, which cause fractures, delirium, and confusion; increased risk of cognitive impairment; and anterograde amnesia. In addition, paradoxical disinhibition with increased excitement, irritability, aggression, and impulsivity may occur in a small proportion of elderly people who take benzodiazepines (26).

Benzodiazepines are also considered a drug of choice in the management of the different stages of alcohol withdrawal, including delirium tremens. In addition to their protective effect against seizures, they are also effective in alleviating the intense anxiety and feelings of impending doom that are frequently associated with delirium tremens and alcohol withdrawal. This result is explained by the GABA enhancing effects of benzodiazepines similar to alcohol. Long-acting agents such as diazepam and chlordiazepoxide provide relatively stable plasma levels. Thus they facilitate a smooth alcohol withdrawal, with minimal rebound symptoms. But a disadvantage of these agents is that they depend largely on hepatic metabolism, which is commonly impaired in chronic alcohol users. Benzodiazepines with shorter half-life that do not undergo hepatic metabolism, such as oxazepam and temazepam, may be more suitable for patients with hepatic impairment or for older patients, whom heavy sedation could predispose to serious medical conditions such as respiratory failure.

Antidepressants

Although their use is not free of complications, antidepressants, particularly SSRIs, are usually considered the first-line pharmacological treatment of anxiety disorders in older people; such disorders include GAD, panic, social phobia, OCD, and PTSD. Unlike benzodiazepines, antidepressants have slower onset of action. This is due to the time required to lower the sensitivity of serotonin autoreceptors, and thus to increase synaptic serotonin. As a general rule, in elderly patients antidepressants are usually started at half the usual starting dose for younger adults, and dose titration goes up slowly.

Introducing SSRIs is commonly associated with initial anxiety, which may exacerbate a pre-existing anxiety. This is particularly significant in older people, who are known to be sensitive to medication effects. There are a few good strategies to deal with initial anxiety, including a very slow up-titration of the dose, or adding benzodiazepines in the first few weeks, then tapering them. There seems to be little difference between the available SSRIs in point if efficacy. Citalopram, escitalopram, and sertraline are thought to have the best safety profiles for older people; this is due to their low cytochrome P450 interactions, and thus lower drug–drug interaction profile. However, citalopram and escitalopram are dose-dependently associated with prolonged QT corrected interval. Thus they should be used with caution, and in doses lower than 20 mg for citalopram and 10 mg for escitalopram (27). Paroxetine is generally used less in older people because of its anticholinergic side effects, potent P450 inhibition, and short half-life, which causes significant withdrawal symptoms. Fluoxetine has the longest half-life of the SSRIs and is therefore associated with fewer withdrawal symptoms upon discontinuation. However, it is not generally considered the first choice for older people, as it is a potent inhibitor of hepatic cytochrome P450 and is thus associated with a high drug–drug interaction profile.

Further prescribing warnings are about older age, female gender, concomitant use of diuretics, low body weight, and lower baseline serum sodium concentration, all of which are considered risk factors for SSRI-induced hyponatremia. Older people on anticoagulation or antiplatelet drugs who receive SSRI are at an increased risk of bleeding. SSRIs can also cause sexual dysfunction and gastrointestinal upset. Regarding the SSRI-related risk of suicide, treatment with SSRIs in older adults is associated with a reduced suicide risk, unlike in the younger age groups, where higher risk is reported (28).

Buspirone is a 5 HT1A receptor partial agonist that has been used to alleviate moderate to severe GAD in the elderly. Generally it has a favourable risk-to-benefit profile. Compared to benzodiazepines, buspirone has a slower onset of action (typically two to four weeks) and is not effective when used as needed. There is no associated risk of physical dependence or withdrawal with buspirone. However, it may not be effective in patients who have had previous treatment with benzodiazepines. Buspirone is metabolised by cytochrome P450, CYP3A4, and has a number of potential drug–drug interactions. Most common side-effects are nausea and headache. These effects are usually alleviated with the continuation of therapy and with slower dose titration. Buspirone has minimal sexual side effects and may even be used in augmentation with SSRIs, to relieve their common sexual side effects. Buspirone is contraindicated in patients who use monoamine oxidase inhibitors, including the antibiotic linezolid, as it poses a high risk of serotonin syndrome.

The atypical antidepressant mirtazapine is generally well tolerated in older people. Its anxiolytic, sedative, and appetite-promoting actions make it a good choice when anxiety is associated with insomnia or appetite loss. It undergoes hepatic metabolism via cytochrome P450. Its clearance is markedly reduced in older people and in patients with moderate to severe hepatic or renal impairment. In these patient groups, it is advisable to start with lower, initially adjusted doses. Side effects include drowsiness, weight gain, elevated serum cholesterol, and the less common but more serious agranulocytosis.

Other classes of antidepressants include the selective noradrenaline reuptake inhibitor (SNRIs) (e.g. venlafaxine, desvenlafaxine and duloxetine). Venlafaxine has been found effective for treating anxiety symptoms in older people. It is associated with a side effect profile similar to that of SSRIs. In addition, it is associated with dose-dependent elevation of the diastolic blood pressure (29), and the rate of discontinuation is higher with venlafaxine than with escitalopram (30). These findings may suggest that SSRIs are better tolerated as first-line agents for the management of anxiety in older adults. Another class of antidepressants that has been shown to be effective in the treatment of anxiety are tricyclic antidepressants. However, their high side effect profile, anticholinergic load, and cardiac side effects make them less suitable for use in older adults.

Vortioxetine is a relatively novel antidepressant, which enhances serotonergic transmission and acts as a serotonin receptor modulator. On the basis of the available data, it is thought to be well tolerated by older adults, and has relatively few side effects that impact cognitive functions, wakefulness, and metabolic and electrocardiogram parameters (31, 32). Moreover, data from three randomised clinical trials point out its potential benefits for cognition in patients with cognitive impairment (33). However, further evidence is required in this regard. The usual starting dose in the older people is 5 mg, which is half the adult starting dose.

Other Medications

There is limited evidence for the use of second-generation antipsychotics, particularly risperidone and quetiapine, in the management of anxiety in older adults and in cases of dementia complicated with behavioural and psychological symptoms (25). However, atypical antipsychotics have a black box warning for increased mortality in elderly patients with dementia. They are also associated with an increased risk of cerebrovascular events (34). Anticonvulsants such as pregabalin and gabapentin show some evidence for use in GAD and social phobia (35). However, they lack evidence for use in older adults. Beta blockers, particularly propranolol, have been used to control physical symptoms of anxiety such as tremors, sweating, and palpitations, but prescribers should be aware of the risk of postural hypotension and of the subsequent risk of falls and fractures.

References

1. Simning, A., Fox, M.L., Barnett, S.L., Sorensen, S., and Conwell, Y. Depressive and anxiety symptoms in older adults with auditory, vision, and dual sensory impairment. *J Aging Health* 2019, 31(8): 1353–75.

2. Silwanowicz, R.M., Maust, D.T., Seyfried, L.S., Chiang, C., Stano, C., and Kales, H.C. Management of older adults with dementia who present to emergency services with neuropsychiatric symptoms. *Int J Geriatr Psychiatry* 2017, 32(12): 1233–40.

3. Zisberg, A. Anxiety and depression in older patients: The role of culture and

acculturation. *Int J Equity in Health* 2017, 16(1): 177.

4. Putsch, R.W. III, and Joyce, M. Dealing with patients from other cultures. In Walker, H. K., Hall, W.D., Hurst, J.W. (eds), *Clinical Methods: The History, Physical, and Laboratory Examinations* (3rd ed.). Boston, MA: Butterworths, 1990. www.ncbi.nlm.nih .gov/books/NBK340.

5. Grenier, S., Préville, M., Boyer, R., O'Connor, K., Béland, S.-G., Potvin, O. et al. The impact of DSM-IV symptom and clinical significance criteria on the prevalence estimates of subthreshold and threshold anxiety in the older adult population. *Am J Geriatr Psychiatry* 2011, 19(4): 316–26.

6. de Beurs, E., Beekman, A.T., van Balkom, A.J., Deeg, D.J., van Dyck, R., and van Tilburg, W. Consequences of anxiety in older persons: Its effect on disability, well-being and use of health services. *Psychological Medicine* 1999, 29(3): 583–93.

7. Moscati, A., Flint, J., and Kendler, K.S. Classification of anxiety disorders comorbid with major depression: Common or distinct influences on risk? *Depression and Anxiety* 2016, 33(2): 120–7.

8. Tully, P.J., Harrison, N.J., Cheung, P., and Cosh, S. Anxiety and cardiovascular disease risk: A review. *Curr Cardiol Rep* 2016, 18(12): 120.

9. Murphy, B., Le Grande, M., Alvarenga, M., Worcester, M., and Jackson, A. Anxiety and depression after a cardiac event: Prevalence and predictors. *Front Psychol* 2019, 10: 3010.

10. Li, W., Xiao, W.M., Chen, Y.K., Qu, J.F., Liu, Y.L., Fang, X.W. et al. Anxiety in patients with acute ischemic stroke: Risk factors and effects on functional status. *Front Psychiatry* 2019, 10: 257.

11. World Health Organization. *International Statistical Classification of Diseases and Related Health Problems: Tenth Revision* (ICD10). WHO, 2014. www.who.int/ health-topics/#C.

12. Flint, A.J. Generalised anxiety disorder in elderly patients: Epidemiology, diagnosis and treatment options. *Drugs Aging* 2005, 22(2): 101–14.

13. Lenze, E.J. Comorbidity of depression and anxiety in the elderly. *Curr Psychiatry Rep* 2003, 5(1): 62–7.

14. Schoevers, R.A., Deeg, D.J., van Tilburg, W., and Beekman, A.T. Depression and generalized anxiety disorder: Co-occurrence and longitudinal patterns in elderly patients. *Am J Geriatr Psychiatry* 2005, 13(1): 31–9.

15. Forsell, Y., and Winblad, B. Feelings of anxiety and associated variables in a very elderly population. *Int J Geriatr Psychiatry* 1998, 13(7): 454–8.

16. Kant, G., D'Zurilla, T., and Maydeu-Olivares, A. Social problem solving as a mediator of stress-related depression and anxiety in middle-aged and elderly community residents. *Cognitive Therapy and Research* 1997, 21: 73–96.

17. Sinoff, G., and Werner, P. Anxiety disorder and accompanying subjective memory loss in the elderly as a predictor of future cognitive decline. *Int J Geriatr Psychiatry* 2003, 18(10): 951–9.

18. Sinoff, G., Ore, L., Zlotogorsky, D., and Tamir, A. Short Anxiety Screening Test: A brief instrument for detecting anxiety in the elderly. *Int J Geriatr Psychiatry* 1999, 14(12): 1062–71.

19. Pachana, N.A., Byrne, G.J., Siddle, H., Koloski, N., Harley, E., and Arnold, E. Development and validation of the Geriatric Anxiety Inventory. *International Psychogeriatrics / IPA* 2007, 19(1): 103–14.

20. Byrne, G.J., and Pachana, N.A. Development and validation of a short form of the Geriatric Anxiety Inventory: The GAI-SF. *International Psychogeriatrics / IPA* 2011, 23(1): 125–31.

21. Papadopoulos, A., Biggs, S., and Tinker, A. Wellbeing in later life: A proposed ecosystematic framework. *British Journal of Wellbeing* 2011, 2: 22–31.

22. Neidhardt, E.R., and Allen, J.A. *Family Therapy with the Elderly*. Newbury Park, CA: SAGE, 1993.

23. Baltes, P.B., and Baltes, M.M. *Successful Aging: Perspectives from the Behavioral Sciences*. New York: Cambridge University Press, 1993.

24. Hilton, L., Hempel, S., Ewing, B.A., Apaydin, E., Xenakis, L., Newberry, S. et al. Mindfulness meditation for chronic pain: Systematic review and meta-analysis. *Ann Behav Med* 2017, 51(2): 199–213.

25. Goncalves, D.C., and Byrne, G.J. Interventions for generalized anxiety disorder in older adults: Systematic review and meta-analysis. *J Anxiety Disord* 2012, 26(1): 1–11.

26. Sachdeva, A., Choudhary, M., and Chandra, M. Alcohol withdrawal syndrome: Benzodiazepines and beyond. *Journal of Clinical and Diagnostic Research* 2015, 9(9): VE01–VE7.

27. Medicines and Healthcare Products Regulatory Agency. Citalopram and escitalopram: QT interval prolongation: New maximum daily dose restrictions (including in elderly patients), contraindications, and warnings. *Drug Safety Update*, 2014. www.gov.uk/drug-safety-update/citalopram-and-escitalopram-qt-interval-prolongation.

28. Barbui, C., Esposito, E., and Cipriani, A. Selective serotonin reuptake inhibitors and risk of suicide: A systematic review of observational studies. *CMAJ* 2009, 180(3): 291–7.

29. Thase, M.E. Effects of venlafaxine on blood pressure: A meta-analysis of original data from 3744 depressed patients. *J Clin Psychiatry* 1998, 59(10): 502–8.

30. Bose, A., Korotzer, A., Gommoll, C., and Li, D. Randomized placebo-controlled trial of escitalopram and venlafaxine XR in the treatment of generalized anxiety

disorder. *Depression and Anxiety* 2008, 25 (10): 854–61.

31. Kelliny, M., Croarkin, P.E., Moore, K.M., and Bobo, W.V. Profile of vortioxetine in the treatment of major depressive disorder: An overview of the primary and secondary literature. *Ther Clin Risk Manag* 2015, 11: 1193–212.

32. McIntyre, R.S., Lophaven, S., and Olsen, C.K. A randomized, double-blind, placebo-controlled study of vortioxetine on cognitive function in depressed adults. *International Journal of Neuropsychopharmacology* 2014, 17(10): 1557–67.

33. Miskowiak, K.W., Ott, C.V., Petersen, J.Z., and Kessing, L.V. Systematic review of randomized controlled trials of candidate treatments for cognitive impairment in depression and methodological challenges in the field. *Eur Neuropsychopharmacol* 2016, 26(12): 1845–67.

34. Sacchetti, E., Turrina, C., and Valsecchi, P. Cerebrovascular accidents in elderly people treated with antipsychotic drugs: A systematic review. *Drug Saf* 2010, 33(4): 273–88.

35. Mula, M., Pini, S., C and Cassano, G.B. The role of anticonvulsant drugs in anxiety disorders: A critical review of the evidence. *J Clin Psychopharmacol* 2007, 27 (3): 263–72.

36. Bancroft, S.L., Weiss, J.S., Libby, M.E., and Ahearn, W.H. A comparison of procedural variations in teaching behavior chains: Manual guidance, trainer completion, and no completion of untrained steps. *J of Applied Behavior Analysis* 2011, 44(3), 559–69.

37. Cooney, G.M., Dwan, K., Greig, C.A., Lawlor, D.A., Rimer, J., Waugh, F.R., McMurdo, M., and Mead, G.E. Exercise for depression. *Cochrane Database of Systematic Reviews* 2013, 9. CD004366. doi: 10.1002/14651858.CD004366.pub6.

Late-Onset Psychosis and Related Disorders

Simon Thacker and Katie Ward

Introduction

The presentation of psychotic symptoms in an older patient in a general hospital raises a wide range of diagnostic possibilities. The risk of physical factors predisposing, precipitating, or perpetuating psychotic symptoms is greater compared to patients presenting in the community. Primary psychosis (that which is not caused by physical illness or other psychiatric conditions such as depression) can occur across the age range. The classification of primary psychosis of late onset has been especially contested because of a debate as to whether schizophrenia has specifically neurodevelopmental origins and, as a consequence, a variety of terminologies have emerged (1). Secondary psychosis arises within delirium (itself triggered by a plethora of possible physical conditions), dementia, adverse drug reactions, sensory deprivation, and mood disorders. The exclusion of secondary psychosis is necessary before primary psychosis can be concluded. However, as is so often the case in medicine for older adults, multimorbidity is common and the skills of the old age liaison psychiatrist are required for disentangling aetiological factors, producing a diagnostic formulation, and assisting in the construction of a plan of care. This chapter proceeds by:

1. describing the types and correlates of psychotic symptoms associated with aging;
2. outlining the illnesses that are characterised by psychotic features in late life, their differential diagnosis, and various treatment strategies;
3. describing the particular challenges of assessing, diagnosing, and treating psychotic disorders of late onset within the general hospital setting; and
4. anticipating what resources for managing late-life psychosis in the general hospital and beyond might look like over the coming years in the NHS.

Psychotic Symptoms in Late Life

Psychotic phenomena lying outside mental illness may be looked upon as debatable psychotic experiences. Whether healthy ageing is associated with increasing hallucinatory experiences is questionable. However, disclosure may be influenced by older people seeking to avoid negative stereotypes (2). Of course, the reality in the general hospital is that the psychiatrist does not meet those who are aging healthily. However, psychotic symptoms are common; they occur in around 20 per cent of non-demented adults aged over 60 without overt psychotic illness; and minor symptoms such as illusions rise in prevalence with increasing age (3). They include a sense of presence, passage (a powerful sensation of someone walking past), and illusions. Patients will often not tell clinicians of these phenomena, for fear of being thought of as 'mad' (2), but when they are divulged an inexperienced clinician may infer a pathological process, because illusions and hallucinations are associated with both physical morbidities (e.g. poor vision and hearing) and mental disorder.

Charles Bonnet syndrome (CBS) arises in patients who have impaired peripheral vision. It is a cerebral reaction to the resultant sensory deprivation. Patients with CBS can be surprisingly tolerant of their visual hallucinations, but one third of patients find them to be distressing (4). It is not a psychotic *disorder* because insight is preserved and there is no delusional elaboration, but distinguishing CBS from mental illness may be difficult, especially if cognitive deficits are independently eroding the 'understandability' of the phenomenon. Charles Bonnet syndrome has a variable course: spontaneous remission may occur, or ongoing tolerance to the strangeness of the experience may emerge. Treatment options, beyond explanation and reassurance, are limited; but, for those patients who are distressed by CBS, the psychiatrist will need to work collaboratively with the ophthalmology department. Charles Bonnet hallucinosis does not respond to antipsychotic drugs (4, 5).

The auditory hallucination known by some clinicians as tinnitus, often accompanied by hearing impairment, is described in the literature as a distressing experience, correlating strongly with depression and anxiety. Simple sounds such as buzzing, ringing, or sizzling are common descriptions of tinnitus, although occasionally more elaborate, emotive musical sounds are experienced. Treatments for tinnitus are of limited effect and there is scanty randomised-controlled trial evidence of the value of antipsychotic medication.

Antidepressant treatment may salve depressive comorbidity, and anticonvulsants have been used with reported success in case series (6). Musical hallucinations are not rare in hearing-impaired populations, occurring in 2.5 per cent of patients aged over 60 who attend an audiology clinic (7). Working closely with colleagues in audiology is essential if treatment is to be optimised (8).

Secondary Psychosis in Late Life

Physical Disease States

The identification of the causes of secondary psychosis (a type that is caused by other medical or psychiatric illness) is of vital importance because of the risk of missing treatable physical lesions or omitting to treat an affective disorder. The nature of the psychotic features offers some clue as to aetiology. Visual, tactile, and olfactory hallucinations are more closely associated with psychosis related to physical illness. Vague, poorly systematised, or fleeting delusions suggest an organic brain dysfunction. However, no psychotic features are pathognomonic for primary psychosis, which is therefore a diagnosis of exclusion (9).

A Finnish study considered patients aged above 60 presenting over a year to psychiatric services with a first episode of psychosis outside the context of an established neurological disease. The study employed a chart review and expert panel consensus to draw diagnostic conclusions and found medical conditions to be the precipitant in 49 per cent of cases, while depressive psychosis, very late onset schizophrenia-like disorder, and delusional disorder constituted 20 per cent, 19 per cent, and 13 per cent of the cohort, respectively. Overall yearly incidence for late-onset psychosis was estimated at 48/ 100,000 in this population (10).

Integrated Assessment

The exclusion of an organic cause for late-onset psychosis should be incorporated in a full biopsychosocial assessment that brings to bear the skills of physicians, nurses, occupational therapists, physiotherapists, pharmacists, and social workers. Comprehensive Geriatric Assessment (on which see Chapter 19) is a useful framework for biopsychosocial assessment and should function in the general hospital as a lingua franca into which psychiatrists can integrate their assessments (11).

MINE is a useful mnemonic for checking for physical disease states that can cause - late-life psychosis (see Table 15.1).

Dementia and Delirium

Around half of older people admitted to acute wards in the general hospital will be experiencing dementia, delirium, or both (13). It should not be inferred that referrals from medical and surgical colleagues describing the 'confusion' indicate dementia or delirium. Often this term is used imprecisely within the general hospital, to describe patients (particularly older ones) who act or behave 'strangely'. On the other hand, the patient presenting with delusions or hallucinations and who may appear cognitively

Table 15.1 Common medical causes of psychosis in older persons

Metabolic	Abnormal levels of: sodium calcium magnesium phosphate vitamin b12/folate deficiency hepatic encephalopathy uraemia hypoxia
Infection	meningitis encephalitis neurosyphilis HIV/AIDS
Neurological	Parkinson's disease epilepsy stroke subdural haematoma brain tumour multiple sclerosis limbic/autoimmune/paraneoplastic encephalitis lupus and other vasculitides
Endocrine	hyper/hypothyroidism hyper/hypoadrenalism hyper/hypoglycaemia hyper/hypoparathyroidism

Reinhardt and Cohen (12).

intact may be harbouring dementia and delirium. This can be particularly problematic with patients of high intellectual and social attainment, who can perform misleadingly well on cognitive tests as a result of ceiling effects (14).

Psychotic features often emerge as part of dementia. Careful history taking and triangulation with carers are required to separate confabulation from true delusions. Hallucinosis is often visual in nature, although other modalities are not uncommon (15). Separating cognitive misapprehension in the form of illusions and misidentification from true hallucinations – that is, perceptions that lack any real-world stimulus – can be challenging.

Dementia with Lewy bodies is commonly seen in psychiatric practice in the community and may present with prominent hallucinations and delusions before the extent of the cognitive deficit is realised. Dementia with Lewy bodies may be embedded within cerebrovascular disease and drug side effects when patients present to the general hospital. The separation of existing dementia from emergent delirium requires skilled history taking. New-onset psychotic symptoms should always raise the alarm for a delirium, while persistent ones that predate hospital admission should mandate scrupulous history taking and cognitive examination, to ensure that a decline commensurate with dementia is identified. When chronic cognitive decline is not found, the possibility of a non-organic psychotic illness is thereby raised.

Affective Disorder in Late Life

Mood disorder is an important differential when assessing a patient who presents with psychosis. Mood may be lowered in reaction to a primary psychosis, and therefore the temporal relationship between onset of mood and psychotic features should be ascertained by careful history taking. A history of prior mood disorder is a useful indicator. Furthermore, the nature of the paranoia is an important guide: guilt and a sense of deserved punishment suggest a depressive psychosis, whereas fear of the undermining of grandiose achievements points to mania rather than to a primary psychotic illness (16).

Drug Use and Psychosis in Later Life

The use of illicit drugs such as cannabis is an increasing issue among baby boomers – the generation born between 1946 and 1964. The assumption of adherence to strictly legal routes of acquiring drugs needs to be challenged in the case of a generation that was exposed to illicit drugs during its youth (17). Psychogenic drug use may exacerbate or trigger psychotic features in younger people (18), and continued use may lower thresholds for psychosis in later life. Psychotic sequelae may arise from the use of prescription drugs that are not uncommonly prescribed in later life, such antiparkinsonian medication(19), anticonvulsants (20), steroids (21), and biologics (22).

Alcohol

Rates of alcohol misuse among the elderly, especially women, are rising (17). Confabulation associated with alcohol-related brain damage needs to be distinguished from delusion, through detailed examination of cognition and circumstance. Cognitive assessment is not a routine part of assessment in alcohol services and must not be overlooked in presentations to the general hospital (23).

Primary Psychoses of Late Onset

The emergence of non-affective, non-organic psychotic illness in later life against the background of possible alternative aetiologies poses both a diagnostic and technical challenge for clinicians.

Considering prevalence, an American study that used a definition of schizophrenia that restricted the diagnosis to age of onset before 45 reported one-year prevalence rates of 0.6 per cent among individuals aged 45–64 and 0.2 per cent among individuals aged 65 years and older (24). In a Dutch study of a population aged 60 and over, the emergence of schizophrenia-like conditions in later life was described. The one-year prevalence of early-onset schizophrenia (EOS) was 0.35 per cent, of late-onset schizophrenia (LOS) (40 years and over) 0.14 per cent, and of very late onset schizophrenia-like psychosis (VLOSP) (60 years and over) 0.05 per cent (25).

Very Late Onset Schizophrenia-Like Psychosis

On the basis of published prevalence figures, VLOSP is probably underdiagnosed in routine psychiatric practice. This is possible for a number of reasons, which are described in the following subsections.

Nosological Uncertainty

The term VLOSP is relatively new; it has taken many years to achieve consensus and the process has left a number of confusing terminologies in its wake. Kraepelin introduced the term 'paraphrenia', to distinguish a form of psychosis not associated with the lack of volition and disintegration of personality seen in dementia praecox (1). Kay and Roth introduced the term 'late paraphrenia', to highlight a schizophrenia-like state emerging in late life and associated with the preservation of intellect, communication skills, and personality (26). The fifth edition of APA's *Diagnostic and Statistical Manual of Mental Disorders* (DSMV) and the tenth revision of WHO's *International Statistical Classification of Diseases and Related Health Problems* (ICD10) do not recognise a separate, age-defined form of schizophrenia, but consensus guidelines recommend that the age of onset be used to delimit LOS and VLOSP disorders. Criticism has been levelled at these age-defined syndromes because it is more usual in nosology to set criteria for syndromes and then examine the demographic associations than to use age cut points to define the syndrome (27).

Ascertaining the Problem

Psychosocial factors that are associated with VLOSP militate against psychiatric consultation. Social isolation, persecutory delusions, and lack of insight mean that the presentation of psychosis may be to non-psychiatric services such as the emergency department (ED), the police, or a housing and environmental health department. While these issues are not peculiar to psychosis in late life, services may take a more relaxed view of risk. When psychosis emerges in an older person, once physical disorder is excluded, the psychiatric aspects of care often remain unaddressed (more on this later in the chapter).

Assertiveness of Care

The absence of negative symptoms and of formal thought disorder (28) could mean that mental health practitioners are drawn to conclude that the patient may not be 'sectionable' and little can therefore be done. Ageist assumptions leading to the acceptance of 'strange' and distressed behaviour in older people may underpin this inaction (29). When limited insight is allied to an absence of thought disorder, or possibly even to a fluent assertiveness, the patient with VLOSP may be able to argue persuasively for a non-medical approach to the problem as they perceive it. Indeed, to highlight the point, fewer than one half of older patients experiencing VLOSP receive antipsychotics and, after one year or at point of discharge, that figure drops to less than one third (30).

Distinctive Features of VLOSP

The psychotic features in VLOSP are distinctive. Persecutory delusions allied to the belief that people, radiation, or objects are passing through walls were found in 68 per cent of late-onset cases; this compares to only 20 per cent among younger people who experience schizophrenia (29). Affective response and the ability to communicate fluently are often well preserved, even in the face of intense psychotic experiences (28). This can create a mismatch between the 'science fiction' world of psychotic illness and a surprising domestic order.

The role of sensory impairment in VLOSP is disputed. Classically VLOSP has been associated with hearing loss. Visual impairment may also be a risk factor (31). A review of combined LOS and VLOSP cohorts found no association with hearing loss, but the association with visual impairment remained (32). A Swedish record linkage study failed to confirm the association of VLOSP with either hearing or visual impairment (33).

Migrant patients are more likely to develop VLOSP. Migrants may be at risk of developing VLOSP at a younger age than their indigenous counterparts (34). Remarkable differences in the incidence of VLOSP were found in a London population: 328 (172) female (male) Afro-Caribbean older people compared to 25 (7) female (male) British-born older people, per 100,000 per annum (35). Likewise, a Swedish record linkage study supports the migration theory (33). The mechanisms by which migration may predispose to VLOSP have not been researched systematically but plausibly include both factors related to leaving the country of origin and factors related to adjustment to the host country. The link between migration and psychosis does not appear to be a feature of age, and similar associations between migration and schizophrenia exist across the adult age range (36). Adversities such as gestational exposure to the Second World War, loss of a child in infancy, social isolation, and low income also appear to increase the probability of receiving a diagnosis of VLOSP (33).

Older age increases the risk of receiving a diagnosis of VLOSP, and the incidence of VLOSP accelerates with age more rapidly for women than for men (37). The female gender is consistently associated with a high likelihood of receiving a diagnosis of VLOSP (33, 37). This compares strikingly to the fact that, in the case of EOS, the association with the female gender is the inverse (36).

Early-Onset Schizophrenia

There are notable differences between VLOSP and EOS. People presenting with VLOSP demonstrate female preponderance, lack of affective blunting, absence of thought disorder, less genetic loading, better educational achievement, and greater likelihood of non-auditory hallucinosis (olfactory, tactile, visual) (1, 38). These differences are summarised in Table 15.2. Cognitive deficits arise in both VLOSP and EOS, often in the

Table 15.2 Summarises the key differences between VLOSP, EOS, and DD.

	VLOSP	EOS	DD
Gender	F>M	F=M	F=M
Delusions	Present	Present	Present
Hallucinations	Present	Present	Absent
Sensory impairment	Present	Absent	Absent
Affect	Intact	Impaired	Intact
Intellect	Intact	Impaired	Intact
Thought disorder	Absent	Present	Absent

realm of executive function, working memory, and motor and verbal ability; but they are distinct from the impairments seen in dementia, since recall is relatively well preserved (39, 40).

The aging of patients who experience long-standing psychotic illness creates the phenomenon of the 'graduate' – the person who enters later life and whose chronic psychotic vulnerability meshes with his or her acquired physical morbidities. Life expectancy is diminished in EOS, and the outcome for those who survive into later life is variable; 50 per cent have favourable outcomes. Persistent psychotic features at the onset and the absence of affective features predict a poor outcome (41).

Psychotic features may have been in remission for many years or, conversely, may have been persistently troublesome at the point of presentation to the general hospital. Declining physical health before acute hospitalisation may have meant that adjustments in psychiatric medication have already taken place before admission, or psychotropic drugs may be suspected as the culprit in triggering the admission. It can be tempting to adjust or stop psychiatric drugs in the face of falls, worsening bradykinesia, tremor, hypotension, or cardiac abnormalities that can perhaps be too readily attributed to long-standing and previously well-tolerated psychotropic medication. Balancing such interventions against the risk of a decompensation of mental well-being must be undertaken carefully and in consultation with the patient, his/her family, and the community psychiatric team, whose members can provide a longitudinal perspective, as opposed to the 'snapshot' witnessed by the general hospital staff.

Delusional Disorder

Delusional disorder (DD) is a rare condition that is often well hidden from psychiatrists, as otherwise well-adjusted and capable patients eloquently assert their delusions in the face of counterfactual evidence. The ascertainment of delusion as opposed to overvalued ideas or just eccentric beliefs can be complex, requiring triangulation with family, other health and social care professionals, police, and the housing department (42).

Delusional parasitosis is a variant of DD found in the elderly that can cause significant distress – for example a fixated belief about infestation by bugs, worms, and the like, or professional scepticism about the reality of the experience. Persecutory delusions about 'neighbours from hell' are not uncommon, for example beliefs about drug dealers and prostitution racketeers. A hallmark of DD is that the delusions are not bizarre but rooted in a horrible plausibility. Although presentation may occur in late life, careful history taking may reveal years of dispute with the authorities about allegedly troublesome neighbours. There is a paucity of evidence for the treatment of DD. Although antipsychotic medication is a plausible proposal, the limited randomised control trial evidence that exists supports the use of cognitive behavioural therapy (CBT) (43).

For a quick reference to the differences between EOS, VLOSP, and DD, please refer to Table 15.2.

Personality Features and Life Events

The distinction between paranoid personality and psychotic illness can be difficult to make, and a paranoid personality provides fertile ground for an emergent VLOSP or delusional disorder (44). Late life may be associated with bereavement and increased social isolation, thereby contributing to the decompensation of a schizoid–paranoid personality into psychosis. But the research remains inconclusive. Kay and Roth described that specific precipitants explaining the emergence of late-onset psychosis were not the norm (26), but a Swedish cohort study found strong associations between the loss of a partner or child and the onset of VLOSP (33). Persecution in earlier life has also been associated with late-onset psychotic illness (45).

Presentations to a Liaison Service

Personality Problems Merging into VLOSP

An 80-year-old Polish widow found wandering the streets, escaping from drug dealers who pumped fumes into her flat, is brought to the ED by police when she refused to re-enter her home. She was annoyed and seeking the arrest of her neighbours. She was angry and insisted on leaving ED. Her daughter was at end of her tether: 'She will not listen to me!' The patient reportedly never trusted strangers after her detention in a Soviet concentration camp and had a suspicious view of government authorities. She had become more isolated since the death of her spouse five years earlier. The use of the Mental Health Act (MHA) was associated with much protest and distress, but she stabilised on amisulpride (50 mg, once daily) and agreed to move in with her daughter after their reconciliation.

Postoperative Delirium and Relapse of EOS Paranoid Schizophrenia

An 85 year-old Asian man had been on depot fluphenazine for decades. Over the past year he had poor mobility, which was attributed to drug-induced parkinsonism, and his community psychiatrist switched him to aripiprazole. The patient was admitted to the general hospital after a fall and hip fracture. On the orthopaedic ward he was visually hallucinating Teddy Boys and was in fear for his life. Because of improving performance on cognitive tests and family willingness to support him, he was promptly discharged home with a diagnosis of resolving delirium. He was admitted to a psychiatric ward two weeks later, when found wandering the streets seeking refuge from Teddy Boys; his mobility had improved markedly. It was concluded that he had relapsed into schizophrenia, where restoration of his depot effected a resolution of his psychosis.

Delusional Disorder

A 93-year-old Holocaust survivor and widow living alone had become increasingly litigious vis-à-vis health services over the past 20 years, after the death of her husband from what she always considered to have been a medical error. This culminated in a complaint that a locum general practitioner had given her a wrong injection. No evidence was found for this error. The patient received support from a community psychiatric nurse but declined antipsychotic medication. There were no signs of self-neglect, and she remained cognitively plausible although she refused formal testing. She was admitted to the general hospital with lung sepsis. She was fearful, protesting assault by staff and resisting care. She presented a picture of agitated delirium coloured by her pre-existing, untreated DD.

Cannabis Psychosis/VLOSP

A 72-year-old 'ex-hippie' and former heroin addict with no children had been widowed for five years. He experienced numerous bereavements and was socially isolated. The patient was registering increasing protests to authorities about neighbours stealing his electricity and water and talking about him as the 'mark' and a 'stooge'. He was admitted with a hip fracture and referred to liaison psychiatry because of 'confusion' but no evidence of delirium. He wanted the hospital authorities to deal with his neighbours. He admitted to smoking cannabis daily. He agreed to commence risperidone (1 mg) daily and to receive follow-up from the community mental health team while still protesting the activities of his neighbours and maintaining that cannabis help to soothe him. Follow-up revealed ongoing complaints about neighbours, but he was concordant with the risperidone and believed that his neighbours had found another 'mark' and were now leaving him alone.

Assessment

History is essential to reaching the correct diagnosis and management plan. The referral note from the treating medical team is only the start of information gathering. Cross-referencing with previous psychiatric notes, staff views of the attitude and behaviour of the patient on the ward or in the ED (acceptance of advice, food, fluids, personal care, etc.), and summary notes from other services such as the police or the ambulance services are invaluable in building up a picture, particularly if there is no family informant available.

The mental state examination may reveal suspiciousness against the authorities and indignation that the protests of the patient are not being taking seriously. Careful and diplomatic examination of cognition (the patient may think that you are trying to undermine the credibility of his or her testimony) is important, and especially looking for inattention and disorientation that might suggest organic brain disorder.

Although the MHA operates on risk thresholds, the assessment of the patient's capacity to consent to an ongoing admission to the general hospital, psychiatric transfer, or community options is a crucial pillar of any patient-centred care plan. It is easy to overestimate capacity when psychosis is occurring in the context of plausibly intact cognition and the absence of formal thought disorder. The ability to weigh up care options may be impaired because, even if the patient portrays understanding of your clinical concerns, they may not think that it applies to them, given their delusional interpretation of events.

Management

In the general hospital setting, comprehensive geriatric assessment leading to a biopsychosocial care plan should be the approach employed to ensure that essential medical and functional morbidities are not left unaddressed amid the 'drama' that might accompany a psychotic presentation. The treatment of physical triggers for psychosis does not prohibit the use of antipsychotic medication, but a successful resolution of physical problems may allow antipsychotic therapy to be withdrawn promptly.

For patients with enduring psychotic symptoms that accompany VLOSP, DD and E/LOS engagement with mental health services is the key to successful management. However, rates of concordance with antipsychotic treatment for VLOSP are low, 27 per cent at one year (29). Liaison consultation is an opportunity for engagement with mental health services but the brevity of an acute hospital stay may limit what can be achieved without prompt handover to a well-resourced, proactive community team (46). Depot medication can sometimes be well tolerated in VLOSP, but depot antipsychotics should be deployed as part of a person-centred care plan and not as a means to ration engagement with community services (46, 47).

The use of the MHA may be necessary in the short term, but may not improve long-term outcome (46). Patients whose persecutory delusions have arisen on a background of real-life persecution by malign authorities may cause much professional soul-searching when the use of the MHA is being considered. Close collaboration with family members, friends, community services, and the multidisciplinary liaison team should take place in order to ensure that the best interests of the patient remain paramount.

Insight is on a continuum and, even with successful treatment, may be only partially achieved. Indeed, it is surprising how concordance with antipsychotic medication and community services can exist alongside delusional persecution, which is now merely rendered more tolerable while the perpetrators remain at large.

Choice of Antipsychotic Medication

The ATLAS double-blind, randomised, placebo-controlled study enrolled participants with VLOSP. It demonstrated symptom reduction at 12 weeks on amisulpride (100 mg, once daily), and this was sustained for a further 12 weeks of treatment. Drop-out rates in the treatment arm were 37 per cent between weeks 12 and 24. The number of reported side effects was double in the treatment arm compared to the placebo arm of the trial, and many clinicians would advocate a lower starting dose of amisulpride because of the risk of extrapyramidal side effects. Nevertheless, these results are encouraging and show how an effective drug treatment of people with VLOSP is possible (48).

The international consensus on VLOSP concluded that, while antipsychotics are the mainstay of treatment, doses may need to be as low as one tenth of those given to young patients (1). In an American survey of expert opinion, atypical antipsychotics, including risperidone, olanzapine, and quetiapine, were the favoured treatment for 'late-life schizophrenia' (49).

Depot medication is often invoked as a means to ensure concordance with antipsychotic therapy, but doses may have to be as much as five times lower in VLOSP than in early-onset schizophrenia (47).

Future Directions

Liaison psychiatry will only ever be a brief moment in the course of the experience of chronic psychosis, but it has the potential to intervene and assist the patient in shifting towards a more favourable trajectory. Amisulpiride is effective in VLOSP, but caution about side effects is required. We know little about the long-term management of this and related conditions, but an effectively resourced and assertive approach in the community is likely to improve outcomes. Timely and effective communication between liaison and community psychiatric teams will assist in maintaining engagement with a group of patients who are likely to have limited insight. Detention and treatment under the MHA may be a necessary platform from which to shape a plan of community care, but the extension of the work of crisis and home treatment teams to older adults is important in the pursuit of the least restrictive care. Whether post-hospital care is managed through an age-inclusive community team or through a specific older adults service is less important than the team's appreciation of the suffering that undertreated psychosis can wreak in this vulnerable and often overlooked group of patients.

References

1. Howard, R., Rabins, P.V., Seeman, M.V., Jeste, D.V., and the International Late-Onset Schizophrenia Group. Late-onset schizophrenia and very-late-onset schizophrenia-like psychosis: An international consensus. *Am J Psychiatry* 2000, 157(2): 172–8.

2. Badcock, J.C., Dehon, H., and Laroi, F. Hallucinations in healthy older adults: An overview of the literature and perspectives for future research. *Front Psychol* 2017, 8: 1134.

3. Soulas, T., Cleret de Langavant, L., Monod, V., and Fenelon, G. The prevalence and characteristics of hallucinations, delusions and minor phenomena in a non-demented population sample aged 60 years and over. *Int J Geriatr Psychiatry* 2016, 31(12): 1322–8.

4. Teunisse, R.J., Zitman, F.G., Cruysberg, J.R.M., Hoefnagels, W.H.L., and Verbeek, A.L.M. Visual hallucinations in psychological normal people: Charles Bonnet's syndrome. *Lancet* 1996, 347 (9004): 794–7.

5. Jacob, A., Prasad, S., Boggild, M., and Chandratre, S. Charles Bonnet syndrome: Elderly people and visual hallucinations. *Br Med J* 2004, 328(7455): 1552–4.

6. Fornaro, M., and Martino, M. Tinnitus psychopharmacology: A comprehensive review of its pathomechanisms and management. *Neuropsychiatr Dis Treat* 2010, 6: 209–18.

7. Cole, M.G., Dowson, L., Dendukuri, N., and Belzile, E. The prevalence and phenomenology of auditory hallucinations among elderly subjects attending an audiology clinic. *Int J Geriatr Psychiatry* 2002, 17(5): 444–52.

8. Pinto, P.C.L., Marcelos, C.M., Mezzasalma, M.A., Osterne, F.J.V, de Melo Tavares de Lima, M.A., and Nardi, A.E. Tinnitus and its association with psychiatric disorders: Systematic review. *J Larynogol Otol* 2014, 128(8): 660–4.

9. David, A., Fleminger, S., and Kopelman, M. *Lishman's Organic Psychiatry: A Textbook of Neuropsychiatry*, 4th ed. Oxford: Wiley Blackwell, 2009.

10. Louhija, U.M., Saarela, T., Juva, K., and Appelberg, B. Brain atrophy is a frequent

finding in elderly patients with first episode psychosis. *Int Psychogeriatr* 2017, 29(11): 1925–9.

11. Thacker, S., Skelton, M., and Harwood, R. Psychiatry and the geriatric syndromes creating constructive interfaces. *BJPsych Bull* 2017, 41(2): 71–5.

12. Reinhardt, M.M., and Cohen, C.I. Late-life psychosis: Diagnosis and treatment. *Curr Psychiatry Rep* 2015, 17(2): 1–13.

13. Whittamore, K.H., Goldberg, S.E., Gladman, J.R.F, Bradshaw, L.E., Jones, R.G., and Harwood, R.H. The diagnosis, prevalence and outcome of delirium in a cohort of older people with mental health problems on general hospital wards. *Int J Geriatr Psychiatry* 2014, 29(1): 32–40.

14. Stern, Y., Albert, S., Tang, M.X., and Tsai, W.Y. Rate of memory decline in AD is related to education and occupation. *Neurology* 1999, 53(9): 1942.

15. Ropacki, S.A., and Jeste, D.V. Epidemiology of and risk factors for psychosis of Alzheimer disease: A review of 55 studies published from 1990 to 2003. *Am J Psychiatry* 2005, 162(11): 2022–30.

16. Lake, C.R. Hypothesis: Grandiosity and guilt cause paranoia: Paranoid schizophrenia is a psychotic mood disorder: A review. *Schizophrenia Bulletin* 2008, 34(6): 1151–62.

17. Rao, T., and Crome, I. *Our Invisible Addicts*. London: Royal College of Psychiatrists, 2018.

18. Moore, T.H., Zammit, S., Lingford-Hughes, A., Barnes, T.R., Jones, P.B., Burke, M., et al. Cannabis use and risk of psychotic or affective mental health outcomes: A systematic review. *Lancet* 2007, 370(9584): 319–28.

19. Zahodne, L.B., and Fernandez, H.H. Pathophysiology and treatment of psychosis in Parkinson's disease: A review. *Drugs Aging* 2008, 25(8): 665–82.

20. Chen, Z., Lusicic, A., O'Brien, T.J., Velakoulis, D., Adams, S.J., and Kwan, P. Psychotic disorders induced by antiepileptic drugs in people with epilepsy. *Brain* 2016, 139(10): 2668–78.

21. Robinson, D.E., Harrison-Hansley, E., and Spencer, R.F. Steroid psychosis after an intra-articular injection. *Ann Rheum Dis* 2000, 59(11): 926.

22. Atigari, O.V., and Healy, D. Schizophrenia-like disorder associated with etanercept treatment. *Br Med J Case Reports* 2014, 13 January: bcr2013200464.

23. Wadd, S., Randall, J., and Thake A.. *Alcohol Misuse and Cognitive Impairment*. Alcohol Research UK, 2013. https://s3.eu-west-2.amazonaws.com/files.alcoholchange.org.uk/documents/FinalReport_0110.pdf.

24. Robins, L.N., and Regier, D. *Psychiatric Disorders in America*. New York: Free Press, 1991.

25. Meesters, P.D., de Haan, L., Comijs, H.C., Stek, M.L., Smeets-Janssen, M.M.J., Weeda, M.R., et al. Schizophrenia spectrum disorders in later life: Prevalence and distribution of age at onset and sex in a Dutch catchment area. *Am J Ger Psychiatry* 2012, 20(1): 18–28.

26. Kay, D.W.K., and Roth, M. Environmental and hereditary factors in the schizophrenias of old age and their bearing on the general problem of causation in schizophrenia. *J Ment Sci* 1961, 107: 649–86.

27. Cohen, C.I. Very late-onset schizophrenia-like psychosis: Positive findings but questions remain unanswered. *Lancet Psychiatry* 2018, 5(7): 528–9.

28. Almeida, O.P., Howard, R.J., Levy, R., and David, A.S. Psychotic states arising in late life (late paraphrenia): Psychopathology and nosology. *Br J Psychiatry* 1995, 166: 205–14.

29. Howard, R., Castle, D., O'Brien, J., Almeida, O., and Levy, R. Permeable walls, floors, ceilings and doors: Partition delusions in late paraphrenia. *Int J Geriatr Psychiatry* 1992, 7(10): 719–24.

30. Lam, C.C.S.F., Reeves, S.J., Stewart, R., and Howard, R. Service and treatment

engagement of people with very late-onset schizophrenia-like psychosis. *BJPsych Bull* 2016, 40(4): 185–6.

31. Prager, S., and Jeste, D.V. Sensory impairment in late-life schizophrenia. *Schizophrenia Bull* 1993, 19(4): 755–72.

32. Brunelle, S., Cole, M.G., and Elie, M. Risk factors for the late-onset psychoses: A systematic review of cohort studies. *Int J Geriatr Psychiatry* 2012, 27(3): 240–52.

33. Stafford, J., Howard, R., Dalman, C., and Kirkbride, J.B. The incidence of nonaffective, nonorganic psychotic disorders in older people: A population-based cohort study of 3 million people in Sweden. *Schizophrenia Bull* 2018, suppl_1: S377–378.

34. Mitter, P., Reeves, S., Romero-Rubiales, F., Bell, P., Stewart, R., and Howard, R. Migrant status, age, gender and social isolation in very late-onset schizophrenia-like psychosis. *Int J Geriatr Psychiatry* 2005, 20(11): 1046–51.

35. Reeves, S.J., Sauer, J., Stewart, R., Granger, A., and Howard, R.J. Increased first-contact rates for very-late-onset schizophrenia-like psychosis in African and Caribbean-born elders. *Br J Psychiatry* 2001, 179: 172–4.

36. Jongsma, H.E., Turner, C., Kirkbride, J.B., and Jones, P.B. International incidence of psychotic disorders: A systematic review and meta-analysis. *Lancet Public Health* 2019, 4(5): 229–244.

37. Stafford, J., Howard, R., and Kirkbride, J.B. The incidence of very late-onset psychotic disorders: A systematic review and meta-analysis. *Psychol Med* 2018, 48(11): 1775–86.

38. Chen, L., Selvendra, A., Stewart, A., Castle, D. Risk factors in early and late onset schizophrenia. *Comp Psychiatry* 2018, 80: 155–62.

39. Ting, C., Rajji, T.K., Ismail, Z., Tang-Wai, D.F., Apanasiewicz, N., Miranda, D., et al. Differentiating the cognitive profile of schizophrenia from that of Alzheimer disease and depression in late life. *PLoS ONE* 2010, 5(4): e10151.

40. Van Assche, L., Morrens, M., Luyten, P., Van de Ven, L., and Vandenbulcke, M. The neuropsychology and neurobiology of late-onset schizophrenia and very-late-onset schizophrenia-like psychosis: A critical review. *Neuroscience & Biobehavioral Reviews* 2017, 83: 604–21.

41. Harrison, G., Hopper, K., Craig, T., Laska, E. Siegel, et al. Recovery from psychotic illness: A 15- and 25-year international follow up study. *British Journal of Psychiatry* 2001, 178: 506–17.

42. Fear, C.F. Recent develpoments in the managment of delusional disorder. *Adv Psychiatr Treat* 2013, 19(3): 212–20.

43. Skelton, M., Khokhar, W.A., and Thacker, S.P. Treatments for delusional disorder. *Cochrane Database of Systematic Reviews* 2015, 5.

44. Kay, D.W., Cooper, A.F., Garside, R.F., and Roth, M. The differentiation of paranoid from affective psychosis by patient's premorbid characteristics. *Br J Psychiatry* 1976, 129(3): 207–15.

45. Reulbach, U., Bleich, S., Biermann, T., Pfahlberg, A., and Sperling, W. Late-onset schizophrenia in child survivors of the Holocaust. *J Nerv Ment Dis* 2007, 195(4): 315–9.

46. Reeves, S., Stewart, R., and Howard, R. Service contact and psychopathology in very-late-onset schizophrenia-like psychosis: The effects of gender and ethnicity. *Int J Geriatr Psychiatry* 2002, 17(5): 473–9.

47. Thacker, S. The use of Depot neuroleptics in the elderly: A survey. *Int J Geriatr Psychiatry* 1996, 11(5): 423–7.

48. Howard, R., Cort, E., Bradley, R., Harper, E., Kelly, L., Bentham, P., et al. Antipsychotic treatment of very late-onset schizophrenia-like psychosis (ATLAS): A randomised, controlled, double-blind trial. *Lancet Psychiatry* 2018, 5(7): 553–63.

49. Alexopoulos, G., Streim, J., Carpenter, D., and Docherty, J. Using antipsychotics on older patients. *Journal of Clinical Psychiatry* 2004, 65(suppl 2): 5–99, 100–2 (discussion), 103–4 (quiz).

Drug and Alcohol Misuse in Older People

Tony Rao and Cathy Symonds

Introduction

Alcohol and drug misuse is no longer confined to younger people: older people in the baby boomer cohort, born between 1946 and 1964, show the fastest rise in rates of both mortality and misuse of drugs and alcohol by comparison with all other age groups (1). In the setting of liaison psychiatry, this has relevance for the increased likelihood of comorbid medical disorders, polypharmacy, cognitive impairment, and special considerations to bear in mind when it comes to older people, such as mental incapacity and safeguarding. Older people are also more likely to show atypical presentations of drug and alcohol misuse, and an increasing number of them are admitted with alcohol-related brain damage.

Definitions

The misuse of drugs and alcohol is collectively termed 'substance misuse'. Substance refers to any psychoactive compound that is taken for its pleasurable effects and that acts on the brain to alter one's mood, thought processes, or behaviour. When the use of substances is associated with harm to health and to social function, it is termed 'misuse'. The most severe form of misuse is called 'dependence', a state in which both health and social function are affected. Alcohol, tobacco, opioids, benzodiazepines, and Z drugs are the substances most commonly misused by older people. The misuse of cannabis and gabapentonoids is also becoming more common among older people.

Although the traditional definition of older people has been people aged 65 and older, it should be noted that some younger people with substance misuse have an accelerated biological ageing that can interact adversely with comorbid mental and physical disorders such as depression, dementia, liver disease, and cardiovascular risk factors.

There is also a distinction to be made between early and late onset in drug and alcohol misuse. Up to a third of 65+-year-olds with alcohol misuse will have developed this habit after the age of 50. In the United Kingdom, the definition of alcohol misuse is now based on drinking more than the lower-risk level, which is 14 units or fewer, for both men and women of any age.

Epidemiology

Between 2016 and 2017, people aged 65+ formed 30 per cent of hospital admissions related primarily to alcohol in England. This proportion has risen by more than 100 per cent since 2010–11, when this age group formed 14 per cent of hospital admissions. Alcohol misuse has been found in up to 15 per cent of referrals to liaison old age psychiatry services (2).

In the United Kingdom, lifetime use of cannabis in people aged between 65 and 74 rose from less than 1 per cent in 2000 to 7 per cent in 2014, while lifetime use of amphetamines rose from 0.4 to 0.8 per cent over the same period.

Between 2001 and 2015, the number of alcohol-specific deaths rose by 45 per cent among people aged 50+ but remained the same among 15–49-year-olds. The age group with the highest rate of such deaths changed from 50–54-year-olds in 2001 to 60–64-year-olds in 2015. Over the past ten years, the number of deaths related to poisoning from all drugs has more than doubled among people aged between 50 and 69, in England and Wales (3).

Prescription drug misuse is also rising among older people, largely through over-prescribing for a medication that is not clinically indicated or mis-prescribing for a clinically indicated medication. The most commonly prescribed drugs with the potential for misuse are benzodiazepines; Z drugs, zaleplon, zolpidem and zopiclone; opioids (for pain); and gabapentinoids. Older people may also use opioids for cough and diarrhoea.

Rates of dual diagnosis (mental disorders that coexist with substance misuse) as high as 66 per cent have been found in hospital settings. In older people, depression and cognitive impairment are the most common types of mental disorder in dual diagnoses, the latter referring mainly to alcohol-related brain damage.

Depression has a strong association with alcohol misuse. Older people with depression are three to four times more likely to have alcohol-related problems than those without; and this is accompanied by a higher risk of suicide and social–functional impairment. Depression is associated with a higher risk of past-year cannabis and cocaine use in people aged 50 and older. Alcohol misuse in older people is also associated with anxiety, antisocial personality disorder, and post-traumatic stress disorder (3).

Heroin and methadone users aged 50+ have considerable physical comorbidity, which ranges from 11 per cent for diabetes mellitus to 54 per cent for hypertension. Other comorbid disorders within this prevalence range associated with substance misuse are arthritis, cirrhosis, hepatitis C, lung disease, and cardiac disease. With the ageing of heroin users, the numbers of older people with comorbid physical disorders such as lung and heart disease and hepatitis are likely to increase, adding to the public health burden.

Drug Interactions

Alcohol has adverse interactions with both prescription and non-prescription drugs. Women are at higher risk than men, because their higher body fat to water ratio leads to a higher blood alcohol concentration for any given amount of alcohol consumed. Polypharmacy is also common in older people, 40 per cent taking five or more prescription drugs.

The main types of adverse reactions occur (1) from the potentiation of side effects at a receptor level (i.e. pharmacodynamically) and (2) by either increasing or decreasing the metabolism of other drugs (i.e. pharmacokinetically).

The most common alcohol-related adverse pharmacodynamic interactions are with benzodiazepines and amitriptyline, whose sedative effect gets increased and this in turn increases the risks of falls. There is a risk of oversedation and respiratory depression with opioids (morphine and codeine). Chronic alcohol consumption increases the metabolism

Box 16.1 Barriers to the identification of substance misuse in older people (Royal College of Psychiatrists, 2011)

Practitioner Barriers	Individual Barriers
• Ageist assumptions • Failure to recognise symptoms • Lack of knowledge about screening • Discomfort with the topic • Lack of awareness of substance misuse in older people ('If you don't think about it, you won't see it') • Misuse traditionally considered to be rare in old age • Symptoms may mimic, or be hidden by, symptoms of physical illness • Unwillingness to ask • Absence of informants	• Attempts at self-diagnosis • Symptoms attributed to the ageing process or to screening • Reluctance to report (shame, denial, pessimism about using, pessimism about recovery) • Many do not self-refer or seek treatment • Perceived stigma of the word 'addiction' • Cognitive problems – substance-induced amnesia, underlying dementia • Unwillingness to disclose • Collusion of informant(s) • Screening

of paracetamol, such that toxic metabolites from paracetamol are likely to be associated with liver damage. This is particularly relevant for paracetamol overdose in older people. Benzodiazepines increase the risk of respiratory depression when taken with opioids.

Antibiotics such as ciprofloxacillin, clarithromycin, erythromycin, itraconazole, ketoconazole, and ritonavir all increase the adverse effects of buprenorphine, methadone, and loperamide through pharmacokinetic interactions. Similarly, drugs such as fluoxetine and metoclopramide increase the adverse effects of oxycodone, codeine, dihydrocodeine, and tramadol.

Assessment

Successful screening and a comprehensive assessment require an approach that maximises the therapeutic relationship. A non-judgemental and non-ageist approach, with respect for dignity, privacy, and autonomy, is essential. Fluency in the patient's first language will influence the validity of the assessment, hence an interpreter may be required. The pacing of the interview needs to take into account factors such as seating comfort, sensory impairment, clouding of consciousness, level of comprehension, cognitive impairment, and privacy. Assessors should also be aware of underreporting of substance use through denial, stigma, lack of awareness, or memory impairment. A slower pace is needed, as more than one assessment is often required.

There may be barriers to assessment in older people (Box 16.1), and they may be present for both assessor and patient.

Screening instruments for substance misuse in older people are confined to those that identify alcohol misuse (4). The CAGE questionnaire – felt that you should Cut down;

Annoyed by others criticising your drinking; felt Guilty about drinking; had an Eye-opener / felt the need to drink first thing in the morning to steady nerves or get rid of a hangover – allows a rapid screen meant to detect the core features of alcohol dependence. However, it is relatively insensitive to the difference between harmful and hazardous drinking and does not distinguish between current and prior alcohol problems.

The Alcohol Use Disorders Identification Test (AUDIT) (Box 16.2) is the most commonly used screening tool for alcohol misuse. It contains ten questions that explore alcohol use over the past year. The total score indicates a drinking risk category, ranging from lower risk to possible dependence. The AUDIT also serves as a clinical decision tool, as the score provides an indication of appropriate interventions. It can also be used as an outcome measure. A lower cut-off for increasing risk of drinking is recommended for older people.

Screening should be followed by a comprehensive assessment of substance misuse (3). Greater attention should be given to physical illness, drug interactions, social functioning, and social networks in older people than in younger adults. In older people there is comparatively less emphasis on forensic history and occupational history than in younger people. Social pressures such as debt – or even substance-using 'carers', or open drug dealing – may impact on the older person's welfare. Vigilance about safeguarding is essential. Functional ability in the activities of daily living has greater relevance when assessing older people. Neuropsychological evaluation is also relevant. Both these areas require multidisciplinary assessment.

A diagnosis of alcohol dependence is made when three or more of the criteria listed in Box 16.3 are fulfilled (5).

Acute Presentations of Alcohol Misuse and Dependence

Older adults with alcohol misuse and dependence may present acutely to healthcare services with a variety of physical and mental health complaints, without initially disclosing their alcohol intake. These presenting complaints can by cardiovascular (e.g. atrial fibrillation, heart failure), gastrointestinal (e.g. weight loss, dyspepsia, ulceration, liver disease), orthopaedic (e.g. osteoporosis, fractures), and neurological (e.g. peripheral neuropathy) – as well as of many others types (6).

Falls in the elderly are a significant public health issue and cost the NHS an estimated £2.3 billion per year (7). Alcohol misuse can cause falls either as a direct result of acute intoxication or indirectly, through its long-term sequelae (e.g. peripheral neuropathy and/or cerebellar dysfunction). Older adults who misuse alcohol may suffer more serious consequences in the form of falls due to alcohol-induced osteoporosis (leading to more significant fractures) and clotting dysfunction caused by alcohol-related liver disease (leading to increased morbidity from head injuries and more significant traumas). Because of ageist assumptions and lack of disclosure from the patient, the role of underlying alcohol misuse may be overlooked, and thus an opportunity for intervention may be missed.

Alcohol Withdrawal

As with younger patients, the onset of delirium tremens (DT) typically occurs two to five days after cessation of drinking alcohol or a significant reduction in alcohol intake. Delirium tremens is a medical emergency; alcohol withdrawal seizures are a risk twenty-

Box 16.2 Alcohol Use Disorders Identification Test

Questions	Scoring system				
	0	1	2	3	4
1. How often do you have a drink containing alcohol?	Never Go to Q9&10	Monthly or less	2–4 times per month	2 – 3 times per week	4+ times per week
2. How many units of alcohol do you drink on a typical day when you are drinking?	1–2	3–4	5–6	7–8	10+
3. How often have you had 6 or more units if female, or 8 or more if male, on a single occasion in the last year?	Never	Less than monthly	Monthly	Weekly	Daily or almost daily
4. How often during the last year have you found that you were not able to stop drinking once you had started?	Never	Less than monthly	Monthly	Weekly	Daily or almost daily
5. How often during the last year have you failed to do what was normally expected from you because of your drinking?	Never	Less than monthly	Monthly	Weekly	Daily or almost daily
6. How often during the last year have you needed an alcoholic drink in the morning to get yourself going after a heavy drinking session?	Never	Less than monthly	Monthly	Weekly	Daily or almost daily
7. How often during the last year have you had a feeling of guilt or remorse after drinking?	Never	Less than monthly	Monthly	Weekly	Daily or almost daily
8. How often during the last year have you been unable to remember what happened the night before because you had been drinking?	Never	Less than monthly	Monthly	Weekly	Daily or almost daily
9. Have you or somebody else been injured as a result of your drinking?	No		Yes, but not in the last year		Yes, during the last year
10. Has a relative or friend, doctor, or other health worker been concerned about your drinking or suggested that you cut down?	No		Yes, but not in the last year		Yes, during the last year

Score	Drinking categorization
0–7	Lower risk (0–4 for 65+ age group)
8–15	Hazardous/increasing risk
16–19	Harmful/higher risk
20+	Possible/dependence

> **Box 16.3** Diagnostic criteria for alcohol dependence syndrome (World Health Organisation 1992)
>
> A strong desire or compulsion to drink alcohol
>
> Difficulties in controlling use in terms onset, termination, or levels of use
>
> Physiological withdrawal state when use ceases or reduces
>
> Evidence of tolerance (increased amounts required to achieve effects originally produced by lower amounts)
>
> Progressive neglect of alternative pleasures or interests because of increased amount of time necessary to obtain alcohol or to recover from its effects
>
> Persistence with substance use despite clear evidence of overtly harmful consequences (physical or mental)

four to forty-eight hours after cessation (8). Recognising alcohol withdrawal syndrome and delirium tremens in the elderly is vitally important and must be considered as a differential diagnosis of any delirium presentation. Delirium tremens occurs in about 5 per cent of the patients who undergo alcohol withdrawal and, if left untreated, it may be fatal in up to 15–20 per cent of this population. But early detection and prompt initiation of treatment usually prevent the onset of symptoms and reduce mortality to around 1 per cent (9).

The Clinical Institute Withdrawal Assessment of Alcohol Scale, Revised (CIWA-Ar) is used to aid the diagnosis of delirium tremens and to gauge the severity of withdrawal (Box 16.4). Older adults may not show the same symptoms of withdrawal, especially those with comorbid diabetes or neuropathic dysfunction. They may not exhibit the characteristic signs of tremor, sweating, tachycardia, or rise in body temperature. For this reason, the CIWA-Ar) should be used with caution (10, 11). A diagnosis of delirium, with or without physical symptoms, in an older adult with alcohol dependency syndrome should prompt the clinician to consider a diagnosis of delirium tremens. The CIWA-Ar alone may lead to the underestimation of symptoms, a late diagnosis, and an increased risk of alcohol-related brain injury, including Wernicke-Korsakoff syndrome.

The treatment of alcohol withdrawal in the elderly is the same as in younger adults, with high-dose intravenous B vitamins (e.g. Pabrinex). Older adults may require lower doses of benzodiazepines than younger adults, and shorter-acting lorazepam or oxazepam may be considered an alternative to chlordiazepoxide in patients with alcohol-related liver disease, advanced age, or other comorbidities.

Suicide and Self-Harm

Multiple studies have demonstrated that older age and substance misuse are risk factors for suicide and self-harm (12). Comorbid mood disorders combined with relationship difficulties, social isolation, and financial problems associated with alcohol dependency can further increase risk. Both intoxication and alcohol-induced brain injury can increase impulsivity and thereby the risk of acting on suicidal thoughts. Adequate risk assessment of alcohol-dependent patients should be undertaken when they are not acutely intoxicated.

Box 16.4 Clinical Institute Withdrawal Assessment–Alcohol Revised (CIWA-Ar)

Signs of withdrawal monitored every 1–2 hours for 24 hours.

Problem	Range
Nausea and vomiting	0–7
Tremor	0–7
Paroxysmal sweats	0–7
Anxiety	0–7
Agitation	0–7
Tactile disturbances	0–7
Auditory disturbances	0–7
Visual disturbances	0–7
Headache fullness in head	0–7
Orientation and clouding of sensorium	0–4
Total CIWA-Ar Score	0–67

Acute Presentations of Drug Misuse: Opioids/Cannabis/Stimulants

Intoxication and Overdose

As with alcohol, acute intoxication with substances – most commonly opiates and benzodiazepines (3) – may not be recognised in older adults, given the prevalent ageist assumptions. Patients may present with acute confusional states, drowsiness, falls, and cognitive impairment. Accidental overdose is possible in older adults for a variety of reasons, including the physiological changes that accompany ageing (e.g. reduced renal function and increased body fat), other comorbidities, and polypharmacy. Signs of opioid overdose include respiratory depression (made worse in patients with a comorbid pathology, e.g. chronic obstructive pulmonary disease), reduced levels of consciousness, and pinpoint pupils. Patients exhibiting such signs require emergency treatment. Opioid toxicity can be effectively reversed with naloxone; nevertheless, care needs to be taken with patients requiring opiates for pain relief. Flumazenil can be used to reverse benzodiazepines, but may precipitate withdrawal seizures.

Recreational cannabis users who previously used cannabis without ill effect may find themselves suffering unexpected adverse reactions to the drug, including acute confusion and psychosis, because of changes in the strength of the cannabis currently available. Within only a ten-year period (1998–2008), the tetrahydrocannabinol (THC) potency of confiscated cannabis has increased by 103 per cent (13). It has been suggested that cannabis has a wide variety of medicinal uses but taking so-called medicinal cannabis could lead to acute intoxication, which may include confusion, paranoia, and disinhibition; and it could also impair cognitive function. The long-term use of cannabis by the elderly and its effect on cognition has not been studied.

Spice is one of several names for a group of synthetic cannabinoids, and is a novel psychoactive drug that typically contains tetrahydrocannabinol and cannibicyclohexanol, plus a variety of different compounds. It is usually smoked and produces a sedative, anxiolytic, and dissociative effect. Spice use in older adults tends to be seen in the street-drinking population. Acute intoxication can lead to psychotic symptoms, and some individuals present as extremely violent. The use of spice alongside alcohol dependency may complicate alcohol withdrawals.

Stimulant use is less common among the elderly, yet lifetime cocaine and amphetamine use has increased ten-fold in the baby boomer population in England from 1993 to 2012 (14). Certain subcultures (e.g. Northern soul and dance culture) were associated with the use of amphetamines, and there is a general trend in older people to return to the patterns of substance misuse of their youth. This means that acute intoxication with stimulants should not be discounted merely on account of age. A careful, non-judgemental history should be taken, and urine drug screening should be used if there is any doubt.

Drug-Induced Psychosis

Drug-induced psychosis can present at any age and may be a result of misuse of any drug, prescribed or not. Older adults are more at risk of psychoactive substances that cause delirium and psychosis. History taking is key to diagnosis, as is the use of urine drug-screening kits. Common presentations are clouding of consciousness, agitation, suspiciousness, aggression, and autonomic changes such as with heart rate, blood pressure, and breathing.

Withdrawal

Patients may develop a withdrawal syndrome from benzodiazepines or opiates for a number of reasons, as in-patients. A patient may not disclose or be able to disclose his or her use of prescribed and non-prescribed medication. A patient may be nil by mouth and have no alternative route prescribed, which leads to the omission of long-term benzodiazepines or opiates. Withdrawal may be precipitated by an overly rapid, intentional reduction in medication. Withdrawal from benzodiazepines may cause confusion, insomnia, irritability, anxiety, sweating, tremor, nausea, and myalgia. In some individuals, benzodiazepine withdrawal may precipitate seizures and psychosis (15). Withdrawal from opiates can be assessed using the Clinical Opiate Withdrawal Scale (COWS) (16), which rates symptoms such as autonomic arousal and abdominal pain. Benzodiazepine, opiate, and nicotine withdrawal in the elderly may precipitate delirium.

Alcohol-Related Brain Damage

The aetiology of alcohol-related brain damage in multifactorial. There may be accompanying traumatic brain injury, cerebrovascular disease and stroke, cerebellar degeneration, as well as Wernicke's encephalopathy (WE) and Korsakoff's syndrome (KS).

Amnestic Syndromes

Amnestic syndromes comprise WE and KS. Wernicke's encephalopathy is associated with haemorrhage into the dorsomedial nucleus of the thalamus and mammillary bodies.

> **Box 16.5** Diagnosis of alcohol-related dementia
>
> Evidence of cognitive impairment
>
> Significant alcohol use, defined by a minimum average of 35 standard drinks (> 52 UK units) per week for men and 28 (> 42 UK units) for women, for a period longer than five years.
>
> The period of significant alcohol use must occur within three years of the clinical onset of cognitive impairment.

The aetiology of this microvascular damage is deficiency of vitamin B1 (thiamine). Thiamine deficiency in chronic alcohol misuse is associated with inadequate nutritional intake, decreased absorption of thiamine from the gastrointestinal tract, and impaired thiamine utilisation in cells.

Although WE has a classic triad of oculomotor abnormalities, cerebellar dysfunction, and altered mental state, only 20 per cent of patients present with the full triad. A more common presentation is mental sluggishness, apathy, disorientation, poor attention, agitation, and hallucinations. Only 25 per cent of patients have cerebellar dysfunction.

Repeated episodes of WE that are not treated with parenteral thiamine progress to KS, with more permanent impairment of memory. Korsakoff's syndrome is characterized by severe anterograde amnesia and retrograde amnesia extending for years before brain damage. Confabulation occurs in the form of events made up to fill in absent memories.

There is preserved short-term memory, as the neuroanatomical impairment results in faulty encoding of information from short-term to long-term memory. Amnestic syndromes are confined to memory and are not classified as dementias.

Alcohol-Related Dementia

Alcohol-related dementia (ARD) arises after several years of heavy drinking. A diagnosis of probable ARD is made using three diagnostic criteria shown in Box 16.5 (17).

Alcohol-related brain damage (ARBD) shows better performance than Alzheimer's disease on semantic and verbal memory but poorer performance on visuospatial tasks (18). Unlike in many other forms of dementia, some people with ARBD have partial reversibility, for instance in frontal white matter integrity, particularly for late-onset alcohol misuse (19). This may occur as early as after a month of abstinence.

Alcohol use disorders frequently complicate primary dementia too, increasing the cognitive decline. Frontal lobe damage is particularly common in ARBD (20).

Comorbidity

Acute gastric mucosal damage can happen even with lower-risk drinking. Alcohol can inhibit gastric and intestinal motility and cause upper gastrointestinal bleeding; this is due to gastric erosions or peptic ulceration. Mallory–Weiss tears (haematemesis from a tear in the mucosa of the oesophagus) can occur because of alcohol-related vomiting. The initial stage of alcohol-related liver damage is fatty liver, which can progress to alcoholic hepatitis and then to cirrhosis.

Tobacco smoking is associated with bronchitis, emphysema, pneumonia, chronic obstructive pulmonary disease, and lung cancer. Smoking cannabis is associated with chronic obstructive pulmonary disease (COPD), but many cannabis smokers also smoke tobacco.

Drug misuse increases the likelihood of cardiovascular events and deaths. Hypertension, cardiomyopathy, and stroke are associated with substance misuse. Cardiac arrhythmias like atrial fibrillation can result from increasing and higher-risk alcohol consumption, as well as from cannabis. Intravenous cocaine and heroin use increase the risk of endocarditis. Alcohol, amphetamines, and cocaine are also associated with an increased risk of stroke.

Older people are more likely than others to experience falls. This presentation is multifactorial, with loss of balance, autonomic neuropathy, peripheral neuropathy, cardiac disease, osteoporosis, and myopathy all implicated. The systemic effects of substances mean that substance misuse should always be considered when an older person presents with a fall.

Integrated Care

Providing integrated care for patients who misuse of alcohol has been shown to be cost-effective and life-saving. Hospital alcohol teams, combined with assertive outreach services, have been demonstrated to prevent frequent reattending at emergency departments and emergency alcohol detoxifications. Hospital alcohol teams should be led by a consultant gastroenterologist with input from liaison or addiction psychiatry, mental health nurses, and specialist liver nurses. These teams should offer a seven-day alcohol specialist nurse-led service, providing expert assessments of patients who appear to be at risk of alcohol withdrawal (21).

Integrated work can help to identify areas of unmet physical healthcare needs (e.g. alcoholic liver disease and hepatitis from historic intravenous drug use) as well as mental health needs. This approach allows appropriate signposting, communication with primary care, and use of assertive outreach teams if necessary.

Medico-Legal Aspects

Older people with substance misuse should not be assumed to lack capacity, even if they make an unwise decision. Substance misuse should always be considered a possible cause in any older person with fluctuating mental capacity, or where there is evidence of elder abuse. If a healthcare professional suspects substance misuse in an older person, joint work with other teams and social care involvement should be undertaken in order to assess capacity and proactively identify any associated safeguarding concerns.

Deprivation of Liberty Safeguards (DoLS) may concern people with substance misuse, if they lack capacity. This applies to hospitals and care homes. The code of practice for DoLS in the Mental Capacity Act (MCA) states that depriving a patient of liberty may be justifiable if it is in that patient's best interest, to protect him or her from harm; it is a proportional response when compared with the harm faced by the person and if there is no less restrictive alternative.

There may be circumstances in which either the MCA or the Mental Health Act (MHA) may apply, and the question which act applies will be for the judgement of the health professional. However, if the patient retains capacity, the MCA cannot be used.

Box 16.6

Alcohol use and the legal entitlement to drive

Alcohol misuse – defined by medical enquiry and/or abnormal blood results
Group 1 – license revoked until had 6/12 period abstinence or controlled drinking
Group 2 – license revoked until had 1 year abstinence or period of controlled drinking
Alcohol dependence – defined by medical enquiry and/or abnormal blood results
Group 1 – license revoked until 1 year of abstinence and normal blood results
Group 2 – license revoked until 3 years abstinence

Alcohol-related seizure(s)

Group 1 – after one alcohol-related seizure need 1 year after event before driving again, and 1 year abstinence and normal bloods
Group 2 – need 5 years without seizure and must have been off antiepileptic meds for 5 years (+group 1 rules)

If the treatment is for a physical condition, then the MHA does not apply unless there is a direct relationship between the mental disorder and the physical condition, as for example in poor nutrition from a depressive disorder. If the treatment is for a mental disorder and the patient retains capacity, the MCA cannot be used. Where detention is deemed necessary, the MHA must be used, provided that the relevant criteria are met.

Substance Misuse and Driving

The United Kingdom has one of the lowest rates of road traffic accidents in the world (2.4 per 100,000), but 17 per cent of these accidents are alcohol-related (22). Older people are involved only in 15 per cent of all accidents where alcohol is a contributing factor (23). However, aging is associated with greater impairment in divided attention, visual search problems, poor judgement of vehicle approach speed and slow post turn decision maneuvering (24).

In the United Kingdom, there are specified rules around alcohol use and entitlement to drive. These are shown in Box 16.6.

Discharge Planning

Discharge planning for older adults with substance misuse should get the whole multi-disciplinary team (MDT) involved in establishing their current and predicted social, medical, and psychiatric care needs. Discharge planning should be supportive and collaborative with the patients, should take into account their wishes and values, and should consider whether or not they have capacity to make the necessary decisions themselves. The presence of any cognitive impairment, including frontal lobe dysfunction, should be established. Frontal lobe dysfunction is often overlooked and underestimated by traditional measures of cognitive testing but can impact heavily on the risk of self-neglect and accidental self-injury, including accidental fires. Assessment of function therefore needs to be broader than a mere bed-side testing.

Occupational therapy and physiotherapy assessment are an integral part of the MDT assessment. This should include real-world examples specific to the individual and his or her environment (e.g. crossing the road, making a hot meal). Through these assessments, recommendations can be made of aids and adaptions that should help patients to live as safely and as independently as possible (e.g. compliance aids for medication). For patients who are at risk of accidental fires, community fire safety officers can provide home safety checks designed to prevent accidental injury.

Careful consideration should be given to the assessment of carer needs for older adults with substance misuse. Addiction, by its very nature, can strain the relationship between patients with substance dependency and their loved ones. Carers may need specific support from charities such as Al-Anon and from substance misuse services.

The carer may feel under pressure to supply alcohol to a patient who is unable to stop drinking, and damage limitation measures may need to be considered (e.g. modifying alcohol intake after discussion with the multidisciplinary team, in the best interest of a cognitively impaired patient, to slowly reduce alcohol intake). Consideration should be given to safeguarding concerns, if the patient with substance dependence has responsibility for children or vulnerable adults (e.g. a partner with dementia).

The discharge planning process should aim to establish what support is needed to enable the patient to remain free of substance misuse or, if that is not possible, what support can be put in place to limit harm. This may include assertive outreach support and follow-up with substance misuse services, as well as follow-up with mainstream physical and mental health services.

References

1. Rao, R., and Roche, A. Substance misuse in older people. *Brit Med J* 2017, 358: j3885.

2. Rao, R. 'Sadly confused': The detection of depression and dementia on medical wards. *The Psychiatrist* 2001, 25: 177–9.

3. Crome, I., Dar, K., Janikiewicz, S., Rao, T., and Tarbuck, A., 2018. *Our Invisible Addicts: Second Report of the Older Persons' Substance Misuse Working Group of the Royal College of Psychiatrists (CR211)*. London: Royal College of Psychiatrists, 2018.

4. Royal College of Psychiatrists. *Substance Misuse in Older People: An Information Guide. Cross Faculty Report FR/OA/A)/01.* London: Royal College of Psychiatrists, 2015.

5. World Health Organization. *The Tenth Revision of the International Classification of Diseases and Related Health Problems (ICD-10)*. Geneva: WHO, 1992.

6. Blow, F.C., Gillespie, B.W. et al. Brief screening for alcohol problems in elderly populations using the Short Michigan Alcoholism Screening Test–Geriatric Version (SMAST-G). *Alcoholism: Clinical and Experimental Research (Suppl.)* 1998, 16: 372.

7. Nayional Institute of Clinical Excellence. *Falls in Older People: Assessing Risk and prevention. Clinical Guideline (CG161).* London: NICE, 2013.

8. Adinoff, B., Bone, G.H., Linnoila, M. Acute ethanol poisoning and the ethanol withdrawal syndrome: Medical toxicology. *Adverse Drug Exp* 1988, 3: 172–96.

9. Pompei, P., Foreman, M., Rudberg, M.A., Inouye, S.K., Braund, V., and Cassel, C.K. Delirium in hospitalized older persons: Outcomes and predictors. *J Am Geriatrc Soc* 1994, 42: 809–15.

10. Roffman, J.L., and Stern, T.A. Alcohol withdrawal in the setting of elevated blood alcohol levels. *Primary Care Companion to the Journal of Clinical Psychiatry* 2006, 8: 170–3.

11. Sullivan, J.T., Sykora, K., Schneiderman, J., Naranjo, C.A., and Sellers, E.M. Assessment of alcohol withdrawal: The revised clinical institute withdrawal

assessment for alcohol scale (CIWA-Ar). *Br J Addict* 1989, 84: 1353–7.

12. Ness, J., Hawton, K., Bergen, H., Cooper, J., Steeg, S., Kapur, N., Clarke, M., and Waters, K. Alcohol use and misuse, self-harm and subsequent mortality: An epidemiological and longitudinal study from the multicentre study of self-harm in England. *Emerg Med J* 2015, 32: 793–9.

13. El-Sohly, M.A., Mehmedic, Z., Foster, S., Gon, C., Chandra, S., and Church, J.C. Changes in cannabis potency over the last 2 decades (1995–2014): Analysis of current data in the United States. *Biological Psychiatry* 2016, 7: 1–7.

14. Fahmy, V., Hatch, S.L., Hotopf, M., and Stewart, R. Prevalences of illicit drug use in people aged 50 years and over from two surveys. *Age and Ageing* 2012, 41: 553–6.

15. Pétursson, H. The benzodiazepine withdrawal syndrome. *Addiction* 1994, 89: 1455–9.

16. Tompkins, D.A., Bigelow, G.E., Harrison, J.A., Johnson, R.E., Fudala, P.J., and Strain, E.C. Concurrent validation of the Clinical Opiate Withdrawal Scale (COWS) and single-item indices against the Clinical Institute Narcotic Assessment (CINA) Opioid Withdrawal Instrument. *Drug Alcohol Depend* 2009, 105: 154–9.

17. Oslin, D., Atkinson, R.M., Smith, D.M., and Hendrie, H. Alcohol-related dementia: Proposed clinical criteria. *Int J Geriatr Psychiat* 1998, 13: 203–12.

18. Ridley, N.J., Draper, B., and Withall, A. Alcohol-related dementia: An update of the evidence. *Alzheimers Res Ther* 2013, 5: 3.

19. Gazdzinski, S., Durazzo, T.C., Studholme, C., Song, E., Banys, P., and Meyerhoff, D.J. Quantitative brain MRI in alcohol dependence: Preliminary evidence for effects of concurrent chronic cigarette smoking on regional brain volumes. *Alcohol Clin Exp Res* 2005, 29: 1484–95.

20. Rao, R. Cognitive impairment in older people with alcohol use disorders in a UK community mental health service. *Adv Dual Diag* 2016, 9: 154–8.

21. National Confidential Enquiry into Patient Outcome and Death. *Measuring The Units: A Review of Patients Who Died with Alcohol-Related Liver Disease.* London: NCEPOD, 2013.

22. World Health Organization. *Global Status Report on Road Safety, 2015.* Geneva: World Health Organization, 2015.

23. Department of Transport. *Reported Drinking and Driving (RAS51).* London: Department of Transport, 2018.

24. Clarke, D.D., Ward, P., Bartle, C., and Truman, W. Older drivers' road traffic crashes in the UK. *Accident An Prev* 2010, 42(4): 1018–24.

25. *Drug or Alcohol Misuse or Dependence: Assessing Fitness to Drive: Advice for Medical Professionals to Follow When Assessing Drivers with Drug or Alcohol Misuse or Dependence.* London: Department of Transport, 2018.

17

Perioperative Medical Management of Older People

Lessons from Hip Fracture Patients

Atef Michael and Nonyelum Obiechina

Introduction

The population of the world is ageing (1). Although this is particularly true in developed countries, some developing countries are beginning to follow this trend (1). This shift in demographics, together with medical advances, has led to more older patients having surgery and other invasive procedures, many of which would have been unthinkable fifty years ago (2). Among these surgical procedures are emergency surgery for hip fracture patients (2). Although the principles discussed in this chapter would apply to most surgical procedures in older patients, hip fracture surgery is frequently referred to here and used as a case in point.

Hip fractures are common in older patients with an observed median age of 83 years in women and 84 years in men (3). They frequently result from a combination of bone fragility, frailty, and falls (3, 4). Many patients who sustain hip fractures have multiple comorbidities and are on multiple medications (polypharmacy), some of which can increase the risk of falls (3, 4). Comorbidities commonly include cardiovascular disease, previous strokes and transient ischaemic attacks (TIAs), respiratory disease such as chronic obstructive pulmonary disease (COPD), and chronic kidney disease; they all impact adversely on surgical and functional outcomes (3, 4). In addition, many older patients have underlying dementia, which is the strongest independent predictor of postoperative delirium. Post-operative delirium itself is associated with increased mortality, length of hospital stay, and increased risk of institutionalization (4). Conversely, it also increases the risk of dementias. Depression has also been shown to occur commonly after hip fracture and is a further contributor to poor functional outcomes (6). Hip fractures carry a high mortality and morbidity rate in older patients (4, 7, 8) (see Box 17.1). Some propose to refer to it as a 'hip attack', by analogy to a 'heart attack', and recommend that the intervention should have a similar degree of urgency (4, 7, 8).

Surgery remains the best option for getting patients mobile again and for reducing the risks of immobility-associated conditions such as pneumonia, venous thromboembolism (VTE), and pressure sores. Moreover, surgery offers the best chance of reducing pain, improving quality of life, and improving overall outcomes (3, 4, 7, 8). It is recommended that surgery be carried out, preferably, within the first twenty-four to thirty-six hours of the hip fracture and no later than after forty-eight hours (3, 4, 7, 8). Unfortunately, surgery carries its own risks, which are due to potential anaesthetic complications and the risks of the operative procedure itself (3, 4). The overall mortality from hip fractures remains high even with surgery and is about 7–10 per cent within the first thirty days and 20–30 per cent within the first year (3, 8). Less than 50 per cent of survivors regain the level of functioning they had before their hip fracture (3, 4). It is

Box 17.1   Factors contributing to increased mortality of hip fracture patients, in the first three months

Post-operative complications
Pneumonia (aspiration or hospital-acquired), acute kidney injury
Cardiovascular events, thromboembolic disease, delirium
Comorbid conditions, major surgery
The major trauma that caused the fracture

Box 17.2   Lack of physiological reserve in the major organs in older people:

- 50 per cent decline of left ventricular filling by the age of 80
- 50 per cent decline of lung function by the age of 70
- 50 per cent decline of renal function by the age 70
- one third decline of liver weight by the age of 90
- 5 to 10 per cent shrinkage in size of the brain after age 60

thought that comorbidities contribute significantly to postoperative mortality but that up to a third of the mortality is due to the effect of the fractures themselves, including the trauma that led to them (2, 4).

It has been known for some time that optimal management of elderly patients with hip fractures requires integrated, multidisciplinary team work across anaesthetists, orthopaedic surgeons, geriatricians, nurses, pharmacists, physiotherapists, occupational therapists, and dieticians (9). Orthogeriatric support has transformed the care of hip fracture patients. The collaborative models vary from country to country (9). In the United Kingdom, the orthogeriatrics liaison service has shown significant benefit, not only in terms of reducing mortality but in other outcome measures too, such as reduced pressure sores and addressing secondary prevention through falls assessments and bone protection designed to reduce the risk of future fractures (2, 9). Different hospitals have different levels of collaboration and models of service provision. In some countries, such as the United States, cardiologists and respiratory physicians are also involved in pre-operative assessments of these patients (9). The recommended pre- and postoperative approaches to patient management that these collaborations have developed over time are discussed in what follows.

Pre-Operative Management

General Considerations

Older patients lack physiological reserve, and this is important to bear in mind during the pre-operative assessment (10, 11). By the age of 70 years, the left ventricular filling, the lung function, and the renal function have declined in most cases by as much as 50 per cent by comparison to their counterparts in a 30-year-old (see Box 17.2) (10, 11). By the time clinical signs of failure occur in any organ system, it is likely that any remaining functional reserve has been compromised (10, 11). In addition, anaesthetic and surgical stressors can take up significant functional reserve (11). Pre-operative management aims to identify high-risk patients, especially those with limited cardior-espiratory reserve, with dementia, and with a significant number of comorbidities (11).

The aim is also to identify treatable conditions in these patients, so they can be optimised before surgery (11). The Comprehensive Geriatric Assessment (CGA) which is a multidisciplinary, multimodal assessment of physical, cognitive, nutritional, and functional aspects of an older patient, is now the recommended assessment tool for the perioperative screening of hip fracture patients (3, 11).

Dementia is an important risk factor for post-operative delirium (5, 11). Enhanced care pathways used to identify patients at risk of post-operative delirium have identified neurocognitive diseases such as dementia and Parkinson's disease, emergency surgery, and complex procedures as high predictors of post-operative delirium (3, 5, 11). Identifying patients at high risk of delirium and intervening to reduce the risk in these patients are the most effective treatment strategies (5, 11). Treating conditions that cause delirium – for example infections, electrolyte abnormalities, metabolic complications such as hypoglycaemia, hyperglycaemia, and hypercalcaemia, anaemia, constipation, and pain – is a very important part of managing post-operative delirium or reducing its risk (3, 5, 11).

It is essential to strike a delicate balance between the need to treat the acute medical conditions that the patients present with and the necessity to operate on the patients as soon as possible, in order to reduce pain and facilitate early mobilisation (4, 7). Time-to-surgery after hip fracture affects the outcome; many studies have shown that operating on patients within the first thirty-six hours of sustaining a hip fracture is associated with a better outcome and lower mortality (12, 15). Operating after forty-eight hours was shown to be associated with poorer outcomes and greater risk of pneumonia, pressure sores, and VTE (14, 16).

The guidelines of the Association of Anaesthetists of Great Britain and Ireland (AAGBI), 2011 recommend the use of a protocol-driven pathway to reduce the logistical barriers to achieving a timely operation while also ensuring an adequate optimisation of the patients (16). Close work among orthopaedic surgeons, anaesthetists, orthogeriatricians, and trauma coordinators is essential to facilitating timely interventions and reducing avoidable delays of surgery (16). These medical problems include hypovolaemia, dehydration with acute kidney injury, electrolyte imbalance, infections such as pneumonia and other infections, delirium, patients on antiplatelet agents, anticoagulants, and patients with pacemakers and implantable cardiac defibrillators (16, 1, 9).

Although reasons to delay surgery may be justified, for instance in patients who remain unwell despite efforts to optimise their medical condition, there are some potentially avoidable reasons for delaying surgery (16). They include suboptimal planning for theatre spaces, delays in reversal of warfarin, uncomplicated hyperglycaemia, asymptomatic and mild to moderate electrolyte imbalance, and patients with infections who are already on antibiotics and are stable (16, 17). Other reasons are unnecessary requests for echocardiograms, for example in patients found to have faint ejection systolic murmur but are otherwise asymptomatic (1, 6).

In addition to the guidelines published by the AAGBI, many units now have local pathways with recommendations for the treatment of hip fracture patients from their arrival in accident and emergency department through their entire hospital journey, up until discharge (16, 20). In the United Kingdom, hip fracture management in all National Health Service (NHS) hospitals is audited regularly by the national hip fracture database (NHFD), and the units are benchmarked against national standards. Performance is also used to determine eligibility for tariff payments on each patient (20).

Pain Control in Hip Fracture Patients

Pain is a common symptom in hip fracture patients. Patients living with dementia may not always be able to communicate their needs verbally (21). Poorly controlled pain is one of the risk factors for post-operative delirium, and it is already common in patients with pre-existing cognitive impairment (22). Furthermore, untreated pain in dementia is associated with agitation and distress (21, 22).

The assessment of pain may not always be straightforward in people living with dementia who have an impaired ability to understand their needs or to communicate verbally (21, 23). For this reason, pain assessment tools are recommended (21, 23).

The World Health Organisation (WHO) analgesic ladder advocates the use of a three-step process for pain control (23) (see Box 17.3). This is done as a stepped-up sequence from non-opioids to weak opioids and up to strong opioids, according to the severity of pain (23). A patient's treatment should start at the step appropriate for the severity of the pain (23). There are perioperative techniques for achieving good post-operative pain management. They include neuro-axial opioid analgesia, patient acti-vated analgesia (PCA) with systemic opioids, and peripheral regional analgesic tech-niques (16, 23). It is recommended that patients have regular analgesia prescribed, in addition to analgesics being prescribed for when requested by patients (PRN). Regular intravenous paracetamol is used in many units alongside PRN oramorph (16, 23). Some clinicians favour oxycodone over morphine because of its versatility and rela-tively favourable side effect profile (23). Ilio-fascial block administered on admission can also reduce the requirement for opiates and may reduce the risk of post-operative delirium (23, 24).

Box 17.3 Pain Control in Hip Fracture Patients

The WHO analgesic ladder advocates the use of a three-step ladder for pain control:

- non-opioids
- weak opioids
- strong opioids

For mild pain:

paracetamol 1g QDS {regular)
+/− adjunct

For moderate pain:

paracetamol 1g QDS {regular)

+ weak opioid {codeine or tramadol)
+/− adjunct for severe pain

strong opioid {morphine or pethidine)

+/− paracetamol 1g QDS
+/− adjunct

Adjuvants include:

NSAID
oramorph PRN
other opiates

> **Box 17.4** Anaemia and hip fracture
>
> Pre-operatively: up to 50 per cent of hip fracture patients are anaemic on admission.
> Perioperatively: patients lose about 20 gm/L of haemoglobin.
> Post-operatively: more than 90 per cent of hip fracture patients are anaemic.
> Patients with pre-operative haemoglobin < 90 g/L should have blood transfusion before surgery.

Optimising Anaemia before Surgery

Pre-operative anaemia is common in older patients and is associated with increased mortality (25). Up to half of hip fracture patients are anaemic on admission to hospital, and more develop anaemia post-operatively (16, 25). The causes are, frequently, multifactorial; common reasons include a reduction in the production of erythropoietin, a reduction in viable stem cells in the bone marrow, and specific deficiencies in haematinics such as iron, B12, and folic acid (25). Certain disease conditions, particularly inflammatory ones, can cause anaemia of chronic disease, as can chronic kidney disease (25). Blood loss intra- and post-operatively contributes significantly to post-operative anaemia (16, 25).

The AAGBI recommends that older patients with pre-operative haemoglobin of less than 90 g/l should have two units of blood transfusion before surgery and that, in patients with Ischaemic heart disease, the threshold for transfusion should be 100 g/l (16). The cause of the anaemia should be investigated and blood samples for serum iron, ferritin, B12, and folic acid levels should be taken before transfusion (16) (see Box 17.4).

Pneumonia and Other Infections

Older patients can have pneumonia, urinary tract infection, or other infections in the pre-operative period (26). The incidence of pneumonia in pre-operative hip fractures has been estimated at 0.3–3.2 per cent, depending on the cohort studied (26). In hip fracture patients, ore-operative pneumonia is associated with poorer outcomes (26). Infections, when identified pre-operatively, should be treated according to the local antibiotic policy and the guidelines of the hospital. As long as the patient is not septic, is haemodynamically stable, and is able to maintain his or her target oxygen saturation with or without oxygen, surgery can still be performed after the first dose of antibiotic (16, 26). Particularly in the case of pneumonia, spinal anaesthesia may be the preferred anaesthetic option (16). Chest physiotherapy may be indicated post-operatively in some cases, particularly for patients with chronic respiratory diseases.

These patients need to be monitored closely and, should they become septic or haemo-dynamically unstable, require urgent escalation – ideally to a high dependency unit (HDU) or an intensive care unit (ICU) (16, 26).

Optimising Fluid Balance before Surgery

It is crucial to ensure that hypovolaemia is corrected before surgery with intravenous fluids and that acute kidney injury is treated (27). The intravenous fluids used should also be able to correct any concomitant electrolyte imbalance (27). For instance, in the case of hyponatremia – provided that it is not severe (i.e. sodium is more than 120 mmol/l (millimoles per litre)) and that the patient does not have neurological symptoms – 0.9 per cent normal saline can be used in this situation (27, 28). Fluid balance charts to monitor fluid intake and hourly urine output are important in the perioperative period. In addition, heart rate, blood pressure, respiratory rate, and oxygen saturation need to be monitored as part of the National Early Warning Score (NEWS) (16, 27, 28). Older patients are particularly vulnerable to the risk of acute kidney injury if they do not have adequate fluids. Conversely, they can easily become fluid-overloaded because of their reduced cardiac reserve (29). The right balance needs to be achieved. As a safety guide, older people should not be given more than one litre intravenously per twelve hours, unless clinically indicated, and in that case close monitoring for signs of fluid overload should be undertaken (29, 30). Serum urea, creatinine, and electrolytes should be monitored carefully in the peri-operative period (2, 9). A blood urea greater than 18 mmol/l or serum creatinine larger than 230 micromol/l without a history of chronic kidney disease can be a justifiable reason to delay surgery for optimisation (16, 29).

Optimising Electrolyte Imbalance before Surgery

Ideally, electrolyte imbalance should be corrected before surgery. However, attempting to strike the balance between an early surgery (preferably within thirty-six hours and no longer than forty-eight hours) and biochemical optimisation means that achieving the ideal electrolyte balance is not always feasible (12, 16). Provided that no concomitant cardiac or neurological problems are associated with the electrolyte imbalance and, in the case of hyponatraemia, provided that it has not occurred acutely, many anaesthetists will accept patients for theatre with a sodium of 120–150 mmol/l and a potassium of 2.8–6.0 mmol/l, with close monitoring and ongoing corrective treatment (16, 28, 30). The serum bicarbonate should ideally be in the range of 18–36 mmol/l (16 (see Box 17.5 for a summary)).

Hyponatraemia and the Older Hip Fracture Patient

Hyponatraemia is common in older patients. It is also one of the most common electrolyte imbalances in the peri-operative period and may present a real clinical challenge (21, 29). It is defined as a sodium level of less than 135 mmol/l. It can be acute or chronic (27, 28). Patients with hyponatraemia are hypovolemic, euvolemic, or hypervolemic (27, 28).

Acute hyponatraemia occurs when there is a drop in sodium levels of 12 mmol/l or more in less than forty-eight hours (16, 27, 28). It can be classified as mild when the

---

Box 17.5 Electrolyte balance (the allowed pre-operative range):

Sodium	120–150 mmol/l
Potassium	2.8–6.0 mmol/l
Bicarbonate	18–36 mmol/l
Urea	< 18 mmol/l (without history of CKD)
Serum creatinine	< 230 μμmol/l (without history of CKD)

sodium level is between 128 and 134 mmol/l, moderate when the level ranges between 120 and 127 mmol/l, and severe when the level falls below 120 mmol/l (27, 28).

The immediate management of hyponatraemia is determined by whether it is acute or chronic and mild, moderate, or severe, and by the severity of the patient's symptoms (28). Patients with acute severe hyponatraemia, especially in the presence of neurological symptoms such as seizures and depressed level of consciousness, need to be managed in a HDU. It is important not to correct the hyponatraemia too rapidly, as this may cause central pontine myelinolysis (28). The recommendation is to increase the sodium level by 8–12 mmol/l in twenty-four hours, and no more than 18 mmol/l in forty-eight hours in acute hyponatraemia, and 6 mmol/l in twenty-four hours for chronic severe hyponatraemia (16, 28).

Essentially, the underlying cause of the hyponatraemia should be sought and treated (28). For instance, in hypovolaemic hyponatraemia, culprit medications such as thiazide diuretics and angiotensin-converting enzyme (ACE) inhibitors may need to be stopped, and a normal saline infusion may help (27, 29). Hypervolemic states such as congestive cardiac failure may require loop diuretics; these can excrete more water than sodium and improve the hyponatraemia in this situation, while also treating the congestive cardiac failure (30, 31). Fluid restriction to 1–1.5 litres a day may help both the hyponatraemia and the congestive cardiac failure (30, 31). Sometimes the administration of a vasopressin receptor antagonist such as tolvaptan or conivaptan may help, if initial measures fail to improve the sodium levels 31. Euvolemic hyponatraemia can be caused by a wide range of conditions that result in the syndrome of inappropriate ADH secretion (SIADH). SIADH may also be caused by medications, for example antidepressants such as fluoxetine and sertraline and antiepileptics such as carbamazepine (31). In these instances, stopping the offending agent where possible and fluid restriction to 500 ml in less than the twenty-four hour urinary output may help (28, 31). Where there is no significant response, a vasopressin receptor antagonist may help by inhibiting the binding of the ADH to the collecting tubules in the nephrons (31).

Atrial Fibrillation before Surgery

Most anaesthetists are happy to take to surgery patients with atrial fibrillation, provided that the ventricular rate is between 60 and 90 per minute and that the patient has normal blood pressure and is not in heart failure (16). When the ventricular rate is more than 100 per minute, rate control with a beta blocker is recommended, on condition that there are no contraindications (32). If beta blockers are contraindicated, a loading dose of digoxin may be given to slow down the ventricular rate (32). Alternatives include intravenous amiodarone, given as 300 mg over one hour and followed by 900 mg administered over 23 hours (32). Where concerns remain, it may be prudent to involve a cardiologist.

Antiplatelet Treatments before Surgery

Many elderly patients are on antiplatelet agents such as aspirin or clopidogrel for secondary prevention after coronary stents in ischaemic heart disease (33). There are concerns about increased blood loss intra-operatively and bleeding at the site of a spinal block with these drugs (33). Although aspirin can be withheld pre-operatively, the recommendation to stop or continue clopidogrel is less clear (33, 34). There is some concern that stopping it, especially in patients with drug-eluting stents for ischaemic heart disease, may increase mortality (33, 34). A recent systematic review of the evidence for the management of antiplatelet therapy in non-cardiac surgery found that it was difficult to draw any specific conclusions because of significant methodological flaws and widespread heterogeneity in the study designs (33). Its authors therefore recommended that each case should be evaluated and decided in a collaboration between cardiologists, anaesthetists and surgeons (33). The general consensus by the Scottish Intercollegiate Guidance Network (SIGN) and the AAGBI is that clopidogrel should not be discontinued and platelet transfusion is not warranted unless patients need it for other reasons (34). The decision to continue or discontinue antiplatelets therapy in the perioperative period depends on several factors, including the original indication for the antiplatelet, the potential consequences of discontinuation, and the bleeding risk with continuation (16, 34). In any event, this is likely to affect the choice of the anaesthetic used, since clopidogrel may, for instance, increase the risk of spinal haematoma with neuro-axial anaesthesia (16, 34).

Anticoagulants before Surgery

Some older patients are on long-term anticoagulation for different indications (35, 37). The most common indications for long-term anticoagulation in older people are atrial fibrillation and mechanical prosthetic heart valves (36, 37). In some cases, the patients are on long-term anticoagulation for a recurrent or unprovoked venous thrombo-embolic disease (VTE) such as deep vein thrombosis (DVT) or pulmonary embolism (37). Some of the anticoagulants are vitamin K antagonists such as warfarin, phenindione, or synthrone (38).

Newer oral anticoagulants (NOACs), also called direct oral anticoagulants (DOACs), are increasingly being used in VTE and atrial fibrillation (39). Vitamin K antagonists can be reversed with vitamin K and prothrombin complex concentrate (PCC) (40). Dabigatran, a DOAC that is a direct thrombin antagonist, has also got a reversal agent, etaracizumab (41, 44). More recently, a reversal agent called 'andexanet alfa' has become approved by the Federal Drug Agency (FDA) for the factor Xa antagonists apixaban and rivaroxaban (39, 41, 44). Unfortunately, this is, currently, prohibitively expensive. For warfarin, the current recommendation is to reduce the international normalised ratio (INR) to less than 1.5 before surgery (41). As regards the DOACs, the National Institute of Clinical Excellence (NICE) Clinical Knowledge Summaries site has advised that, for procedures with a high risk of bleeding such as hip fracture surgery, apixaban, edoxaban, or rivaroxaban should be stopped forty-eight hours before the procedure and dabigatran may need to be stopped seventy-two (if CrCl is 50–80 ml/min) or even ninety-six hours (if CrCl is 30–50 ml/min) before the intervention (42, 44). Different hospitals may adopt variations on this scheme after consultation with their local haematology team.

In patients with prosthetic heart valves or recurrent or recent VTE, or in patients with active malignancy, bridging anticoagulation with low molecular heparins (LMWH) or unfractionated heparin can be used for the period during which the INR is less than 2 when warfarin is withheld (43, 44). The aim is to reduce thrombotic and thrombo-embolic events (43, 44). When in doubt, enlisting the help of a haematologist can be useful.

Pacemakers and Implantable Cardiac Defibrillators

Some patients may have permanent pacemakers (PPMs) related to a previous heart block. It is important that they are checked and deemed to be working satisfactorily before surgery (45). A small number of patients may have an implantable cardiac defibrillator (ICD) from a previous ventricular fibrillation (46). The ICDs may increase the risk of shock to the patient when diathermy is used during surgery and may need to be deactivated before certain operative proce dures (47).

Generally, cardiac devices such as PPMs and ICDs should be assessed pre-operatively, to decide whether there is any need to change the mode of the PPM or to deactivate the ICD (45, 47). It is also important to check the devices post-operatively, to readjust or reactivate them and to ensure functionality (45, 47). These issues need to be clarified pre-operatively with the cardiology team.

The Diabetic Elderly Patient and Surgery

Diabetes mellitus in the elderly patient can adversely affect post-operative outcomes (48). Trauma and surgery can increase the stress response in diabetic patients and worsen their hyperglycaemia (49). Patients do need to be fasted before surgery, and it is therefore imperative that there are protocols in place to prevent hypoglycaemia and to keep it to a minimum (48).

Most guidelines advise trying to achieve 'reasonable' normoglycaemia with a majority of glucose readings below 11.0 mmol/l (6, 48). Different protocols currently exist for managing diabetes in the perioperative period; a common theme is prioritising the patients so that they are the first on the theatre list, in a bid to avoid unnecessary prolonged fasting (16, 48). It is recommended that all diabetic medications be taken as usual on the day before surgery (16, 48). Patients may need to have their blood glucose monitoring hourly while they are fasted (48). Capillary blood glucose should be checked hourly during surgery and until the patient wakes up and starts to eat. If the blood glucose drops below 4 mmol/l, 150 ml of dextrose 10 per cent can be given intravenously (16, 48). Hypoglycaemia is more immediately serious than hyperglycaemia.

Many type 2 diet-controlled diabetic patients do not require any therapy peri-operatively (16, 48). For type 2 diabetics on oral hypoglycaemics, on the morning of the operation the oral hypoglycaemics are withheld (48). They can have dextrose or saline infusions, and if their blood glucose rises, variable-rate intravenous insulin infusion (VRIII) is used (48). After surgery, the oral hypoglycaemic regime can be resumed when patients start to eat (48).

For patients on insulin, basal insulin should continue. Short-acting insulin for mealtimes should be omitted while the patient is nil by mouth (48, 49). Pre-mixed insulin should have 50 per cent of the morning dose reduced (16, 48). Variable-rate intravenous insulin infusion should be used if the glycaemic control is poor or if the patient is insulin-treated and is expected to miss more than one meal post-operatively. These patients need hourly monitoring of their blood glucose (48).

If serum ketones are more than 1.0 mmols/l, this should be corrected before surgery and patients should be screened for diabetic ketoacidosis (48, 49). Patients with type 1 diabetes are more likely to become ketotic, particularly if they are starved for a long time before surgery (50). They need blood glucose, serum ketones, and acid–base status monitoring (50). If they develop diabetic ketoacidosis, they need to be on fixed-dose

---

Box 17.6 The Diabetic Elderly Patient and Surgery

General rules:

- Try to achieve a majority of glucose readings below 11.0 mmol/l.
- Hypoglycaemia is more serious than hyperglycaemia.
- Try to avoid unnecessarily prolonged fasting.
- If the blood glucose drops to below 4 mmol/l, dextrose can be given intravenously.
- All diabetes medications should be taken as normal on the day before surgery.
- Capillary blood glucose should be checked hourly during surgery and until the patient wakes up and starts to eat.
- Many type 2 diet-controlled diabetic patients do not require any therapy peri-operatively.
- If the blood glucose rises, VRIII is used.
- Basal insulin should continue in the perioperative period as usual.
- Mealtime insulin should be omitted when patient is nil by mouth.

---

insulin infusions and dextrose or saline infusions while fasted (50). Their glucose, ketones, and acid–base status should be normalised before surgery (50). Once they are able to eat and drink post-operatively, they can go back on their usual Insulin regime (50). (See Box 17.6 for a summary.)

The Parkinson's Disease Patients and Surgery

Patients with Parkinson's disease are at risk of falls and osteoporosis and therefore their risk of sustaining fractures is significant (51). Not surprisingly, therefore, a substantial number of patients with hip fractures have Parkinson's disease (52). More than 50 per cent of Parkinson's disease patients are not adequately managed when they are hospitalised for operative interventions (53). Moreover, the presence of Parkinson's disease increases the risk of post-operative complications, as a result of both the effect of the disease itself and the potential interruption of anti-Parkinsonian treatment during the perioperative period (53). Possible complications include aspiration pneumonia, urinary tract infections, and rigidity if the anti-Parkinsonian treatment is delayed because of prolonged peri-operative fasting (53). In extreme cases, patients can develop neuroleptic malignant syndrome if they suddenly stop taking their dopamine or agonist medications (54). The syndrome is characterised by a high temperature, rigidity, and a rise in muscle enzymes such as creatine kinase; and it can be fatal (54). Minimising these risks requires accurate and timely identification of patients with Parkinson's disease, increasing awareness of the importance of timely dopaminergic medications, and planning the hip fracture pathway with this in mind (53, 54). Prioritising the patients for early morning surgery may also help to reduce disruption to their drug schedule (53, 54). Involving the hospital pharmacists to help with information on an appropriate non-oral alternative such as a patch (rotigotine) or a subcutaneous injection of apomorphine is also recommended (55, 59). Both rotigotine and apomorphine are dopamine receptor agonists (DAs) (55, 59).

Medications for Parkinson's disease include levodopa, DAs, cathecol-o-methyltransferase inhibitors (COMT inhibitors), and monamine oxidase inhibitors (MAO inhibitors) (57). These medications are commonly used in combination (57). The regime used will vary from patient to patient, depending on patient tolerability and on how advanced the disease is; many patients are on complex regimes (57). Ideally, a Parkinson's disease specialist or a Parkinson's disease nurse should be involved in the peri-operative period, particularly in the more complex patients (53). A full review on Parkinson's disease please can be found in Chapter 18.

Dopamine receptor agonist patches (rotigotine) can be used in the perioperative period, and the doses are based on calculation charts designed to convert different treatments into near equivalent doses of rotigotine (58). Patients who are on doses that exceed the maximum dose of rotigotine may need to have subcutaneous a pomorphine (53, 59). It is preferred that in these cases a review of the patient by a Parkinson's disease specialist or nurse is expedited, as apomorphine is a specialised drug and has side effects that include excessive vomiting (53, 59). Patients need to have anti-emetics before they receive apomorphine, while bearing in mind that most anti-emetics can exacerbate the Parkinsonian symptoms (59). Exceptions include ondansetron (60). Domperidone was used extensively in the past, but concerns about an increased risk of ventricular arrhythmia limit now its use (61). Post-operatively, once the patients are able to eat and drink, they can be restarted on their usual oral regimens (53).

Reasons to Delay Hip Fracture Surgery

Although it is generally recommended that rapid optimisation of patients' condition and surgery be achieved as soon as possible in order to improve the outcomes of hip fracture surgery, there are some medical conditions where delay of surgery is the safer option (16). Surgery may need to be delayed in any serious medical condition that cannot be treated, managed, or improved within a few days (62, 63). In these instances, successful treatment of the medical condition takes precedence over surgery (16, 62, 63). In some cases the medical condition may be a contraindication to surgery; examples include recent acute myocardial infarction and recent acute strokes (63, 64). In other cases surgery may need to be delayed pending optimisation; patients with decompensated congestive cardiac failure, patients with persistent hypotension, and patients with severe respiratory failure fall in this category (16, 30, 63). Arrhythmias such as ventricular tachycardia or severe bradyarrhythmia and heart block may also delay surgery until they have been appropriately treated and the patient stabilised (16, 63). Most anaesthetists and surgeons delay surgery if INR is greater than 1.6, if haemoglobin is less than 70 gm/l, or if the blood glucose is more than 33 mmol/ l (16).

Post-Operative Management of Hip Fractures

Anaemia, acute kidney injury, delirium, and urinary tract and chest infections are common medical post-operative complications after hip fracture surgical repair (16, 63). Acute left ventricular failure, acute coronary syndrome, and stroke or TIA account for up to 5 per cent of post-operative complications. Vascular complications tend to occur earlier than infections (4, 63, 64). We will briefly discuss post-operative anaemia, acute kidney injury, delirium, and prevention of VTE, as well as post-operative depression and cognitive dysfunction and their impact on post-operative outcomes.

Post-Operative Anaemia

Post-operative anaemia is common, mostly as a result of blood loss during surgery, and occurs in more than 90 per cent of patients (65). It is important to screen for and reduce pre-operative anaemia in order to limit the degree of post-operative anaemia that may result from intra-operative bleeding. Pre-operative anaemia has been identified as a predictor of increased mortality and morbidity in these patients (65).

It is recommended that patients with post-operative haemoglobin of less than 100 g/l receive blood transfusion if they have ischaemic heart disease or if they are symptomatic with the anaemia (16, 65). Patients without ischaemic heart disease and patients who are not symptomatic may require blood transfusion if their post-operative haemoglobin is less than 90 g/l (65). Some guidelines adopt a more restrictive approach to blood transfusion and have a much lower threshold for transfusing asymptomatic patients: 80 g/l in some cases, or even 70 g/l in patients with good cardiorespiratory reserve (65, 67). Each case should be considered in the context of the full clinical picture and associated comorbidities (16, 65). An alternative to blood transfusion is iron infusions, provided that the patient is not actively bleeding and is haemo-dynamically stable (66, 67).

Post-Operative Acute Kidney Injury

Many elderly patients who sustain hip fracture have chronic kidney disease (CKD) (16, 29). Pre-operative dehydration, intra-operative blood loss, and the haemo-dynamic instability caused by cement in some operations can result in acute kidney injury (AKI) (16, 29). Other causes include infections and nephrotoxic medications such as frusemide and ACE inhibitors that the patient may already be on for their comorbid conditions (16, 29). Many hip fracture patients have a degree of deterioration of their estimated glomerular filtration rate (eGFR) post-operatively (29). Patients undergoing a hemiarthroplasty tend to experience more post-operative decline in eGFR than patients who had dynamic hip screw (DHS) (16, 29). This may be related to the greater amount of blood loss observed in patients during hemiarthroplasty (65).

To reduce the risk of AKI, patients should be well hydrated pre-operatively. This is crucial also in order to minimise the periods of intra-operative hypotension (16, 29). Where AKI occurs, meticulous medical management and proper fluid balance are vital (16, 29). Management relies mainly on balanced fluid replacement (including blood transfusion, if indicated). Treating team should consider withholding nephrotoxic medications when possible, and referral to the urology team if obstructive uropathy is present for further management (16, 29).

Post-Operative Vascular Complications

Most post-operative vascular complications occur early, within the first week after surgery, and include myocardial infarction, stroke, and congestive cardiac failure (4, 63, 64). They frequently occur in patients who have a predisposition for these complications, for example hypertensive patients and patients with known ischaemic heart disease (IHD), previous stroke or TIA, and peripheral vascular disease (63, 64). Patients with atrial fibrillation may be at increased risk of an ischaemic stroke or TIA as a result of stopping their anticoagulation, and it is important to restart it as soon as it is safe to do so, in most cases after forty-eight hours (16, 64). Some patients with delirium present without the usual symptoms of these vascular complications (63, 64). For example, patients with acute myocardial infarction may not always present with chest pain, but they show general deterioration, features of decompensated heart failure, or delirium (30, 63). It is important to have a high index of suspicion and to do serial electrocardiograms (ECGs) and troponins in such instances (63). These patients should ideally be managed in the coronary care unit (CCU), with cardiology input (16, 63). In the case of stroke patients, they should be seen by a stroke physician and, preferably, managed in the stroke unit (64).

Prevention of Venous Thrombo-Embolism

There is an increased risk of VTE in patients who are immobile and have pelvic and hip fractures (67). Surgery further increases this risk (67, 68). Without VTE prophylaxis, the incidence of objectively confirmed, hospital-acquired DVT in hip fracture patient is 40 to 60 per cent. Prophylactic doses of LMWH are used to reduce the risk of VTE (68). They are given from the day of admission, usually in the evening. For instance, enoxaparin (40 mg) is administered subcutaneously once a day, in the evening (68). Significant renal impairment (creatinine clearance less than 15 ml/minute in the case of enoxaparin) can preclude the use of LMWH, as can concurrent bleeding, severe thrombocytopenia, recent stroke, and subdural haematoma (69). In these cases it is advisable to discuss alternative options with the haematologist. In some cases mechanical thrombo-prophylaxis may be considered, for instance through intermittent pneumatic compression devices (IPC), although the evidence for their efficacy is sparse by comparison with the evidence for medical thrombo-prophylaxis (70). The majority of symptomatic VTEs associated with hospital admissions occur after hospital discharge (6–8, 70). For this reason, thrombo-prophylaxis in hip fracture patients is usually extended for up to thirty-five days after surgery (16, 20).

Post-Operative Delirium

Delirium is an acute disorder of attention and cognitive function (71). It is one of the commonest complications in hip fracture patients (16, 71). It is often precipitated by surgery, dehydration, electrolyte imbalance, medications, infection, or head injury (71). The diagnostic criteria for delirium are derived from the ICD10 (International Classification of Diseases) code and from the fourth edition of the *Diagnostic Statistical Manual* (72, 73). Assessment tools include the Cognitive Assessment Method (CAM) and the 4-Point Assessment Tool Test (4-AT) (74). A full review of delirium will be found in Chapter 11.

The prevalence of post-operative delirium in hip fracture patients ranges between 45 and 70 per cent, depending on age and the cohort studied (75). Delirium in this category of patients is associated with greater mortality, morbidity, and a longer stay in hospital (75). It is therefore important that patients who are at high risk for delirium are identified pre-operatively and measures are taken to prevent post-operative delirium (75). It is also important that the staff that looks after these patients is able to recognise post-operative delirium early and to treat it promptly (75).

Pain increases the risk of delirium; adequate analgesia can lower this risk. It is crucial to identify the underlying cause of the delirium and to treat it (77). This may include correcting electrolyte abnormalities, rehydrating, and treating infections (77). A review of the patients' medications designed to identify and, if possible, stop or reduce the dose of culprit medications is important (77). These include opioids, antihistamines, and anticholinergic drugs (77). For patients who have been on benzodiazepines for a long period, it is important that the medication is not omitted in hospital, as this can precipitate withdrawal symptoms and delirium (78). Proactive involvement of the orthogeriatric team can reduce the risk of delirium.

Strategies specific to the surgical patient that have been shown to work to reduce the incidence of post-operative delirium include depth of anaesthesia monitoring (using the bispectral index), intra-operative dexmedetomidine infusion, use of non-opioid analgesia, and iliac fascia femoral block, which reduces the need for opioid analgesics (79). Obviously, as the pathophysiology of delirium becomes better understood, especially at the molecular level, it is hoped that more specific strategies will become available to target the different pathways involved (79, 80). That said, it is important to identify known medical causes of delirium and to treat them, in an attempt to reduce both the risk and the duration of delirium in these patients (4, 20, 79). Evidence for the role of the anaesthesia type in the development of delirium in elderly hip fracture patients remains conflicting (79, 80). The REGAIN (Regional versus General Anaesthesia for Promoting Independence after Hip Fracture) study is an ongoing multicentre clinical trial that looks at the impact of the type of anaesthetic in causing delirium in elderly hip fracture patients (80). It is hoped that the results will add to existing strategies in combating post-operative delirium. Delirium is discussed in more depth in Chapter 11.

Post-Operative Depression in Hip Fracture Patients

Depression is common in hip fracture patients (6, 81, 83). It causes reduced motivation, which in turn results in inability to engage with early rehabilitation and mobilisation after surgery (6, 81). It is also frequently associated with cognitive impairment and dementia, as well as contributing to delirium post-operatively (81, 82). This has been shown in various studies, including a recent one from the John Hopkins Medical Centre (82). Although the findings are still in the preliminary stages, they do raise questions about whether routine screening of hip fracture patients for depression should be undertaken as part of the risk assessment for post-operative complications (82). Depression has been shown to impair T cell lymphocyte function and suppress immunity in older patients (83). It has also been linked to elevated levels of pro-inflammatory cytokines such as interleukin 1 (IL-1), interleukin 6 (IL-6), and tumour necrosis factor alfa (TNF alfa), all of which are associated with delirium (83). There is evidence that depression increases susceptibility to infections such as pneumonia as a result of this described immunosuppression (81, 83).

Patients with depression should be assessed individually on the risk–benefit ratios of using antidepressants (83). Antidepressants, when combined with cognitive behavioural therapy (CBT), have been found to be effective in treating elderly patients with depression (83). Unfortunately, CBT is not always accessible to older patients. Some evidence suggests that nurse-led interventions such as exposure of patients to increased social contact may help to reduce depression in hip fracture patients, but more evidence is needed (6, 81, 83). Further information on the assessment and treatment of depression can be found in Chapter 12.

Post-Operative Cognitive Dysfunction

Post-operative cognitive dysfunction (POCD) is a persistent but stable cognitive impairment that can arise at any time between seven days to twelve months after surgical treatment (84). Unlike delirium, it does not arise acutely; it is insidious and subtle in its presentation and is not associated with fluctuations in lucidity or conscious state and attention (84, 85). It does, however, involve multiple domains of impaired cognition such as memory, executive function, verbal fluency, and visuospatial awareness (84). Neuro-inflammation has been proposed as one of the main mechanisms of action (85). Post-operative cognitive dysfunction is thought to be related to general anaesthesia, and the monitoring of depth of anaesthesia is one of the ways to reduce the risk of this development (84, 85). It is potentially reversible but needs to be recognised in its own right, as distinct from dementia and delirium (84, 85).

Other Considerations and Measures

Nutritional assessment and supplementation in patients who are malnourished or at risk of becoming so, early mobilisation as part of rehabilitation, measures to reduce the infection, for example antibiotic prophylaxis, are other measures undertaken in hip fracture patients (20, 86). Other interventions include the treatment of osteoporosis as part of secondary prevention of future fractures, falls prevention plans, and the prevention of pressure sores (20, 87).

Conclusion

- With the current demographic changes, more older patients are expected to undergo surgery and other invasive procedures.
- Older people have more post-operative complications and higher mortality than younger people because of their diminished physiologic reserve and comorbid conditions.
- Optimising the physical, haematological, and biochemical parameters is important for improving the surgical outcome.
- Fluid balance is of paramount importance; too little fluid causes acute kidney injury, too much fluid causes fluid overload and left ventricular failure.
- Post-operative complications depend on the surgery and commonly include acute kidney injury, volume overload, vascular complications, infections, and delirium.
- Dementia is a big risk factor for post-operative delirium, and it is important to identify the relevant patients and intervene to reduce this risk.
- Post-operative depression and cognitive dysfunction should be considered and addressed.
- Pain control is crucial to reducing the patient symptoms, enhancing recovery, and reducing the risk of delirium.
- Early mobilisation after surgery reduces the risk of infections, thromboembolic disease, deconditioning, and institutionalisation.

References

1. United Nations. *World Population Prospects: The 2017 Revision.* New York: United Nations, Department of Economic and Social Affairs, Population Division, 2017.

2. Kyriacou, H., and Khan, W.S. Important perioperative factors, guidelines and outcomes in the management of hip fractures. *Journal of Preoperative Practice* 2021, 3(4): 140–6.

3. National Clinical Guidance Centre. *The Management of Hip Fractures in Adults.* London: National Clinical Guidance Centre, 2011. www.ncgc.ac.uk.

4. Carpintero, P., Caeiro, J.R., Carpintero, R., Morales, A., Silva, S., and Mesa, M. Complications of hip fractures: A review. *World Journal of Orthopaedics* 2014, 5(4): 402–11.

5. Smith, T., Pelpola, K., Ball, M., Ong, A., and Myint, P.K. Preoperative indicators for mortality following hip fracture surgery: A systematic review and meta-analysis. *Age and Ageing* 2014, 43(4): 464–71.

6. Cristandi, P., Lenze, E.J., Avidan M.S., and Rawson, K.S. Trajectories of depressive symptoms after hip fracture. *Psychological Medicine* 2016, 46(7): 1413–25.

7. Klestil, T., Roder, C., Stotter, C., Winkler, B., Nehrer, S., Lutz, M., Klerings, I., Wagner, G., Gartlehner, G., and Nussbamer-Streit, B. Impact of timing of surgery in elderly hip fracture patients: A systematic review and meta-analysis. *Scientific Reports* 2018, 8(1): 13933.

8. HIP ATTACK Investigators. Accelerated surgery versus standard care in hip fracture (HIP ATTACK): An international, randomised, controlled trial. *Lancet* 2020, 395(10225): 698–708. doi: 10.1016/S0140-6736(20)30058-1.

9. Gringoryan, K.V., Javendan, H., and Rudolph, J.L. Orthogeriatric care models and outcomes in hip fracture patients: A systematic review and meta-analysis. *Dtsch Arztebi Int* 2013, 110: 255–62.

10. Alvis, B.O., and Hughes, C.G. Physiology considerations in geriatric patients. *Anesthesia / Clin.* 2015, 33(3): 447–56. doi: 10.1016/j.anclin.2015.05.003.

11. Coccia, F., and Rozzini, R. Goals of surgery and assessment tools for the elderly patients referred for cardiac and non-cardiac surgery. *Monaldi Archives for Chest Disease* 2017, 87: 849.

12. Leung, F., Lau, T.W., Kwan, K., Chow, S.P., and Kung, A.W. Does timing of surgery matter in fragility hip fractures? *Osteoporosis International* 2010, 21(4): s529–s534.

13. Sobolev, B., Guy, P., Sheehan, K.J., Kuramoto, L., Sutherland, J.M. et al. Mortality effects of timing alternatives for hip fracture surgery. *Canadian Medical Association Journal* 2018, 190(3): E923–32.

14. Lee, D.J., and Elfar, J.C. Timing of hip fracture surgery in the elderly. *Geriatric Orthopaedic Surgery and Rehabilitation* 2014, 5(3): 138–40.

15. Bennet, A., Hsin, L., Patel, A., Kang, K., Gupta, P., Choueka, J., and Feierman, D.E. Retrospective analysis of Geriatric patients undergoing hip fracture surgery: Delaying surgery is associated with increased morbidity, mortality and length of stay. *Geriatric Orthopaedic Surgery and Rehabilitation* 2018, 9. 2151459318795260.

16. Association of Anaesthetists of Great Britain and Ireland. Management of proximal femoral fractures. *Anaesthesia* 2012, 67: 85–98.

17. Sheehan, K.J., Sobolev, B., Villan, Y.F.V., and Guy, P. Patients and system factors of time to surgery after hip fracture: A scoping review. *BMJ Open* 2017, 7: e016939. doi: 10.1136/bmjopen-2017-016939.

18. Zehir, R., Zehir, S., and Kocabay, G. Role of pre-operative electro cardiology in predicting cardiovascular complications in proximal femur su rgery. *Current Research Cardiology* 2015, 2(4): 171–4.

19. Bryant, H.C., Roberts, P.R., and Diprose, P. Perioperative management of patients with cardiac implantable electric devices. *British Journal of Anaesthesia Education* 2016, 16(11): 357–61.

20. *Royal College of Physicians. National Hip Fracture Database Annual Report, 2017.* London: RCP, 2017.

21. Mochinski, K., Kurke, S., Andrich, S., Astrid, S., Gnass, I., Sirch, E., and Icks, A. Drug-based pain management for people with dementia after hip or pelvic fract ures: A systematic review. *BMC Geriatrics* 2017, 17(1): 54. doi: 10.1186/s12877-017-0446-2.

22. Sampson, E., White, N., Lord, K., Leurent, B., Vickerstaff, V., Scott, S., and Jones, L. Pain, agitation, and behavioural problems in people with dementia admitted to general hospital wards: A longitudinal cohort study. *Pain* 2015, 156(4): 675–83.

23. Anekar, A.A., and Cascella, M. WHO analgesic ladder. In *StatPearls*. Treasure Island, FL: StatPearls Publishing, 2021.

24. Freeman, N., and Clarke, J. Perioperative pain management for hip fracture patients. *Orthopaedics and Trauma* 2016, 30(2): 145–52.

25. Potter, L.J., Doleman, B., and Moppett, I.K. A systematic review of pre-operative anaemia and blood transfusion in patients with fractured hips. *Anaesthesia* 2015, 70: 483–500.

26. Patterson, J.J., Bohl, D.D., Basques, B.A., Arzeno, A.H., and Grauer, J.N. Does preoperative pneumonia affect complications of geriatric hip fracture surgery? *American Journal of Orthopaedics* 2017, 46(3): E177–E135.

27. O'Neil, L., Williams, D.M., Gallagher, M., Price, D.E., and Stephens, J.W. Investigation and treatment of hyponatraemia in hospital patients. *Intern MedJ* 2018, 48(11): 1416–7. doi: 10.1111/imj.14100. PMID: 30387299.

28. Cumming, K., Mckenzie, S., Hoyle, G.E., Hutchinson, J.D., and Soiza, R.L. Prognosis of hyponatraemia in elderly patients with fragility fractures. *Journal of Clinical Medicine Research* 2015, 7(1): 45–51.

29. Kang, J.S., Moon, K.H., Youn, Y.H., Park, J.S., Ko, S.H., and Jeon, Y.S. Factors associated with post-operative acute kidney injury after hip fractures in elderly patients. *Journal of Orthopaedic Surgery* 2020, 28(1). doi: 10.1177/2309499019896237E.

30. Lazarini, V., Mentz, R. J., Fiuzat, M., Metra, M., and O'Connor, C.M. Heart failure in elderly patients: Distinctive features and unresolved issues. *European Journal of Heart Failure* 2013, 15(7): 717–23.

31. Wang, L.H., Xu, D.J., Wei, X.J. et al. Electrolyte disorders and aging: Risk factors for delirium in patients undergoing orthopedic surgeries. *BMC Psychiatry* 2016, 16(418). doi: 10.1186/s12888-016-1130-0.

32. The Task Force for the Management of Atrial Fibrillation of the European Society of Cardiology (ESC). Guidelines for the management of atrial fibrillation. *European Heart Journal* 2010, 31: 2369–429.

33. Childers, C.P., Maggard-Gibbons, M., Ulloa, J.G., MacQueen, I.J., Miake-Lye, I.M., Shanman, R., Mak, S., Beroes, J.M., and Shekelle, P.G. Perioperative management of antiplatelet therapy in patients undergoing non-cardiac surgery following coronary stent placement: A systematic review. *Systematic Reviews* 2018, 7(1): 4.

34 Scottish Intercollegiate Guidelines Network (SIGN). *Antithrombotics: indications and Management.* Edinburgh: SIGN, 2012.

35. Dhillon, M., Stock, L., Maisie, G.K., and Mir, A. Appropriate anticoagulation in older adults with atrial fibrillation. *Age and Ageing* 2018, 47: ii25–ii39.

36. Carnicelli, A. Anticoagulation for valvular heart disease. *Journal of the American College of Cardiology* 2015, 18 May. www.acc.org/latest-in-cardiology/articles/2015/05/18/09/58/anticoagulation-for-valvular-heart-disease.

37. Flevas, D.A., Megaloikonomos, P.D., Dimopoulos, L., Mitsiokapa, E., Koulovaris, P., and Mavregenis, A.F. Thromboembolism prophylaxis in ort hopae dics: An update. *EFFORT Open Reviews* 2018, 3(4): 136–48.

38. Eichinger, S. Reversing vitamin K antagonists: Making the old new again. *Haematology: Education Program* 2016, 1: 605–11.

39. Sikorska, J., and Uprichard, J. Direct oral anticoagulants: A quick guide. *European Cardiology Reviews* 2017, 12(1): 40–5.

40. Chai-Adisaksopha, C., Hillis, C., Siegal, D.M., Movilla, R., Haddle, N., Iovio, A., and Crowther, M. Prothrombin complex concentrates versus fresh frozen plasma for warfarin reversal: A systematic review and meta-analysis. *Thrombosis and Haemostasis* 2016, 116(05): 879–90.

41. Leitch, J., and Van Vlymen, J. Managing the perioperative patient on direct oral anticoagulants. *Canadian Journal of Anaesthesia* 2017, 64(6): 656–72.

42. Desai, N.R., and Cornutt, D. Reversal agents for direct oral anticoagulants: considerations for hospital physicians and intensivists. *Hosp Pract (1995)* 2019, 47 (3): 113–22. doi: 10.1080/21548331.2019.1643728.

43. Keeling, D., Campbell Tate, R., and Watson, H. Perioperative management of anticoagulation and antiplatelet therapy. *British Journal of Haematology* 2016, 175: 602–13.

44. Rechenmacher, S.J., Fang, J.C. Bridging anticoagulation. *Journal of the American College of Cardiology* 2015, 66(12): 1392–403.

45. See MHRA guidelines for the perioperative management of patients with implantable pacemakers or implantable cardioverter defibrillators, where the use of surgical diathermy or electrocautery is anticipated. For the perioperative management of patients with implantable pacemakers or ICDs where the use of diathermy is anticipated, see also Thomas, H., Plummer, C., Wright, I.J., Foley, P., and Turley, A.J. Guidelines for the peri-operative management of people with cardiac implantable electronic devices: Guidelines from the British Heart Rhythm Society. *Anaesthesia* 2022, 77(7): 808–17. doi: 10.1111/anae.15728.

46. Practice Advisory for the Perioperative Management of Patients with Cardiac Implantable Electronic Devices: Pacemakers and Implantable Cardioverter-Defibrillators. An updated report by the American Society of Anaesthesiologists task force on perioperative management of patients with cardiac implantable electronic devices. *Anaesthesiology* 2011, 114: 247–61.

47. Beinart, R., and Nazarian, S. Effects of external electrical and magnetic fields on pace makers and defibrillators: From engineering principles to clinical practice. *Circulation* 2013, 128: 2799–809.

48. Levy, N., Penfold, N.W., and Dhatariya, K. Perioperative management of the patient with diabetes requiring emergency surgery. *British Journal of Anaesthesia* 2017, 17(4): 129–36.

49. Cheng-Shyuan, R., Shao-Chun, W., Yi-Chun, C., Peng-Chen, C., Hsiao-Yu, H., Pao-Jen, K., and Ching-hua, H. Stress-induced hyperglycaemia in diabetes: A cross-sectional analysis to explore the definition based on the trauma registry data. *International Journal of Environmental Research and Public Health* 2017, 14(12): 1527.

50. Association of Anaesthetists of Great Britain and Ireland. *Perioperative management of the surgical patient with diabetes. Anaesthesia* 2015, 70: 1427–40.

51. Pouwels, S., Bagelier, M.T., de Boer, A., Weber, W.E., Neef, C., Cooper, C., and de Vries, F. Risk of fracture in patients with Parkinson's disease. *Osteoporosis International* 2013, 24(8): 2283–90.

52. Lisk, R., Watters, H., and Yeong, K. Hip fractures outcomes in patients with Parkinson's disease. *Clinical Medicine* 2017, 17(3): s20.

53. Coomber, R., Alshameeri, Z., Masia, A.F., Mela, F., and Parker, M.J. Hip fractures and Parkinson's disease: A case series. *Injury* 2017, 48(12): 2730–35.

54. Simon, L.V., Hashmi, M.F., and Callanan, A.L. Neuroleptic malignant syndrome. In *Stat Pearls*. Treasure Island, FL: Stat Pearls Publishing, 2023. www.ncbi.nlm .nih.gov/books/NBK482282.

55. Chambers, D.J., Sebastian, J., and Ahearn, D.J. Parkinson's disease. *British Journal of Anaesthesia* 2017, 17(4): 145–9.

56. Katzanschlager, R. Apomorphine in the treatment of Parkinson' s disease. *European Neurological Review* 2009, 4(1): 28–30.

57. Brooks, D.J., Calabresi, P., Fox, S., Muller, T., Poevre, W., Rascal, O., and Stocchi, F. *Expert perspectives: Parkinson's disease pathophysiology and management. European Neurological Review* 2018, 13 (2): 3–13.

58. Brennan, K.A., Genever, R.W. Managing Parkins on' s disease during surgery. *British Medical Journal* 2010, 341: c5718.

59. Okun, M.S. Subcutaneous apomorphine subcutaneous infusions and Parkinson's disease. *New England Journal of Medicine Journal Watch* 2017. www.jwatch.org/ na47288/2018/08/22/subcutaneous-apomorphine-infusions.

60. Spencer, R., and Semmaga, B. Prescribing anti-emetics for patients with Parkinson's disease. *Prescriber* 2011: 48–9.

61. Leelakonok, N., Hokombo, A., and Schweizer, M.L. Domperidone and risk of ventricular arrhythmias and cardiac death: A systematic review and meta-analysis. *Clinical Drug Investigation* 2016, 36(2): 97–107.

62. Anghetescu, D., Cursaru, A., Mihakea, D., Ene, R., Cirstoiu, C. Recent myocardial infarction and femoral neck fixation surgery: A single centre retrospective study. *Archives of the Balkan Medical Union* 2017, 52(3): 245–8.

63. Samuel, A.M., Diaz-Collado, P.J., Szolomayer, L.K., Nelson, S.J., Webb, M.L., Lukasiewicz, A.M., and Graver, J.N. Incidence of and risk factors for inpatient stroke after hip fractures in the elderly. *Orthopaedics* 2018, 41(1): e27–e32.

64. Gregerson, M., Borris, L.C., and Damsgaard, E.M. Post-operative blood transfusion strategy in fr ail, anaemic elderly patients with hip fractures: The TRIFE randomized, controlled tiral. *Acta Orthopaedica* 2015, 86(3): 363–72.

65. Clevenger, B., and Richards, T. Pre-operative anaemia. *Anaesthesia* 2015, 70 (1): 20–8.

66. Rowlands, M., Forward, D.P., Sahota, O., and Moppeti, I.K. The effect of intravenous iron on post-operative transfusion requirements in hip fracture patients: Study protocol for a randomized, controlled trial. *Trials* 2013, 14: 288.

67. Pederson, A.B., Ehrenstein, V., Szepligeti, S.K., and Sorensen, H.T. Excess risk of venous thromboembolism in fracture patients and the prognostic impact of comorbidity. *Osteoporosis International* 2017, 28(12): 3421–30.

68. Flavus, D.A., Megalokonomos, P.D., Dimopoulos, L., Mitsiokapa, E., Koulovaris, P., and Mavrogenis, A.F. Thromboembolism prophylaxis in orthopaedics: An update. *EFFORT Open Reviews* 2018, 3(4): 136–48.

69. Mattison, L., Lapidus, J.L., and Enocson, A. Is fast reversal and early surgery (within 24 hours) in patients on warfarin medication with trochanteric hip fractures safe? A case-control study. *BMC Musculoskeletal Disorders* 2018, 19: 203.

70. Saunders, R., Comerota, A.J., Ozols, A., Tonejon Torres, R., and Ho, K.M. Intermittent pneumatic compression is a cost-effective method of venous thromboembolism prophylaxis. *Clinico-Economics and Outcomes Research* 2018, 10: 231–41.

71. World Health Organization. *International Statistical Classification of Diseases and Related Health Problems (ICD).* www.who .int/standards/classifications/ classification-of-diseases.

72. Guo, V., Jig, P., Zhang, J., Wang, X., Jieng, H., and Jieng, W. Prevalence and risk factors of operative delirium in elderly hip fracture patients. *Journal of International Medical Research* 2016, 44 (2): 317–27.

73. Wang, C., Qin, V., Wan, X., Song, L., Li, Z., and Li, H. Incidence and risk factors of post-operative delirium in the elderly patients with hip fractures. *Journal of Orthopaedic Surgery and Research* 2018, 13: 186.

74. Krogseth, M., Wyller, T.B., Eugendal, K., and Juliebo, V. Delirium is a risk for institutionalization and functional decline in older hip fracture patients. *Journal of Psychosomatic Research* 2014, 76(1): 68–74.

75. Numan, T., van der Boogard, M., Kamper, A.M., Rood, P.J.T., Peelen, L.M., and Slooter, A.J.C. Recognition of delirium in post-operative elderly patients: A multicenter study. *Journal of the American Geriatrics Society* 2017, 65 (9): 1932–8.

76. Inouye, S.K., and Westendorp, R.G.J., Saczynski, J.S. Delirium in elderly people. *Lancet* 2014, 383(9920): 911–22.

77. American Geriatrics Society Expert Panel on Post-operative Delirium in Older Adults. Post-operative delirium in older adults: Best practice statement from the American Geriatrics Society. *Journal of the American College of Surgeons* 2015, 220(2): 136–48.

78. Cunningham, J., and Kim, L.D. Post-operative delirium: A review of diagnosis and treatment strategies. *Journal of Xiangya Medicine* 2018, 3(2). doi: 10.21037/jxym.2018.0l.03.

79. Li, X., Wang, V., Liu, J., Xiong, V., Chen, S., Han, J., Xie, W., & Wu, Q. Effects of periope rative interventions for preventing post-operative delirium: A protocol for systematic review and meta-analysis of randomized controlled trials. *Medicine* 2021, 100(29). e26662. doi: 10.1097/M D.0000000000026662.

80. Neuman, M., Ellenberg, S., Sieber, F., Magaziner, J., Feng, R., and Carson, J. Regional versus general anesthesia for promoting independence after hip fracture (REGAIN): Protocol for a pragmatic, international multicentre trial. *BMJ Open* 2016, 6.

81. Broggi, M.S., Oladeji, P.O., Tahmid, S., Hernandez-Irizarry, R., and Allen, J. Depressive disorders lead to increased complications after geriatric hip fractures. *Geriatric Orthopaedic Surgery & Rehabilitation* 2021, 12. doi: 10.1177/21514593211016252.

82. Chan, C.K., Staber, F.E., Biennow, K., Inouye, S.K., Khan, G., Leoutsakos, J.S., Marcantonio, E.R., Neufeld, K.J., Rosenberg, P.B., Wang, N., Zetterberg, H., Lyketsos, C.G., and Oh, E. Association of depressive symptoms with post-operative delirium and CSF biomarkers for Alzheimer's disease among hip fracture patients. *American Journal of Geriatric Psychiatry* 2021, 29(12): 1212–21. doi: 10.1016/j.jago.2021.02.001.

83. Alamo, C., Lopez-Munoz, F., Garcia-Garcia, P., and Garcia-Ramos, S. Risk-benefit analysis of antidepressant drug treatment in the elderly. *Psychogeriatrics* 2014, 14(4): 261–8. doi: 10.1111/psyg.12057.PMID:25495088.

84. Rundshagen, I. Post-operative cognitive dysfunction. *Dtsch Arztebl Int.* 2014, 111 (8): 119–25. doi: 10.3238/arztebl.2014.0119.

85. Safavynia, S.A., and Goldstein, P.A. The role of neuroinflammation in post-operative cognitive dysfunction: Moving from hypothesis to treatment. *Front. Psychiatry* 2019, 9. doi: 10.3389/fpsyt.2018.00752.

86. Bell, J.J. et al. Multidisciplinary, multi-modal nutritional care in acute hip fracture inpatients: Results of a pragmatic intervention. *Clin Nutr* 2014, 33(6): 1101–10.

87. Vaculik, J., Stepan, J.J., Dung I., P. et al. Secondary fracture prevention in hip fracture patients requires cooperation from general practitioners. *Arch Osteoporos* 2017, 12, 49. doi: 10.1007/s11657-017-0346-z.

Parkinson's Disease and Related Disorders in Acute Hospitals

Sally A. Jones

Introduction

Parkinson's is a commonly encountered condition in both acute hospitals and rehabilitation settings, particularly among older adults. Although it tends to be thought of primarily as a movement disorder, Parkinson's is also a true neuropsychiatric condition. There are several Parkinson's-related disorders: the 'Parkinson's plus' syndromes, which are less commonly encountered but are still important to understand. People with Parkinson's have both physical health and mental health morbidity, and the likelihood of a liaison psychiatrist being called to assess someone with Parkinson's is therefore high. However, since this condition is often primarily thought of as a movement disorder rather than a neuropsychiatric disorder, the liaison psychiatrist and other doctors who work with older people may not have had much training in it, particularly in the physical problems that can occur.

It is therefore imperative that all doctors who work with adults in acute hospitals have a good understanding of Parkinson's as well as of the common emergency presentations and problems that may occur during an acute admission, since these are the situations that most doctors are likely to encounter when working with older people.

This chapter aims to provide the reader with a basic overview of Parkinson's and related disorders, particularly by focusing on emergency presentations and problems that may occur during an acute admission.

Parkinsonism or Parkinson's Disease?

The first thing to understand is the terminology. Parkinson's is the same as Parkinson's disease (PD). However, many people get confused between 'parkinsonism' and 'Parkinson's'. The term 'parkinsonism' simply refers to the typical signs and symptoms: bradykinesia (slowness of movement), rigidity, tremor, and gait changes (more about these later). There are many causes of parkinsonism, whereas Parkinson's itself refers to a specific condition. True idiopathic Parkinson's is a condition caused by progressive dopaminergic cell loss within the basal ganglia and is the commonest cause of parkinsonism. Lewy body dementia (LBD) and the rarer Parkinson's plus syndromes are also related to progressive dopamine loss, and hence these conditions have a lot in common.

In addition to Parkinson's itself and Parkinson's plus syndromes, there are other causes of parkinsonism that are *not* primarily related to idiopathic progressive dopamine loss; the treatments for the varieties of parkinsonism are therefore different. These varieties are sometimes called Parkinson's mimics. The commonest are vascular

Table 18.1 Causes of parkinsonism

Related to progressive dopaminergic cell loss*	• idiopathic Parkinson's disease • Parkinson's plus syndromes • multi-system atrophy (MSA) • progressive supranuclear palsy (PSP) • corticobasal degeneration (CBD) • Lewy body dementia (LBD)
NOT related to progressive dopaminergic cell loss *(sometimes referred to as Parkinson's mimics)*	• vascular parkinsonism • drug-induced parkinsonism • normal pressure hydrocephalus (NPH) • severe depression with significant psychomotor retardation • functional • rarer mimics – Wilson's disease, space-occupying lesions

* Parkinsonism related to progressive dopaminergic cell loss may have very different treatment and prognosis from those that do not. Distinguishing correctly between different types of parkinsonism is therefore important.

parkinsonism and drug-induced parkinsonism. Drug-induced parkinsonism is of particular importance to psychiatrists, since anti-psychotic drugs are one of the groups of causative medications. People with normal pressure hydrocephalus (NPH) and people with significant psychomotor retardation as a consequence of severe depression may also appear to look parkinsonian on examination. These are all examples of parkinsonism rather than examples of true Parkinson's disease. Table 18.1 illustrates some of the commoner causes of parkinsonism. This chapter will concentrate primarily on Parkinson's disease itself.

Parkinson's Disease

Parkinson's is an α-synucleinopathy in which abnormal aggregates of this protein, along with other proteins such as ubiquitin, make up what is called 'Lewy bodies'. These Lewy bodies are found, among other places, within the substantia nigra in the basal ganglia, resulting in progressive damage to the dopaminergic pathways. In Parkinson's, damage to the substantia nigra is a hallmark and is thought to be the major cause of motor symptoms (1). Although this phenomenon was traditionally thought of as primarily a movement disorder, it should be noted that dopaminergic pathways are not just involved in motor activity. There are three main loops connecting the basal ganglia to the cortex, namely the motor circuit, the associative circuit, and the limbic circuit, and they deal respectively with the control of movement, behaviour and cognition, the control of reward, and the control of emotions (2). This goes some way towards explaining the neuropsychiatric nature of Parkinson's. But the disorder is not fully understood, and even the well-accepted theory of degeneration of basal ganglia functions does not fully explain the problems that arise in Parkinson's, one example being the involvement of the autonomic nervous system.

Why do some people get Parkinson's and others do not? Again, this is not fully understood, but it is likely that the aetiology of Parkinson's is multi-factorial and that

Parkinson's arises from a complex interaction of age-related and environmental factors in genetically susceptible individuals. It is important to note that, in the vast majority of cases, Parkinson's occurs sporadically. However, families with both autosomal dominant and autosomal recessive forms of Parkinson's have been identified. This has enabled the identification of several gene mutations (e.g. in Parkin and LRRK2 genes) that, through further research, may also enable us to improve our understanding of sporadic forms of Parkinson's. It is also important to note that, while the prevalence of Parkinson's increases with age and there is a mean age of onset of 60 (3) to 70 (4) years, a small proportion of patients will be diagnosed before the age of 40.

Signs and Symptoms of Parkinson's

Although Parkinson's is generally described as a movement disorder, it is very important to note that not all signs and symptoms are related to movement. It is also important to note that, while there are a group of commonly experienced signs and symptoms, each patient will have his or her own combination of symptoms and their severity will differ from person to person. Signs and symptoms in Parkinson's can be divided into motor and non-motor symptoms.

Motor Symptoms

The classical triad of motor symptoms is a combination of bradykinesia, rigidity, and tremor. The essential feature is bradykinesia. Not all patients have rigidity and not all patients have a tremor. Gait and postural disturbance are also common. Signs tend to be unilateral at onset and remain asymmetrical even when symptoms progress to the contralateral side. As the condition progresses, other motor problems may develop, partly as a result of fluctuating dopaminergic levels in a brain that becomes more and more dependent on exogenous dopamine provided through medication, as its levels obviously fluctuate. Table 18.2 lists some of the common motor symptoms seen in Parkinson's, and also explains some of the terminology that patients and their specialist teams may use.

These motor symptoms may affect patients in many ways – from falls due to postural instability and freezing of gait to difficulty rolling over in bed at night, or difficulty with handwriting on account of rigidity and bradykinesia.

Non-Motor Symptoms

In addition to the motor symptoms, there are also many non-motor signs and symptoms in Parkinson's. Interestingly, many patients diagnosed with Parkinson's have experienced non-motor symptoms for years before the development of motor symptoms. Common pre-diagnosis non-motor symptoms include rapid eye movement (REM) sleep behaviour disorder, anosmia (loss of sense of smell), constipation, and depression.

Not all patients will experience all symptoms. Non-motor symptoms that may be experienced include:

- autonomic:
  - postural hypotension
  - bladder and bowel problems
  - erectile dysfunction
  - hyperhidrosis (excessive sweating)

Table 18.2 Motor symptoms in Parkinson's

Akinesia and bradykinesia	Absence and slowness of movement. There is also fatigability of repetitive movement, including amplitude.
Rigidity	Stiffness with sustained resistance to passive movement – usually of the limbs, although head/neck may be affected too. Generally 'lead pipe' rigidity, with 'cog-wheeling' if there is superimposed tremor.
Tremor	Typically a resting tremor, often described as pill-rolling (rhythmic movements of thumb against index finger as if rolling something).
Postural changes	Posture often becomes stooped. There is also postural instability. Patients sometimes develop severe postural changes such as disproportionate antecolis of head/neck and camptocormia (severe forward flexion of trunk).
Gait changes	Patients may have a shuffling gait, with small steps, and may also become faster and faster as they walk (festination). There is reduced arm swing caused by bradykinesia. There may be difficulty with gait initiation and turning, as well as freezing of gait.
Hypomimia	Reduced facial expression, which is produced by a combination of bradykinesia of facial muscles and reduced rate of blinking.
Dyskinesia	Abnormal choreiform movements, sometimes described by patients as 'wriggling'.
Dystonia	Sustained abnormal posture of a body part (often the head/neck, the hand, or the foot), caused by involuntary muscle spasm.
Freezing episodes	Transient but sudden and disabling inability to move. This often affects gait but can affect other actions too.
End-of-dose deterioration	The name given to the wearing off of the beneficial effects of medication before the next dose is due.
Motor fluctuations	Describes motor symptoms that fluctuate from bradykinesia (moving too little) to dyskinesia (moving too much). This is often in relation to changing levels of medication during the course of the day, but can also be unpredictable.
'On and off' symptoms	Similar to motor fluctuations, although 'on' periods may describe periods of near normal movement, not necessarily dyskinesia.

- gastrointestinal:
    - constipation
    - nausea
    - anosmia

- neuropsychiatric:
    - apathy
    - mood disorders – anxiety and depression
    - sleep disorders – including REM sleep behaviour disorder, excessive or sudden-onset daytime somnolence, broken sleep, vivid dreams

- visual hallucinations
- psychosis
- Parkinson's disease dementia (PDD)
- impulse control disorders (eg pathological gambling, hypersexuality, binge eating)
- dopamine dysregulation syndrome (an addictive overuse of Parkinson's medication)
- dopamine agonist withdrawal syndrome (similar to other drug withdrawal states)
- punding (complex repetitive behaviours, often in relation to a hobby that goes out of control)

- speech and swallowing problems
  - hypophonia (low voice volume)
  - dysarthria
  - drooling and difficulties with saliva control
  - dysphagia – which may result in recurrent aspiration pneumonia

Staging of Parkinson's

Parkinson's typically progresses over the years. Patients early into their diagnosis are often well controlled with simple regimens of medication and remain active and independent, even working and driving. At the other end of the spectrum, patients with advanced disease may be immobile, living with dementia and swallowing difficulties, in a palliative stage of their lives. Having some way of describing the stage of a person's Parkinson's can therefore be helpful.

There are several instruments for staging Parkinson's. The first is the Hoehn and Yahr Scale, which stages patients predominantly by their motor symptoms and disability level and goes from stage 1, for people with mild unilateral symptoms only, to stage 5, for people who are wheelchair- or bed-bound. Another commonly used tool or method is the Unified Parkinson's Disease Rating Scale (UPDRS), which looks at several domains rather than just motor symptoms. This is longer, taking some time to complete, and is perhaps most commonly used in research settings. Of greater practical use in the daily clinical setting is the scale suggested by MacMahon and Thomas (5), which simply places each patient in one of the following four groups, essentially by using clinical judgement:

- diagnostic phase
- maintenance phase
- complex phase
- palliative phase.

The priorities for patients and their carers change as each person moves through the different stages of the condition; and knowing which phase a person is in can help to guide clinical decisions as well as prompt discussions around advanced care planning.

Parkinson's Medications

Parkinson's medications can be complicated for non-specialists. The main thing to remember is that, in general, Parkinson's drugs given for motor symptoms all aim to increase the presence of dopamine. These drugs can be divided into three main groups:

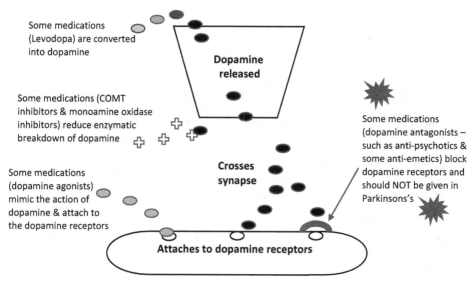

Figure 18.1 Parkinson's drugs and how they work

1. drugs that are converted into dopamine itself: levodopa-containing preparations;
2. drugs that inhibit enzymes in order to reduce dopamine breakdown: the COMT inhibitors and the monoamine oxidase inhibitors;
3. drugs that mimic the action of dopamine and stimulate dopamine receptors: the dopamine agonists.

Figure 18.1 illustrates these basic classes of dopaminergic medication in a schematic diagram, which also demonstrates why dopamine antagonists can be so harmful in patients who already have pre-existing dopamine deficiency.

Levodopa-containing preparations are all combined with a de-carboxylase inhibitor (benzeride or carbidopa) in order to prevent a peripheral breakdown of levodopa before it crosses the blood brain barrier. For this reason, levodopa-containing preparations may be prescribed in a way that reflects this combination. For example, co-careldopa 25/100 indicates a tablet containing 25 mg of carbidopa and 100 mg of levodopa.

Although there are now many different Parkinson's medications, preparations containing levodopa remain, for many patients, the most effective ones in terms of motor symptoms, and just a look at Figure 18.1 indicates why this may be: levodopa is essentially converted into dopamine itself.

Although dopaminergic drugs are the mainstay of pharmacological treatment in Parkinson's, there are also a number of other medications that people with Parkinson's may be taking. The commonest of these are summarised in Table 18.3.

Each person with Parkinson's will be on different preparations, combinations, and timings of their medication – depending on individual assessments of people's motor and non-motor symptoms, timings of their motor fluctuations during a typical waking day, and other comorbidities. These regimens can be complex. The initiation of Parkinson's medication – or changes to it – should only be made by specialists.

Table 18.3 Medication used in Parkinson's

Dopaminergic Drugs	
Levodopa – All with Decarboxylase Inhibitor	
Co-beneldopa Co-careldopa Levodopa/carbidopa intestinal gel	Often still prescribed as brand names in view of the multiple types of preparation and release available. All given orally, except levodopa/carbidopa gel, which is administered via a pump, via percutaneous endoscopic gastrostomy, or via jejunostomy.
COMT inhibitors	
Entacapone Opicapone Tolcapone	All given orally. Administered alongside levodopa preparations (combination products are available), to reduce end-of-dose deterioration.
Monoamine Oxidase Inhibitors	
Rasagiline Selegeline Safinamide	All given orally. Usually an adjunct to other treatments, although some patients may be on this as monotherapy.
Dopamine Agonists	
Apomorphine Pramipexole Ropinirole Rotigotine	Pramipexole and ropinirole are given orally. Apomorphine is given subcutaneously, via injection or continuous infusion. Rotigotine is given transdermally, via an adhesive patch.
Other Drugs – Specialist Input Advised	
Amantadine	Sometimes prescribed to dampen dyskinesia.
Midodrine Fludrocortisone	May be prescribed for symptomatic postural hypotension.
Domperidone	Common anti-emetic of choice in Parkinson's. Note cardiac risks.
Glycopyrronium	Can be used for drooling in Parkinson's – no UK licence at the time of writing, so prescriber's responsibility. Note anti-cholinergic side effect profile.
Rivastigmine	Can be used for Parkinson's dementia. Other cholinesterase inhibitors can be given, or memantine can be considered if cholinesterase inhibitors are not tolerated. At the time of writing, only rivastigmine has a UK license for this indication, so prescribers take responsibility.
Quetiapine Clozapine	Can be used for psychosis in Parkinson's, under specialist supervision only, using lower doses than for the non-Parkinson's population.
Melatonin Clonazepam	Can be used in REM sleep behaviour disorder.

Emergency Presentations in Parkinson's

People with Parkinson's present as emergencies for a number of different reasons. These can be directly due to the Parkinson's itself – for example, an aspiration pneumonia caused by Parkinson's related dysphagia – or else the Parkinson's may complicate unrelated issues: for example, pre-existing autonomic problems will make the assessment of cardiovascular status more difficult in patients who present with sepsis or a gastrointestinal bleed.

Liaison psychiatrists may be called to assess the mental health of people with Parkinson's on any acute medical or surgical ward. In addition, people with Parkinson's may become acutely unwell while on a mental health ward. It is therefore helpful for psychiatrists to have a basic understanding of common emergency presentations in Parkinson's, whether physical or psychiatric.

Emergencies and Common Problems in Hospital

Missed Medication

Parkinson's medication is *time-critical*. Patients may deteriorate very rapidly in terms of their ability to move, to speak, and to swallow if their medications are missed or even just delayed, particularly if their Parkinson's is at the complex stage. This deterioration can lead to life-threatening complications. The same can happen if these patients are given a dopamine antagonist.

It should also be noted that Parkinson's is a gradually progressive condition and does NOT get worse overnight. Therefore, if a Parkinson's patient suddenly deteriorates,

- either it's not the Parkinson's (look for other causes); or
- they've missed medication; or
- they've been given a dopamine antagonist (e.g. an anti-psychotic or the anti-emetics metoclopramide and prochlorperazine).
  - If an anti-emetic is needed, give domperidone (if low cardiac risk) or cyclizine (short term).
  - In severe agitation, give benzodiazipine rather than an anti-psychotic and speak to a specialist if problems persist (low dose quetiapine is sometimes given on specialist advice, if benefits are felt to outweigh risks)

Consequences of missed or delayed medications include:

1. neuroleptic malignant syndrome (sometimes called parkinsonism-hyperpyrexia syndrome);
2. aspiration pneumonia due to deterioration in swallow;
3. falls;
4. immobility and its consequences (e.g. deconditioning, pressure damage, increased risk of venous thromboembolism and hypostatic pneumonia);
5. distress;
6. complaints and other medicolegal consequences.

Swallowing Difficulties and Nil by Mouth Patients

Just as may occur in people who have missed or delayed their Parkinson's medication, similar problems can arise if the patient is either unable to swallow or has been made nil

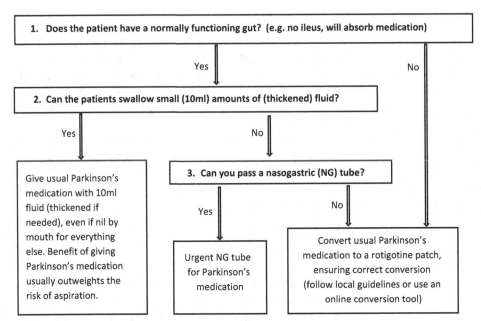

Figure 18.2 Nil by mouth and swallowing problems in Parkinson's

by mouth for other reasons. Figure 18.2 shows a suggested flowchart for the management of these patients, although clinicians should consult local guidelines if these are in place.

The key thing to remember is that patients should NOT miss their medication. If the usual oral administration is not possible, then an alternative route should be sought as a matter of urgency. It is tempting for the non-specialist to convert all patients to a rotigotine patch, which is less invasive and time-consuming than the insertion and management of a nasogastric tube. However, if you refer back to Figure 18.1 and the discussions around medication, you will remember that the medications that tend to have the greatest motor benefit for many patients are the ones that contain levodopa. When well, people with Parkinson's often take several different classes of Parkinson's medications, including levodopa. Converting all to a rotigotine patch means that patients lose the levodopa (which is often giving them the greatest motor benefit) and all classes of medication, except dopamine agonist. This is justified if it is not possible or appropriate to continue patients' usual medications by another route; but it should not be the first option. One should also bear in mind that dose conversion to rotigotine can be complex. One should follow local guidelines if these are in place, or use an online conversion tool.

Falls

People with Parkinson's are prone to falls. There are Parkinson's specific risk factors for falls – for example postural instability, postural hypotension, freezing and festination of gait, dyskinesia, axial rigidity, and cognitive impairment (6). In addition to the risk factors specific to Parkinson's, people with it may also experience the generic risk factors that can affect any other person: inappropriate polypharmacy and sedative medication, arrhythmia, visual impairment, daily alcohol use, improper use of walking aids, environmental hazards, and other comorbidities (6).

When people are in hospital or in other health care settings, the difficulty is that they are generally acutely unwell in addition to all the above risk factors. A fall is a symptom, not a diagnosis, and it is important that clinicians do not miss the fall because of an underlying acute illness and mistakenly attribute the fall simply to Parkinson's.

Helpful questions to ask yourself when a person has fallen are:

1. Why this patient?
2. Why today?

Answering the first question should give the clinician the risk factors for that particular patient, some of which may be modifiable, allowing the clinician to reduce the risk of future falls. Answering the second question should prompt the clinician to explore whether or not there is an acute issue superimposed that may need addressing urgently. For example, someone may always be prone to falls as a result of their pre-existing Parkinson's and visual impairment, but today they are also febrile, confused, and sleepy, which should prompt the clinician to look for an underlying infection and hypoactive delirium as an acute precipitant for the fall.

Postural Hypotension

Postural hypotension is common in people with Parkinson's. Patients may already be taking midodrine or fludrocortisone to help with this symptom. The pitfall, when people are acutely unwell and in hospital, is to assume wrongly that the postural hypotension is normal for them because of their Parkinson's, and thus to miss an acute event such as sepsis or blood loss.

A helpful approach to the hospitalised Parkinson's patient with postural hypotension is to ask the following questions:

- Is there any evidence of sepsis, blood loss, volume loss, or shock? (If yes, address urgently.)
- Is the sodium normal? (Remember, adrenal problems can cause postural hypotension.)
- Is the patient well hydrated? (If not, address this.)
- Is the ECG normal? (If not, address this as required.)
- Is the patient taking any anti-hypertensive medications? (If yes, consider stopping them.)
- If the postural hypotension persists and is symptomatic although the above problems have been addressed, then speak to the medical teams or the Parkinson's team regarding whether medication such as midodrine or fludrocortisone is required.

Gastroenterological Problems

Common acute gastroenterological issues in people with Parkinson's are constipation and nausea. In addition to issues directly related to Parkinson's, people with this disease are also clearly just as likely as the general population to have other acute gastroenterological or surgical issues such as gastroenteritis, obstruction, and perforation.

- Constipation can be severe and can lead to pseudo-obstruction or sigmoid volvulus.
- Some patients with Parkinson's will suffer from recurrent volvulus.

- Nausea is common, and can also be a side effect of dopaminergic medication.
- Remember that some anti-emetics are contra-indicated in Parkinson's (prochlorperazine and metoclopramide).
- Remember that people with vomiting, diarrhoea, or acute surgical issues may not absorb their time-critical Parkinson's medication: follow local guidelines or see Figure 18.2.

Acute Mental Health Issues

Clearly by far the commonest reason for the liaison psychiatrist to be called to see a patient with Parkinson's will be an acute mental health issue. People with Parkinson's may be living with a variety of long-term mental health issues such as apathy, anxiety and mood disorders, PDD, or issues related to behaviour and impulsivity (dopamine dysregulation syndrome and impulse control disorders). When they are admitted to hospital, these (usually) pre-existing problems may become either evident for the first time or more difficult to manage outside the patients' usual home environment, and will probably require help from psychiatry. There may be additional problems, too – such as delirium.

An in-depth exploration of the mental health issues that may occur and how to manage them is beyond the scope of this chapter. But here are a few brief tips and reminders regarding the management of mental health issues arising in people with Parkinson's.

- Delirium
    - The investigation and management of delirium in people with Parkinson's is much the same as for the general population, apart from some additional potential causes and the pharmacological management of severe agitation.
    - Parkinson's medication can cause delirium. Always ask if any of the Parkinson's medication is new or whether there has been a recent dose increase in patients with delirium. However, never stop Parkinson's medication without consultation with the Parkinson's team, particularly as delirium is very often multi-factorial and the medication may only be a contributing factor.
    - Do NOT give antipsychotic medication such as haloperidol, risperidone, or olanzapine for delirium with severe agitation in people with Parkinson's. Local hospital guidelines for delirium may recommend the use of these drugs in the non-Parkinson's population, but they should NOT be used in Parkinson's or in the Parkinson's plus syndromes. If needed, a low dose benzodiazepine may be given instead (for as short a time as possible).

- Hallucinations
    - Hallucinations (particularly visual) are common in people with Parkinson's. They are very common in PDD, but can also occur in the absence of dementia.
    - Exclude delirium as a cause.
    - Did the hallucinations coincide with a new medication or with an increase in dose? Parkinson's medications can be the precipitant, as can medications given for other reasons, such as anticholinergics or opiates.
    - If safe to do so, stop or reduce any non-Parkinson's medication that may be contributing. Always discuss with the Parkinson's team before adjusting Parkinson's medication.

- Try to restore a normal sleep pattern.
- Is there visual impairment with co-existing Charles de Bonnet syndrome?
- Are the hallucinations intrusive or distressing? If not, and if the patient is well, a simple explanation to the patient and carers may be all that is needed to manage the situation.
- Only intrusive or distressing persistent hallucinations require pharmacological management. Rivastigmine can be helpful if the hallucinations are part of a PDD. Low-dose quetiapine or clozapine can be helpful, but their use should be initiated by specialists only, after careful consideration of the risks and benefits. Other antipsychotics are contraindicated.

- Parkinson's disease dementia

  - This is generally dealt with on an outpatient basis rather than by a liaison team during an acute admission. However, it can sometimes be diagnosed for the first time in an in-patient, provided that delirium has been confidently excluded.
  - Hallucinations are a common feature, with management as described above.
  - Rivastigmine has a UK license for use in PDD. Other cholinesterase inhibitors can be used – and memantine can be tried if those are not tolerated – but at the time of writing there is no UK license for the use of these drugs for this indication; prescribers will need to bear this in mind.

- Anxiety and depression

  - In general terms, the management of and approach to people with Parkinson's with these disorders should be the same as for any other person, apart from taking particular care over the choice of medication.
  - Anti-depressants should be used with caution in anyone who takes a monoamine oxidase inhibitor for Parkinson's: this is due to the increased risk of serotonin syndrome.
  - Lithium, valproate, and most antipsychotics can worsen parkinsonism.
  - Sometimes people with Parkinson's experience anxiety and mood symptoms as part of a 'non-motor off' or non-motor symptomatology related to end-of-dose deterioration. Always ask about a pattern to symptoms, particularly in relation to the timing of medication and motor symptoms. Liaise with the Parkinson's team if there appears to be an association of anxiety with the wearing off of Parkinson's medication.

- REM sleep behaviour disorder

  - Management involves practical measures designed to reduce risk (e.g. position of furnishings on which a person may injure themselves), with pharmacological options such as melatonin and low-dose clonazepam. The risk of falls with sedating medications should be discussed with the patient and carers. Advise all parties that the patient must not to drive if there is any somnolence at the relevant times.

- Impulse control disorders

  - Impulse control disorders (ICDs) commonly encountered are pathological gambling, hypersexuality, binge eating, and compulsive shopping.

- The use of both dopamine agonists and levodopa is independently associated with ICDs, but the odds ratio is considerably higher for patients who take dopamine agonists (7).
- The initial management involves practical measures intended to reduce risk (e.g. restricting Internet access) alongside dopamine agonist medication alterations; this is achieved in collaboration with the Parkinson's specialist. Cognitive behavioural therapy may have a role.

- Dopamine dysregulation syndrome
  - Dopamine dysregulation syndrome (DDS) refers to an addictive pattern of dopaminergic medication overuse, usually with levodopa-containing preparations. Management is very difficult and will need close liaison between Parkinson's teams, mental health teams, primary care teams, the patient, and the patient's carers.

The Parkinson's Plus Syndromes

The Parkinson's plus syndromes are a group of neurodegenerative conditions in which there is a clinical picture of parkinsonism combined with additional features. These conditions include multi-system atrophy (MSA), progressive supranuclear palsy (PSP), and corticobasilar degeneration (CBD). Sometimes LBD is also placed within this group. These conditions have a lot in common and there is a degree of overlap between them. All affect the dopaminergic pathways to a greater or lesser extent, and for this reason all can be initially 'misdiagnosed' as idiopathic Parkinson's disease. The clue that the patient may have a Parkinson's plus syndrome are bilateral signs at or near presentation, a poorer than expected response to dopaminergic medication, and the development of additional signs and symptoms, which are summarised in Table 18.4. These additional features can be either the development of signs and symptoms that would not normally be expected in idiopathic Parkinson's at all (such as the 'alien limb' of CBD), or the development of features that do occur in Parkinson's but that, in the Parkinson's plus syndromes, tend to occur much earlier or more severely than would normally be expected. Examples include the presence of early postural instability and falls, as well as dementia or profound autonomic instability early on in the course of the condition. On the whole, these conditions tend to progress more rapidly than idiopathic Parkinson's disease and have a much poorer response to Parkinson's medication.

Why Does the Liaison Psychiatrist Need to Know about These Conditions?

It is not necessary for the non-specialist to have a detailed knowledge of the diagnosis and management of Parkinson's plus syndromes, whose more specialist management should fall under the care of movement disorder specialists, in any case. But, just like patients with Parkinson's, patients with these conditions will present to general wards for a whole number of reasons, some related and some unrelated to their condition, and will therefore require generalists to have a basic understanding of Parkinson's plus syndromes and to be aware of the main difficulties that can arise. There is a great deal of overlap between the Parkinson's plus conditions, but all will have parkinsonism to a greater or lesser degree. All are associated with an increased risk of falls, and all may affect speech and swallowing. Cognitive problems and dementia can be a feature in all

Table 18.4 The Parkinson's Plus Syndromes

Multi-System Atrophy (MSA)

α-synucleineopathy
Two subtypes; both have autonomic failure.
- MSA-P predominantly parkinsonism with autonomic failure.
- MSA-C predominantly cerebellar features (e.g. ataxia, dysarthria) with autonomic failure.
- As disease progresses, patients with MSA-P may develop cerebellar signs and vice versa.

Parkinsonism plus. . .
- early autonomic failure (e.g. postural hypotension, urinary and erectile difficulties);
- postural changes due to dystonia – e.g. disproportionate anterocolis or camptocormia;
- speech and swallow problems;
- cerebellar signs more prominent than parkinsonism in the MSA-C subtype.

Cognition is usually preserved.
Diagnosis usually clinical, DaT scan will be abnormal.
Levodopa sometimes helpful but benefit may not be sustained, can worsen postural hypotension.

Progressive Supranuclear Palsy (PSP)

Tauopathy
Parkinsonism plus. . .
- truncal rigidity and neck dystonia;
- vertical gaze palsy;
- early falls;
- early dementia (frontal);
- speech and swallowing problems;
- may have eyelid dystonia with frontalis overactivity, in an effort to maintain eye opening.

Diagnosis usually clinical, DaT scan will be abnormal.
Typically poor or non-sustained response to levodopa.

Corticobasil Degeneration (CBD)

Tauopathy
Rarer than the MSA and PSP
Parkinsonism plus. . .
- cortical processing problems, including apraxia;
- asymmetrical signs, one limb becoming progressively dystonic or 'having a mind of its own' – the so-called alien limb;
- myoclonus may occur;
- speech problems – patient may become aphasic;
- dysphagia;
- dementia (often frontotemporal).

Diagnosis usually clinical, DaT scan will be abnormal.
Typically poor response to levodopa.

the Parkinsons plus syndromes apart from MSA, where dementia is less commonly found. People with MSA in particular may have significant autonomic instability, which can make assessing cardiovascular status more difficult in acutely unwell patients. In addition, all these patients will be very sensitive to dopamine antagonists – antipsychotics, prochlorperazine, metoclopramide: never give these medications to people with these conditions unless on specialist advice.

Lewy Body Dementia

Some people also group LBD, also called 'dementia of Lewy bodies' (DLB), with the Parkinson's plus syndromes. This is an α-synucleinopathy, as are Parkinson's and MSA. The motor signs and symptoms of parkinsonism may not be evident at presentation, unlike in the other Parkinson's plus conditions. For this reason, LBD may be misdiagnosed both as Alzheimer's dementia (AD) and as Parkinson's. Symptoms pointing towards LBD as a diagnosis rather than AD include prominent visual hallucinations and the presence of REM sleep behaviour disorder, both of which are common features of LBD. Prominent cognitive features include difficulties with executive function, perception, and visuospatial function. Fluctuations in cognition and alertness in the absence of delirium are also common.

There is considerable overlap between LBD and PDD. There is some debate regarding the extent to which these are the same thing or two separate conditions; some clinicians use the terms interchangeably. However, in general, a condition is labelled PDD if the Parkinson's occurs first and the dementia some years later, and LBD if the dementia is the earlier presenting feature.

In practice and from a cognitive perspective, both PDD and LBD are treated similarly. However, treating the motor signs of parkinsonism is generally more difficult in people with LBD than in people with PDD. Patients with PDD will often have much more prominent motor signs, generally having had motor deterioration for some years ahead of the development of dementia. Patients with PDD may therefore take much higher doses of dopaminergic drugs than can be tolerated by patients with LBD. Levodopa and other dopaminergic drugs worsen the hallucinations in people with both conditions, and there can be a fine balance between treating motor and psychiatric symptoms. Cholinesterase inhibitors are the main pharmacological treatment for both types of dementia. These patients are also extremely sensitive to the adverse effects of dopamine antagonists (e.g. antipsychotics and some anti-emetics); such drugs should never be used for patients with LBD, unless at low doses and on specialist advice, after a careful weighing up of the potential risks and benefits.

Other Causes of Parkinsonism

Vascular Parkinsonism

Vascular parkinsonism is due to cerebrovascular disease, and was previously called 'arteriosclerotic parkinsonism' (8). It is unclear why some people with extensive cerebrovascular disease on imaging develop parkinsonism while others do not. However, patients who do develop parkinsonism typically have bilateral and predominantly lower-body signs. This may lead to the typical vascular gait known as *marche à petit pas*, 'walking in small steps', which can look similar to the shuffling gait in Parkinson's.

Postural instability, falls, and cognitive impairment are often present at onset or early in the condition. In contrast, true idiopathic Parkinson's tends to display unilateral upper and lower body signs, while postural instability, falls, and cognitive impairment develop later. Imaging in vascular parkinsonism may show multiple lacunar infarcts, widespread periventricular white matter lesions, or basal ganglia infarcts (9). A subset of patients with vascular parkinsonism do respond to dopaminergic medication, particularly those with lacunae in the basal ganglia (10), and may therefore be prescribed levodopa-containing medications. However, since in vascular parkinsonism the pathology is not restricted to the basal ganglia and the dopaminergic pathways, poor response to dopaminergic medications should not be a surprise (9).

Drug-Induced Parkinsonism

Drug-induced parkinsonism is another commonly seen 'Parkinson's mimic'. In this case, parkinsonism arises not because of dopaminergic cell loss, but because of dopamine receptor blockade. The most commonly encountered dopamine antagonists are the antiemetics prochlorperazine and metoclopramide, along with most antipsychotics. Sodium valproate and lithium are also implicated sometimes. Not only can these drugs cause drug-induced parkinsonism through dopamine receptor blockade; they can also be very harmful in people with Parkinson's, LBD, and other pre-existing dopamine-deficiency states. This is also true of the newer atypical antipsychotics, although quetiapine and clozapine are better tolerated from the Parkinson's perspective and have been recommended by NICE as the antipsychotics of choice in Parkinson's, (11) bearing in mind that much lower doses should be used in this population.

The treatment for drug-induced parkinsonism consists in withdrawing the offending drug. This may be difficult depending on the severity of any underlying mental health issues and may require changing to an alternative antipsychotic agent. For most people, parkinsonism will resolve within three to six months from stopping the offending drug, although for some people symptoms resolve more quickly than this. Occasionally it is impossible to stop the offending drug, or sometimes symptoms may not resolve as expected, possibly because the drug has 'unmasked' a pre-existing but subclinical dopamine deficiency state. In these situations, advice from a specialist in movement disorders should be sought in order to make specialist decisions regarding medication or DaT scanning (or both).

References

1. Edwards, M., Quinn, N., and Bhatia, K. Pathophysiology of Parkinson's disease. In Edwards, M., Quinn, N., and Bhatia, K., *Parkinson's Disease and Other Movement Disorders*. Oxford: Oxford University Press, 2007, 24–5.

2. Obeso, J.A., Rodrigues-Oroz, M.C., Stamelou, M., Bhatia, K.P., and Burn, D.J. The expanding universe of disorders of the basal ganglia. *Lancet* 2014, 384: 523–31.

3. Ishihara, L.S., Cheesbrough, A., Brayne, C., and Schrag, A.. Estimated life expectancy of Parkinson's patients compared with the UK population. *J Neurol Neurosurg Psychiatry* 2007, 78 (12): 1304–9.

4. Hindle, J.V. Ageing, neurodegeneration and Parkinson's disease. *Age and Ageing* 2010, 39(2): 156–61.

5. MacMahon, D.G., and Thomas, S. Practical approach to quality of life in

Parkinson's disease: The nurse's role. *J Neurol* 1998, 245(suppl. 1): s19–22.

6. Van der Marck, M.A., Klok, M.P., Okun, M.S. et al. Consensus-based clinical recommendations for the examination and management of falls in patients with Parkinson's disease. *Parkinsonism and Related Disorders* 2014, 20: 360–9.

7. Weintrab, D., Koester, J., Potenza, M.N., Siderowf, A.D., Stacy, M., Voon, V., Whetteckey, J., Wunderlich, G.R., and Lang, A.E. Impulse control disorders in Parkinson's disease: A cross sectional study of 3090 patients. *Archives Neurol* 2010, 67(5): 589–95.

8. Critchley, M. Arteriosclerotic parkinsonism. *Brain* 1929, 52: 23–83.

9. Thanvi, B., Lo, N., and Robinson, T. Vascular parkinsonism: An important cause of parkinsonism in older people. *Age and Ageing* 2005, 34(2): 114–19.

10. Zjilmans, J.C.M., Katzenschlager, R, Daniel, S.E, and Lees, A.J. The L-dopa response in vascular parkinsonism. *J Neurol Neurosurg Psych* 2004, 75: 545–7.

11. National Institute for Health and Care Excellence (2017). Parkinson's disease in adults. NICE Guideline NG71, 2017. www.nice.org.uk/guidance/ng71.

Chapter 9

Comprehensive Geriatric Assessment in Clinical Practice

Khalid Ali

A History of Comprehensive Geriatric Assessment

The most succinct definition of comprehensive geriatric assessment (CGA) describes it as '[a] multidimensional, multidisciplinary process which identifies medical, social, and functional needs, and the development of an integrated and co-ordinated care plan to meet patient needs' (1). The concept and practice of CGA were based on the foundation of 'geriatrics medicine' when Marjory Warren established this specialty. Beginning in 1936, Marjory Warren advocated the proper assessment of older infirm people in warehouses, offering them tailored rehabilitation interventions and discharge planning. The assessment of needs carried out by a multidisciplinary team (MDT) that worked towards the common target of supporting the health and well-being of older people constituted the essence of CGA in Marjory Warren's time and continues to remain a cornerstone of geriatric medicine as we know it today. The data collected by the MDT are used to formulate immediate and long-term treatments and follow-up plans, to coordinate community and secondary care services, to explore long-term care needs, and to negotiate them with the relevant partners, patients, and their support networks. At the core of these assessments is the older persons' understanding of how these assessments and interventions impact on their activities of daily living. The focus on activities of daily living and state of dependency is a key element in what matters to an older person.

It is believed that, by using an evidence-based standardised assessment approach such as the CGA, we can ensure that frail older patients, who are at increased risk of adverse functional outcomes and death, can be formally assessed and offered tailored interventions. This will result in better functional outcomes, shorter hospital stays, and reduced institutionalisation. The perceived benefits of CGA have been highlighted since the early 1990s; a meta-analysis of twenty-nine controlled trials with a total of 9,871 subjects showed that CGA programmes involving assessment and long-term follow-up plans were superior to standard care and improved survival and function of older people (2). A recent mixed-methods study, the HoW-CGA, which contained a literature review, a national survey, and large qualitative and quantitative dataset analysis, showed that CGA still remains the gold standard mechanism in identifying high-risk patients and, through its use in different formats, produces better outcomes for older patients in acute hospitals (3).

The CGA toolkit covers several domains. It starts by collecting demographic data, then it builds a standard medical, psychiatric, and social history, conducts a physical examination, explores nutritional history, and performs specific blood tests. It also extends into psychosocial domains that affect the older person's life, for instance cognition, mood, and lifestyle factors such as exercise, sleep, sexual activity, recreational activities, substance use. The CGA information list includes financial information, available community services, long-term care facilities, and caregiving arrangements. In some settings, it is customary to summarise all this information in a comprehensive 'problem list', as shown next.

The Concept of Comprehensive Geriatric Assessment

The concept of CGA has been a subject of ongoing debate; it has strong supporters and staunch critics from various stakeholder groups, including clinicians and policy makers. Conceptualising CGA can be a daunting task, as CGA itself is, by definition, a multidimensional and multi-professional undertaking. Understandably, healthcare professionals will have different views on the basic principles of CGA, and their views will also differ from those of patients and their families. The situation is complicated further by the fact that there are a multitude of stakeholders that have a vested interest in applying CGA – health service commissioners, policy makers, and organisations that champion older people's rights, such as the British Geriatrics Society (BGS) in the United Kingdom. The notion of CGA acquires different connotations when applied in different contexts – for example in oncology, in surgical settings, or in the context of hospital discharge (interface geriatrics).

Comprehensive geriatric assessment depends on serious investment and 'buy-in' from the whole network of care organisations and stakeholders to implement it effectively. In 2016, John Gladman and his team highlighted several barriers to CGA implementation: guideline factors, professional factors, patient factors, professional interactions, incentives and resources, organisational structure, and social, political, and legal factors (4).

Available evidence to guide the management of older people does not always address the heterogeneity of the older population; a one-size-fits-all approach is not practical to implement in older people. The ethos of CGA addresses the complexity of older people's cohorts by advocating for an individualised assessment, which should consider the needs and expectations of each older person within her or his social networks.

Some interventions are believed to be clinically cost-effective in older people, but they cannot be offered to all of them without considering each person's specific medical, physical, and social circumstances. In these instances, CGA becomes an effective tool for delivering personalised interventions to older people and their carers. For example, a robust CGA might recommend that an older person is eligible for anticoagulation with warfarin for a compelling clinical indication. However, the patient might not agree with the regular blood tests required for the prescription of the right dose of warfarin. In such instances, the need to explore alternatives to warfarin – for example other direct oral anticoagulants – after discussion with the patient and the family cannot be overemphasised. This initial patient–clinician decision must be accommodated by the financial budget and pay heed to the resource limitations that the clinician operates within.

Comprehensive geriatric assessment provides a holistic knowledge of the older person's cultural and spiritual beliefs – factors that can influence his or her choice of the type of long-term residence. Catering for different faiths and affiliations is one such factor. Similarly, end-of-life discussions and advance care planning for older people are important and constitute frequent areas of debate between patients, their families, and healthcare professionals. A well-informed CGA would highlight the preferences and wishes of older people, with important implications for how to proceed with treatment plans.

An underpinning principle of the CGA approach is to provide better outcomes for older people and their carers in health and well-being. However, if older people and their carers do not fully understand the need for and the rationale of CGA or feel that CGA is done *to them* rather than *with them*, then meaningful involvement and partnership is lost. A qualitative study by Darby and team, published in 2017, identified important views of older people that challenged the holistic nature of CGA, namely a perceived absence of treatment after CGA, an incomplete grasp of the role of the geriatrician in the CGA process, and ongoing health and functional needs after discharge from CGA settings (5).

Effectiveness of CGA

One of the earliest evidence-based evaluations investigating the impact of CGA took place in the Department of Ageing and Health in Guy's and St Thomas's Hospital, London, in 2006. A CGA-based approach for older people pre-operatively showed significant improvements in several domains: fewer post-operative complications (such as pneumonia and delirium), less damage to pressure areas, better pain control, earlier mobilisation, appropriate catheter use, and reduced length of stay (6). An older person assessment and liaison team (OPAL) using CGA techniques also demonstrated better clinical outcomes for patients (fewer falls and better management of delirium, chronic pain, constipation, and urinary incontinence) and a reduced length of stay by a mean of three days after the introduction of the service (7).

The evidence base for CGA effectiveness in reducing the number of hospital admissions has been provided by several systematic reviews; in 2017, Jay and colleagues reviewed five studies with a total of 28,434 participants and reported that a consultant geriatrician-led CGA performed in emergency departments reduced admission rates (8). However, the authors called for further research to investigate the effectiveness of the consultant-led approach in reducing readmission rates or length of stay, and also the financial sustainability and viability of the approach. A systematic review by Deschodt and team, in 2013, showed differing results. The review covered twelve studies with a total of 4,546 participants and explored the impact of geriatric consultation teams in acute hospitals. The authors suggested that CGA-led interventions reduced mortality at 6- and 8-months after discharge, but also demonstrated no effect on length of stay, readmission rates, or functional status (9). It should be noted that this systematic review was based on studies from Belgium, Canada, Germany, Madrid, Chicago, Southern California, North Carolina, and Taiwan. The two systematic reviews cited here provide supporting positive but conflicting evidence for CGA-led interventions. This discrepancy invites speculation about the generalisability of CGA across different settings and countries and calls for further research into identifying target populations for CGA-led interventions and having a consensus on outcome measures.

In surgical settings, CGA approaches were found to be beneficial in reducing delirium after hip fracture (10).

Old Age versus the Ageing Process

A review by Parker and team in 2018 identified key aspects of CGA that make it easy to understand for healthcare professionals and members of the public alike (1). Clarity about the conceptualisation and application of CGA can subsequently facilitate its universal application and acceptance by the public as well as by healthcare professionals. The stated key aspects of CGA are as follows:

- CGA's target population and main beneficiaries are people over 55 years and people who receive acute care.
- The main clinical outcomes after CGA are quoted as mortality, activities of daily living, and dependency (1).

As the term itself implies, CGA is an assessment tool that is tailor-made for older people. Establishing a cut-off age of 55 years has the advantage of focusing the relevant specialists on recognising that they are dealing with a special group of people with complex health and social circumstances. Far from being an 'ageist tool' for discriminating against 'young people', a specified age denotes a natural transition in life and a new phase that comes with different requirements and expectations. Dealing with an older person and her or his formal and informal carers requires skill and experience in identifying what matters to an individual. It is common to hear older people saying that, as they get older, they do not want to be a burden on others, and that they would rather pass away than suffer a life of dependency.

The agenda of 'successful ageing' is important to consider when talking about CGA. A meta-analysis of the attributes of successful ageing grouped them as follows:

1. Avoiding disease and disability.
2. Having high cognitive/mental/physical function.
3. Actively engaging in life.
4. Being psychologically well adapted in later life (11).

Three of these four attributes refer to physical functions, which allow for active participation in social life and for achieving a state of well-being with self and the surroundings. It then becomes clear that the activities of daily living, engagement, and participation, whose assessments are are core components of the CGA tool, are also the key elements that older people care about. It logically follows that it is the responsibility of healthcare professionals, as part of their duty of care, to use measures of function that are meaningful to older people.

Insufficient Evidence in Some Areas Relating to CGA

The benefits of CGA in terms of its clinical effectiveness are well supported by evidence from systematic reviews, meta-analyses informed by international randomised controlled trials (RCT) in various settings (8–14). However, it is important to emphasise the context-specific limitations of CGA for older people in clinical practice. A 2011 systematic review by Conroy and team that covered five trials of sufficient quality found that CGA interventions did not reduce mortality or readmissions for frail older people who were rapidly discharged from acute hospitals within seventy-two hours (15).

In special groups of older people in nursing homes with palliative care needs, various forms of CGA tools have been subjected to scrutiny; in 2014, Hermans and colleagues 2014 identified the interRAI PC Assessment Form and the McMaster Quality of Life Scale as the most comprehensive tools of holistic geriatric assessment in those groups (16).

An important advantage of the CGA toolkit lies in the fact that its individual components can provide relevant prognostic information. A CGA is more than the sum of its parts; certain components of CGA can predict post-operative complications and the discharge destinations for older people who undergo surgical oncology. Thus frailty, limitations in the instrumental activities of daily living, and depression all predict discharge to a care home (17).

It is important for commissioners to be convinced of the economic viability of CGA in certain cohorts, for instance surgical patients; recent evidence suggests that a CGA approach offers a cost-effective care model in dealing with orthogeriatric patients (18).

There is still insufficient evidence for the cost-effectiveness of CGA in settings outside the hospital. The CGA concept has also been criticised for failing to acknowledge frailty and for not paying due attention to patient-reported outcome measures (PROMS) (4). One of the limitations of implementing a robust CGA in a variety of settings is that it relies on a multitude of factors such as the need for several members of the MDT and for effective communication between them, the patient, and their families. A team leader with effective leadership and communication skills is needed to coordinate the team members working towards a unified goal, with objective measures of good outcomes for patients, their families, and institutions in terms of clinical and cost-effectiveness.

Applying Comprehensive Geriatric Assessment in Clinical Practice

Comprehensive geriatric assessment practice and its implementation have been accepted to various degrees into mainstream care for older people in the United Kingdom, in Europe, and internationally. In the United Kingdom, the rise of specialist services for older people – for example acute frailty units and outpatient clinics for older people (rapid access clinics for older people (RACOP) – has inevitably brought CGA into clinical practice, as a routine part of it.

Currently, adopting the principles and ethos of CGA in the emergency department (ED) is mandatory, as increasing numbers of older people present to emergency care settings with challenging multiple comorbidities, functional decline, delirium, and a breakdown of community social support networks. Identifying specific frailty syndromes warrants detailed assessments and referral to specialist services for effective interventions. Having the specialist skills to deliver high-quality CGA becomes part of a front door service with positive outcomes for patients and healthcare settings. The '36 frailty flying squad model at the Royal United Hospital NHS Foundation Trust' in the United Kingdom has showed that a multidisciplinary acute elderly care team based in the ED and delivering effective early CGA can achieve early discharge, reduce length of stay, and reduce readmission within 30 days (12). In this model, two medical nurse practitioners, a physiotherapist, and a consultant geriatrician assessed older frail patients referred from the emergency department and instigated management and discharge plans that were reviewed within twenty-four hours.

Comprehensive geriatric assessment also has potential to help effective communications between healthcare professionals and older people and their families in difficult conversations, such as about end-of-life care planning (13).

Case vignette: An 82-year-old lady was seen by her GP after a fall at home. She lives alone, having been widowed six months ago. She has hypertension, diet-controlled

Table 19.1 A case vignette summarising CGA components, assessment, and intervention

CGA Components	Assessment	Intervention
Medical history	Assess blood pressure control, 24-hour ambulatory monitor; investigate underlying reasons of fall, postural hypotension related to medications, cardiac arrhythmias, 24-hour ECG monitor; check baseline blood tests, FBS, urea, and electrolytes, lipid profile, HbA1C, etc.	Adjust blood pressure medications according to tolerance, efficacy, and acceptability.
Functional assessment	Assess activities of daily living and instrumental activities of daily living using Barthel score and Nottingham activities of daily living measures.	Offer a physical assessment by the physiotherapist in the GP practice MDT team.
Social factors	Assess home circumstances, leisure activities, companionship, etc.	Organise home visit by GP practice occupational therapist.
Nutritional assessment	Check body mass index (BMI), check liver function tests including albumin.	GP to perform and record physical examination and blood test results
Other consideration	Assess mood and cognitive measures using measures such as the Montreal Cognitive Assessment (MoCA).	GP to assess mood and cognition and to refer to specialist services, e.g. old age psychiatry

diabetes mellitus, and mild forgetfulness, as described by her daughter, who lives abroad. She takes amlodipine 5 mg once daily and aspirin 75 mg once daily. She does not smoke and enjoys half a glass of sherry with her meals. She does her own shopping with the help of a neighbour, once a week. She attends the local Age UK centre fortnightly and gets there either by walking or by taking the local bus. She gets a monthly pension, having retired twenty-two years ago from working as an assistant in the local post office in her town. Table 19.1 summarises the CGA approach to assessment and interventions.

Comprehensive Geriatric Assessment and Polypharmacy

The burden of polypharmacy and medication-related harm (MRH) is significant in older people, particularly after a hospital admission (19). In one 2018 study, the incidence of MRH within 30 days of hospital admission ranged from 167 to 500 events per 1,000 individuals discharged (17–51 per cent of individuals) (20). Hence a hospital admission and the immediate period after discharge can be a crucial time. A CGA focusing on medicine rationalisation and optimisation has the potential to reduce MRH. Primary and secondary care professionals (doctors, nurses, pharmacists) should work closely with patients and their families to address MRH in a timely manner, using the CGA so as to include knowledge of their patients' special social and environmental factors. In a CGA context, a deeper understating of patients' issues related to their medications – such as adherence, side effects, and health literacy – is a first step towards reducing MRH. Local medicine guidance such as STOP/ START criteria (21) can then be incorporated into a tailored CGA. Risk-predicting tools such as the one developed from the PRIME study (Prospective study to develop a model to stratify the RIsk of Medication-related harm in hospitalised Elderly patients), which identifies older people at the highest risk of sustaining MRH at the point of hospital discharge, can be another way of targeting interventions at older people who need them most (22).

Required Skills for Delivering Comprehensive Geriatric Assessment

By its nature, CGA is a multi-agency approach. The team delivering a comprehensive geriatric assessment needs to be adequately trained in assessing the needs of older people and in acknowledging multimorbidity, polypharmacy, cognitive decline, and demanding social circumstances. An older person frequently presents with one or more of the 'geriatric giants': cognitive impairment, incontinence, instability, and immobility. Medical training has traditionally been heavily influenced by the single-disease model. As the ageing population increases in number across Europe and worldwide, there is a compelling need to invest in training doctors and allied healthcare professionals in geriatrics. As most of the acute hospital admissions in the United Kingdom are admissions of older people, it becomes essential that emergency physicians should receive basic training in geriatrics and in how to perform CGA. Training non-geriatricians in the assessment and management of older people has the potential to transform service delivery (23).

Specialist education and training are key elements in equipping all healthcare professionals with the required knowledge, behaviour, attitude, and skills, which are all mandatory in caring for an older person. Together, embedding a training in the specialist skills needed for CGA in undergraduate studies and encouraging postgraduate doctors to pursue an academic interest in geriatrics are key components in building a work force that can support older people who live in their own home or in care settings.

It cannot be overemphasised that caring for older people is a multidisciplinary task. It is important to engage creatively with all MDT members and embrace new models of delivering CGA.

Practical Tips for Comprehensive Geriatric Assessment Delivery (Box 19.1)

For healthcare practitioners, learning the specialist language and terminology from the world of geriatrics and CGA is mandatory if they want to deliver evidence-based care that is feasible and acceptable to older people and their families.

Terms such as 'frailty', 'sarcopenia', and 'immune senescence', or even 'CGA', can confuse practitioners. Hence the first step is education and training in the language and concepts that specialist geriatricians use commonly but non-specialists view as 'jargon'.

Box 19.1 Top ten tips for the CGA

1. Know the core team of CGA in your local area.
2. Communicate with the CGA team effectively and share specific responsibilities.
3. Allocate an overall coordinator who is responsible for communicating with the older person, her or his carers, and the rest of the CGA team.
4. Set realistic follow-up plans for the older person who had a CGA in your setting: who is doing what, where, and when?
5. Use language that is easily understood by patients and their carers.
6. Always provide a summary of the consultation using a standard grid (as shown in Table 19.1).
7. Ensure that patients and carers understand you by allowing them ample time to ask questions.
8. Use CGA as an opportunity for medications review. Use locally agreed tools to optimise the review of medications – for example STOP/START criteria (21).
9. Know how to measure frailty by using simple measures that are evidence-based and validated, for example handgrip strength as a proxy-measure (with Southampton guidance) (24).
10. Collect CGA data for your cohort of older people and use these data to develop and improve local service provision for older people.

Summary

CGA has considerable evidence to support its use in the routine care of older people in a variety of settings, in hospital and in the community. There is an agreed operational definition that allows its use in practice and in research. Further work is needed to identify the cohort of older people for whom a CGA will bring about the best patient-centred outcomes.

References

1. Parker, S.G, McCue, P., Phelps, K. et al. What is comprehensive geriatric assessment (CGA)? An umbrella review. *Age and Ageing* 2018, 47: 149–55.

2. Stuck, A.E., Siu, A.L., Wieland, G.D., Adams, J. et al. Comprehensive geriatric assessment: A meta-analysis of controlled trials. *Lancet* 1993, 342(8878): 1032–6.

3. Conroy, S.P., Bardsley, M., Smith, P. et al. *Comprehensive Geriatric Assessment for Frail Older People in Acute Hospitals: The How-CGA Mixed-Methods Study.* Southampton (UK): NIHR Journals Library, 2019.

4. Gladman, J.R.F., Conroy, S.P., Ranhoff, A.H. et al. New horizons in the implementation and research of comprehensive geriatric assessment: Knowing, doing and the 'know-do' gap. *Age and Ageing* 2016, 45: 194–200.

5. Darby, J., Williamson, T., Logan, P. et al. Comprehensive geriatric assessment on an acute medical unit: A qualitative study of older people's and informal carer's perspectives of the care and treatment received. *Clinical Rehabilitation* 2017, 3: 126–34.

6. Harari, D., Hopper, A., Dhesi, J. et al. Proactive care of older people undergoing surgery (POPS): Designing, embedding, evaluating, and funding a comprehensive geriatrics assessment service for older elective surgical patients. *Age and Ageing* 2007, 36: 190–6.

7. Harari, D, Martin, F.C., Buttery, A. et al. The older persons' assessment and liaison

team 'OPAL': Evaluation of comprehensive geriatric assessment in acute medical inpatients. *Age and Ageing* 2007, 36: 670–5.

8. Jay, S., Whittaker, P., Mcintosh, J. et al. Can consultant geriatrician led comprehensive geriatric assessment in the emergency department reduce hospital admission rates? A systematic review. *Age and Ageing* 2017, 46: 366–72.

9. Deschodt, M., Flamaing, J., Haentjens, P. et al. Impact of geriatric consultation teams on clinical outcome in acute hospitals: A systematic review and meta-analysis. *BMC Medicine* 2013, 11: 48.

10. Shields, L., Henderson, V., and Caslake, R. Comprehensive geriatric assessment for prevention of delirium after hip fracture: A systematic review of randomized controlled trials. *JAGS* 2017, 65: 1559–65.

11. Kim, S.H., and Park, S. A meta-analysis of the correlates of successful aging in older adults. *Res Aging.* 2017, 39(5): 657–77.

12. Ballham, S., Buxton, S., Camacho, R. et al. 36 Frailty Flying Squad: An emergency department focussed acute care of the elderly service: Dr Genevieve Robson, Royal United Hospital NHS Foundation Trust. *Emerg Med J* 2017, 34: A885–A886.

13. Baronner, A., and MacKenzie, A. Using geriatric assessment strategies to lead end-of-life care discussions. *Curr Oncol Rep* 2017, 19: 75–80.

14. Ellis, G., Whitehead, M., O'Neill, D. et al. Comprehensive geriatric assessment for older adults admitted to hospital. *Cochrane Database Syst Rev* 2011. doi: 10.1002/14651858.CD006211.pub2.

15. Conroy, S.P., Stevens, T., Parker, S.G. et al. A systematic review of comprehensive geriatric assessment to improve outcomes for frail older people being rapidly discharged from acute hospitals: Interface geriatrics. *Age and Ageing* 2011, 40: 436–43.

16. Hermans, K., Mello, J.D.A., Spruytte, N. et al. A comparative analysis of comprehensive geriatric assessments for nursing home residents receiving palliative care: A systematic review. *JAMDA* 2014, 15: 467–76.

17. Feng, M.A., McMillan, D.T., Crowell, K. et al. Geriatric assessment in surgical oncology: A systematic review. *Journal of Surgical Research* 2015, 193: 265–72.

18. Eamer, G., Saravana-Bawan, B., Westhuizen, B.V.D. et al. Economic evaluations of comprehensive geriatric assessment in surgical patients: A systematic review. *Journal of Surgical Research* 2017, 218: 9–17.

19. Parekh, N., Ali, K., Stevenson, J.M. et al. Incidence and cost of medication harm in older adults following hospital discharge: A multicentre prospective study in the UK. *Br J Clin Pharmacol* 2018, 84(8): 1789–97.

20. Parekh, N., Ali, K., Page, A.J. et al. Incidence of medication-related harm in older adults after hospital discharge: A systematic review. *Am Geriatr Soc* 2018, 66(9): 1812–22.

21. Gallagher, P., Ryan, C., Byrne, S. et al. STOPP (Screening Tool of Older Persons' Prescriptions) and START (Screening Tool to Alert Doctors to Right Treatment): Consensus validation. *Int J Clin Pharmacol Ther* 2008, 46(2): 72–83.

22. Parekh, N., Ali, K., Davies, G.J. et al. Medication-related harm in older adults following hospital discharge: Development and validation of a prediction tool. *BMJ Qual Saf* 2020, 29(2): 142–53.

23. Fisher, J.M., Masud, T., Holm, E.A. et al. New horizons in geriatric medicine education and training: The need for pan-European education and training standards. *European Geriatric Medicine* 2017, 8: 467–73.

24. Roberts, H.C.H. J. Dension, H.J., Martin, H.J. et al. A review of the measurement of grip strength in clinical and epidemiological studies: Towards a standardised approach. *Age and Ageing* 2011, 40: 423–9.

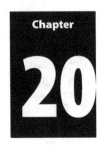

Chapter

20

Interface between Liaison Psychiatry Services for Older People and Wider Community Services

Benjamin R. Underwood, Rosalind Tandy, and Emad Sidhom

Introduction

The liaison psychiatry for older people (LPOP) service looks after older people with mental and physical illness and commonly significant frailty, comorbidity, and legal complexity. Consequently it is one of the most challenging of medical specialties. This is compounded by the fact that the turnover of patients is generally high; in the United Kingdom, the average length of stay for emergency admissions is less than ten days; and few of these admissions will be under LPOP's direct care (1). Given that most mental illnesses and their treatment develop over much longer time spans, ensuring follow-up and continuity of care is essential. Many patients will already be known to psychiatric services outside of the hospital, and assessments or treatments may already have started or be part of long-term care plans. Nearly all patients will be known to general practice. Hence the time spent with LPOP teams is likely to be a single point in the patient journey (albeit often an important one), and a successful interaction with other services, one that produces a smooth handover, is vital for getting the best outcomes for patients. In this chapter we outline the likely services that are available outside the hospital in the United Kingdom, then we go on to explore communication and systems that should help to ensure optimal outcomes.

Services Outside the Hospital

1. Psychiatric services for older people

a. **In-patient services and approved mental health professionals (AMHPs)**
The relationship between psychiatric and acute medical in-patient services is an important one. Psychiatric in-patients commonly require medical intervention in acute trusts during their admission, and for some of the patients who present at acute hospital trusts the optimal outcome will be transfer to an in-patient psychiatric facility. Previous studies have shown that more than a half of the admissions to some psychiatric wards come from the general hospital (2).

A1. Transfer of patients from acute trusts to psychiatric wards. Psychiatric wards may admit patients on the basis of age, geography, sex, or type of mental disorder (organic vs functional), and this can make bed management complex. Make sure you know the local system for identifying beds and their 'gatekeepers'. For patients in England who lack capacity and refuse (or are likely to refuse) broadly defined care and treatment in a psychiatric hospital, a legal basis for authorising their deprivation of liberty is required. This will often mean assessment for detention under the Mental Health Act (MHA), though this legislative position is currently under review. In most parts of the country MHA assessments are coordinated by the Approved Mental Health Professional (AMHP) service.

A2. Transfer of patients from psychiatric wards to the acute trusts. A process should be in place to alert LPOP services at the earliest opportunity when a patient is transferred from the psychiatric hospital and to make sure that all the relevant information is provided. This is particularly important if the patient is detained under the MHA, as proper arrangements for the transfer will need to be in place, including section 17 leave if appropriate and potential change of responsible clinician status if the period of stay in the acute trust is prolonged. Different hospitals will have different arrangements for escorting transferred patients. Clear local arrangements should be in place, and it is worth familiarising yourself with these.

b. **Crisis teams**

Crisis resolution teams, home treatment teams, and dementia intensive support teams have grown in number in the United Kingdom over the past ten years. Despite diverse titles, they share a similar clinical remit: to provide community care for patients who would otherwise require in-patient care. Although in-patient care is sometimes essential, if patients can be treated at home, this is generally preferred by them, has the clinical advantage of avoiding the possible harms of in-patient treatment, and is generally cheaper, allowing for resources to be directed elsewhere. These teams provide safe care and are effective at lowering hospital admission (3). They generally work with patients for a short period of time, usually weeks, until the patient's condition has either resolved or stabilised to a point where they can be safely transferred to other services. The crisis team will often be a point of contact for patients who have been identified as being at high risk in the acute trust and are now leaving hospital. In many trusts, such teams have also become the gatekeepers of admission to in-patient units, on the grounds that admission should be considered only if community care under the crisis team is not possible. This can be a point of discord between teams, for example if there is disagreement on whether a patient requires admission; and this is where building relationships of trust among colleagues is likely to bear fruit. Decisions often need to be made in order to make the best use of the available resources, and the crisis teams will be aware of the available beds and the competing demands on them.

c. **General community services (including memory assessment services)**

These teams provide ongoing care for people with severe and enduring mental illness (such as schizophrenia, bipolar disorder, severe affective disorder, and personality disorder) and, frequently, diagnostic services and follow-up for patients with dementia. In adult services, some of these roles have increasingly become the preserve of specialist teams, for example early-onset psychosis services. Currently this is rarer in older people's services, but age-inclusive services are becoming more common and specialisation may follow suit, even in older people's teams. One area that is already often specialist is that of memory assessment teams, which provide high-volume assessment of patients with cognitive problems. This is, frequently, an area of overlap, where cognitive dysfunction is identified in acute trusts, often as part of delirium, but follow-up is desired to identify any underlying dementia, perhaps after some months, when any delirium has settled. In this case it is helpful for patients and colleagues if the dementia blood screening and any imaging are done while the patient is an in-patient, because getting them for a potentially frail and cognitively impaired elderly person with poor mobility may present a challenge once that person has been discharged. The Improving Access to Psychological Therapy (IAPT) programme teams or the well-being teams do what their name implies by providing psychological therapy – most commonly cognitive behavioral therapy (CBT) – at scale. They are usually age-inclusive and will allow self-referral.

d. **Electroconvulsive therapy**

Electroconvulsive therapy (ECT) consists in the brief passage of an electric current through the brain that is designed to induce seizure under a general anaesthetic and muscle relaxant. It has proven to be effective, well tolerated, and safe for older adults who suffer treatment-resistant depression (4). The remission rate is 73–90 per cent in patients over the age of 65 years, and ECT may be more commonly used in older adults with severe depression and psychotic symptoms.

Electroconvulsive therapy may be particularly relevant to old age liaison psychiatrists – not just because of the age of the patient seen but because patients may deteriorate when seriously mentally unwell, for example through dehydration, and be transferred to the acute hospital for medical care. As ECT is a procedure requiring general anaesthetic, it is often performed in operating theatres, and therefore may be performed on the acute hospital site. The decision regarding ECT should include pre-ECT assessment, a decision on electrode placement, an estimate of the number of sessions, and assessment of efficacy and evaluation of both cognitive and non-cognitive side effects of ECT, as well as the legal basis for its administration. Be aware of how and where ECT is provided in your local area, as delivering this treatment across settings almost always requires close collaboration and organisation. For patients in the acute trust who require ECT, liaising with the ward the patient is on will be important, as it will make sure that the requirements of the procedure (e.g. nil by mouth, bloods, or making the appropriate MHA paperwork go with the patient) are understood so as to avoid cancelled treatments.

2. General practice

In the United Kingdom nearly every patient you see will be registered with a general practitioner (GP). Often there will be an individual doctor who knows the patient well and may have done so for some time. Such doctors can be invaluable sources of longitudinal as well as current information, accurate and up-to-date – on current medical problems, investigations, and medications. The practice admin team may be able to send you a patient summary with this information. General practitioners often constitute a first port of call for patients outside the hospital and can coordinate complex services for an individual. Hence involving them at the point of discharge and ensuring accurate and prompt information about the admission is essential.

General practice teams in the United Kingdom include general GPs, but are increasingly multidisciplinary in their makeup, being made up of nurses, doctors, pharmacists, therapists, paramedics, and physician associates. Such a team provides care for its practice population from cradle to grave and is the gateway to wider health and well-being service provision. Each practice team is now part of a primary care network, which usually includes several practices and covers around 50,000 patients. With the formation of these networks, further extended roles are appearing, for instance that of the embedded mental health worker.

In the United Kingdom, general practice is often demand-led to a significant degree and operates on the basis of the patient's or carer's contacting the practice to ask for support. Most practices will offer a phone or online consultation to triage patients and, where appropriate, individuals will be care-navigated to the most appropriate member of the team or to another service. Appointments are offered for long-term condition management and for some screening activities, but these are in the minority by comparison with response to patient requests. For the frail and cognitively impaired elderly patients who may not proactively ask for help, high-quality communication between hospital and general practice and care planning across them are vital.

A discharge summary from a mental health liaison team should should detail with clarity the likely diagnosis, the investigation results, the medications, and the agreed plan once patients have left the hospital, and all discussions around long-term and future care wishes should be included. It is possible that the GP does not have access to a particular hospital's pathology and radiology results; therefore these should be included, too. If a decision has been made that an onward referral to another specialty, community services, or secondary psychiatric care is required, it should be actioned by the hospital team before discharge, where this is possible. When medications are stopped or changed, there should be a clear rationale and, ideally, a record of discussing this decision, ideally with the patient and, if appropriate, with the patient's carer. Patients can find it difficult when medication that they have been told to take for many years is ceased.

The duty doctor at each practice can be contacted, usually by telephone, if an urgent discussion is required or if any information gathering about the patient's history is needed. Adult and child safeguarding multidisciplinary team (MDT) meetings are held on a regular basis within practices and are attended by other community workers, for example district nurses and social workers. Some practices also have separate, mental health-specific, MDT meetings. If the individual has complex medical or social needs or is frequently attending the hospital, it may be helpful for the liaison team to attend one of these meetings to discuss specific patients, facilitate joint care planning, and optimise communication.

3. Wider community services for older people

To most psychiatrists, these services may seem daunting to interact with because of their size, diversity, and lack of familiarity. However, making the effort is likely to bring benefit to your patients. Increasingly they are part of either mental health or acute trusts. Community resources may include district nursing, community physiotherapy, occupational therapy, and services based on clinical presentation. These include cardiac, respiratory, Parkinson's disease, multiple sclerosis, neurological rehabilitation, continence, speech and language therapy, diabetes, dietetics, and podiatry services, as well as in-patient rehabilitation for older people. Given the frequent need for care after discharge from acute trusts and the potential for ongoing safeguarding or legal concerns, social services are a further important professional group to interact with.

4. **Third-sector services, including charity and voluntary services**
   Although some charities are national in their reach, such as Age UK or the Alzheimer's Society, many more will be local and specific to your area; and even national bodies often have a very localised offer. Often each area will produce a directory of local services, and this will be invaluable as a general guide and a source of reference for individual patient need. An alternative source of advice will be colleagues who have been working in the local community for some time and will have presumably developed excellent local knowledge.

Communication and System Working

For any patient moving between acute care and the community, communication between clinicians is important. Movement between teams can be a high-risk time for patients. A personal call between the hospital clinician and the receiving clinician in the community can help to build relationships, avoid misunderstandings, and promote safe care. Time taken to build relationships, perhaps by sharing educational opportunities or away days, will facilitate care provision in any subsequent difficult clinical situations. Communication is particularly important where an individual is cared for by a number of different services, possibly even for the same condition.

Some issues around communication occur at the level of individual clinicians, while others may be better resolved at a system level. Examples include community and acute services that either use the same electronic record system or at least ensure that clinicians can access the different systems. Where different parts of the system are operating on different electronic healthcare records, verbal handover (perhaps using a validated tool such as SBAR) and sending documents (which can be uploaded) become even more important (5, 6). Uniformity in cognitive testing is generally helpful. If a mini-mental state examination (MMSE) (7) has been done in the community and was followed by a Montreal Cognitive Assessment (MoCA) (8) in the hospital, the results from these tests will be much harder to compare than if a single instrument were used. Multiple-discharge summaries (e.g. separate physical and mental health summaries) or summaries that are very long can be confusing; if detail is required, then including a clear and concise précis at the top of the document could help. With the right systems, behaviours, and communication in place, the challenge of looking after the patients who present at LPOP services can be significantly ameliorated and good outcomes can be ensured.

References

1. Imison, C., Poteliakhoff, E., and Thompson, J. Older people and emergency bed use: Exploring variation. The King's Fund, August 2012. www .kingsfund.org.uk/sites/default/files/field/ field_publication_file/older-people-and-emergency-bed-use-aug-2012.pdf.

2. Edmans, B.G., Wolverson, E. Dunning, R., Slann, M., Russell, G., Crowther, G., Hall, D., Yates, R., Albert, M., and Underwood, B.R. Inpatient psychiatric

care for patients with dementia at four sites in the United Kingdom. *Int J Geriatr Psychiatry* 2021, 37(2). doi: 10.1002/gps.5658.

3. Rubinsztein, J.S. et al. Efficacy of a dementia intensive support (DIS) service at preventing admissions to medical and psychiatric wards: Qualitative and quantitative evaluation. *BJPsych Bull* 2020, 1–5. doi: 10.1192/bjb.2020.24.

4. Jiang, X. et al. Efficacy and safety of modified electroconvulsive therapy for the refractory depression in older patients. *Asia-Pacific Psychiatry* 2020, 12 (4). doi: 10.1111/appy.12411.

5. Alexander, L. Bechan, N., Brady, S., Douglas, L., Moore, S, et al. Quality improvement of clinical handover in a liaison psychiatry department: A three-phase audit. *Ir Med J* 1116(6). https://pubmed.ncbi.nlm.nih.gov/30518203.

6. Glass, O.M., Hermida, A.P., Hershenberg, R., and Schwartz, A.C. Considerations and current trends in the management of the geriatric patient on a consultation–liaison service. *Current Psychiatry Reports* 2020, 22(5).

7. Folstein, M.F., Folstein, S.E., and McHugh, P.R. 'Mini-mental state': A practical method for grading the cognitive state of patients for the clinician. *J Psychiatr Res* 1975, 12, 189–98.

8. Nasreddine, Z.S. et al. The Montreal Cognitive Assessment, MoCA: A brief screening tool for mild cognitive impairment. *J Am Geriatr Soc* 2005, 53: 695–9.

Psychometric Measures in Old Age Psychiatry

Tareq Qassem

In this chapter we will discuss the basics of psychometrics and scales commonly used in depression and dementia, specifically in assessing cognitive functions, activities of daily living (ADLs), and behavioural and psychological symptoms of dementia (BPSD). The scales and tools discussed are only those related to older adults with a focus on those that could be used in hospital settings.

Psychometric Measures

Introduction to Psychometrics

Psychometric tools are formal instruments that measure a specific part of the psychological process. They can assist in screening for specific disorders such as depression or dementia. They can also be used to monitor the progression of disease or response to treatment. They are used in studies and have been increasingly used as clinical outcome measures (1). Psychometric tests are helpful tools but applying them in an acute hospital setting could pose many challenges. This is due to the characteristics of hospital environments: the lack of available private spaces, fast flow in the hospital's admission and discharge process, and the nature of the illness that led to admission.

What Makes a Good Psychometric Test?

Fitzpatrick and colleagues (1) have proposed that a good psychometric tool needs to have good clinical utility and psychometric robustness.

Clinical utility is the usefulness of a psychometric tool to clinical practice, as measured by the following criteria:

1. Acceptability: the degree with which the instrument is acceptable to patients. Several factors can affect the acceptability of a test: its mode of administration, the health condition of respondents, the questionnaire design, its use of language, and the time taken to administer the test (2).

2. Feasibility: the simplicity of administering and processing a test. The staff's views and required training, as well as patients' acceptance of tests, make a great difference, even in self-administered scales (3, 4).

3. Interpretability: how meaningful the test scores are. There are four approaches for a broad interpretation of a tests score:

   a. Variations in instrument scores compared to formerly documented scores generated by the same instrument.

b. The adoption of the minimal clinically important difference (MCID), which is equal to the smallest changes in instrument scores that are identified as beneficial by patients (5).

c. The use of normative data from the general population to interpret scores from generic instruments.

d. The use of an exact cut-off point that differentiates cases from none-cases (1).

4. Psychometric robustness: related to tools performance aspects such as the following:

a. Reliability: reflects how internally consistent or reproducible the test is. It also reflects how free from measurement error a psychometric instrument is (6). A part of the reliability is internal consistency (internal reliability) – a measure of how well the items within a scale correlate to each other. Another part is reproducibility (external reliability), which evaluates whether an instrument yields the same results on repeated administrations with the same respondents. This is assessed by test–retest reliability and inter-rater reliability. Test–retest reliability reflects consistency over time. The closer the accordance between repeated tests, the higher the reliability of the instrument (7, 8). It is worth noting that repeated reliability measures may be influenced by a 'practice effect': repeat testing may lead to higher scores if subjects in the sample 'learn' to answer the same questions, which can be an issue in some cognitive tests (9).

b. Validity: the degree to which a test measures what it is meant to measure. There are several types of validity, which can be assessed both qualitatively and quantitatively. Content validity evaluates whether the test items sufficiently address the domain of interest. Face validity examines whether an instrument is subjectively viewed as measuring the domains of interest. Both are qualitative methods that are used to assess the validity of a psychometric instrument (10). Validity testing involves some quantitative evaluation using statistical inferences. Criterion validity is assessed when an instrument correlates with another instrument or measure that has a recognised validity or a 'gold standard' (1).

Construct validity reflects the quantitative degree to which the test measures a theoretical construct by a specific procedure (11). Predictive validity reflects the degree of correlation of a psychometric test score with future values or events of interest (1).

c. Responsiveness: the capacity of a test to recognise important changes that are due to an intervention or to the passage of time. There is no particular agreed upon method for evaluating responsiveness. However, effect size can be used to evaluate test responsiveness to change (12).

5. Precision: the tool's precision plays a significant role in selecting the right test. For example, in screening tests, it is more important to have a test with the capacity to pick most cases (i.e. a test with great sensitivity) than to have a test that can eliminate non-cases (i.e. a test with high specificity, e.g. a confirmatory test). A perfect diagnostic test should differentiate with 100 per cent accuracy subjects with a disease (test score above a certain cut-off) from subjects without the disease (test score below a certain cut-off). Unfortunately, such a perfect test does not exist in reality. Therefore a diagnostic procedure can distinguish between subjects with and subjects without disease only with varying degrees of precision. Values above the cut-off are

not always indicative of disease, because subjects without the disease can sometimes have higher values too. Such elevated values of a parameter of interest are called false positive (FP) values. On the other hand, values under the cut-off are mainly found in subjects without the disease. However, some subjects with the disease could have a test score below the cut-off. Those values are called false negative (FN) values. Thus we may encounter, in the test population, the following four groups (13):

a. true positives (TPs): subjects with the disease and with test scores higher than the cut-off;

b. false positives (FPs): subjects without the disease but with test scores higher than the cut-off;

c. true negatives (TNs): subjects without the disease and with test scores below the cut-off;

d. false negatives (FNs): subjects with the disease but with test scores below the cut-off.

Practical Guidelines for Using Assessment Tools for Older Adults

Advancing age is associated with increasing sensory impairment. Hence it is essential to maximise the older person's ability to take part effectively in assessment by minimising the effect of sensory impairment, and also the interruptions and distractions. The American Psychological Association (14) has made the following recommendations for conducting a psychological assessment on older adults:

1. Minimise background noise, as individuals with hearing loss have difficulty discriminating between sounds in the environment.

2. Arrange the seating so as to render it conducive to conversation. Try to sit close to the client, face to face, at a table rather than on the far side of a desk.

3. Increase the lighting and reduce the impact of glare from windows.

4. Use material in large print and avoid glossy papers.

5. Ensure that the patient has his or her hearing aid or reading glasses. Have magnifying glasses available on conference tables.

6. Look at the client when speaking. Many individuals with hearing loss read lips to compensate for poor hearing.

7. Speak slowly and distinctly. Older adults may process information more slowly than younger adults.

8. Do not over-articulate or shout, as this can distort speech and facial gestures.

9. Use a lower pitch of voice, because the ability to hear high-frequency tones is the first and most severe impairment experienced by many older adults with compromised hearing.

10. If the cognitive assessment is a part of a long assessment interview, it is preferable to check whether the patient needs to have a short break.

Cognitive Screening Tools

Cognitive assessment is an essential part of diagnosing dementia. Memory complaints are a frequent cause of medical consultation; therefore reliable and validated tools for discriminating between healthy and impaired patients are necessary (15). The cognitive screening tools are different in purpose and scope from the neuropsychological tests, which are more comprehensive and detailed. The main aim of cognitive screening tools is to identify individuals with a high probability of suffering significant cognitive impairment. Such tools need to be of high sensitivity and should not take long to administer. Neuropsychological tests take longer to administer and score and can be handled only by certified staff with extensive training in the use of those tools (16).

Several cognitive tests have been developed and validated to support the diagnosis of dementia. The Mini-Mental State Examination (MMSE) was considered the gold standard (15). However, it has incurred criticism because of the underrepresentation of memory and executive functioning tasks, ceiling and floor effects, and influence of education – as well as on account of copyright restrictions on its use (17). New screening tests have subsequently been developed. Some of them evaluate several cognitive domains; examples are the Addenbrooke's Cognitive Examination III (ACE-III), the Mini-ACE (18, 19), the Montreal Cognitive Assessment (MoCA) (20), and the Rowland Universal Dementia Assessment Scale (RUDAS) (21). Others, such as the Frontal Assessment Battery (FAB) (22), are more specific and limited to assessing certain functions.

The Mini-Mental State Examination

The MMSE is a brief tool that aims to assess cognitive functioning and its change (23). It is probably the most popular cognitive screening tool used, and has been extensively studied in different populations (23). The MMSE has a high test–retest reliability, internal consistency, and high inter-observer reliability (24). It consists of eleven items with a maximum score of 30. At a cut-off score of 24, its sensitivity is 87 per cent and its specificity is 82 per cent (25). The MMSE lacks sensitivity in frontotemporal dementia and in dementia with Lewy bodies (DLB). It does not assess executive functions, and contains a limited number of episodic and semantic memory or visuospatial tasks. The MMSE had a pooled sensitivity of approximately 80 per cent in memory clinics. In mixed specialist hospital settings, the MMSE sensitivity is approximately 71 per cent, while in non-clinical community settings it is approximately 85 per cent (26). It takes a trained, yet non-specialist interviewer approximately ten minutes to administer the MMSE (24).

Addenbrooke's Cognitive Examination-III or ACE-III

The original Addenbrooke's Cognitive Examination (ACE) was developed by Hodges and team as an extended cognitive screening technique designed to detect dementia and differentiate between Alzheimer's dementia and frontotemporal dementia (27). It was subsequently updated as Addenbrooke's Cognitive Examination-Revised, then as ACE-III. The ACE-III is a nineteen-item tool that tests five cognitive domains and can be administered in fifteen to twenty minutes. A total score is given out of 100, with subscores out of 18 for attention, out of 26 for memory, out of 14 for fluency, out of 26 for language, and out of 16 for visuospatial processing (18). The ACE-III has a high sensitivity and specificity at cut-offs previously recommended: 88 (sensitivity = 100 per cent; specificity = 96 per cent) and 82 (sensitivity = 93 per cent; specificity = 100 per cent). The internal consistency of the ACE-III, measured by Cronbach's α coefficient, was 0.88. The ACE-III requires some training for its administration (18).

In addition to English, the ACE-III has been validated in the following languages:

- Arabic (28, 29)
- Chinese (30)
- Indian varieties such as Hindi, Telugu, Kannada, Malayalam, Tamil, and Indian English (31)
- Italian (32)
- Japanese (33)
- Portuguese (34)
- Spanish (35)
- Thai (36)
- Urdu (37)

In addition to validation in different types of dementia, the ACE-III has been validated for mild cognitive impairment (MCI) in English with a sensitivity cut-off of 88 in the range of 75 per cent to 77 per cent and a specificity in the range of 89 per cent to 92 per cent (38). Other studies have validated the ACE-III in MCI in other languages (29).

The Mini-Addenbrooke's Cognitive Examination

The Mini-Addenbrooke's Cognitive Examination (MACE) is a recently described screening instrument, derived from ACE-III by Mokken scaling. This instrument comprises tests of attention, memory, categorical verbal fluency, clock drawing, and memory recall (score range 0–30). The MACE has identified two suggested cut offs: ≤ 25/30 (sensitivity of 85 per cent) and ≤ 21/30 (specificity of 100 per cent) (19). The MACE has also been validated in MCI with a sensitivity ranging from 64 per cent to 95 per cent and a specificity ranging from 46 per cent to 79 per cent at cut-off points of 21 and 25 respectively (38). The MACE takes under five minutes to administer.

The Montreal Cognitive Assessment

The Montreal Cognitive Assessment is a thirty-point cognitive screening test that includes short-term memory recall tasks and visuospatial assessment along with multiple aspects of executive functions and tasks designed to assess attention, concentration, and working memory. The MoCA also includes several language tasks, an abstract reasoning assessment, and tasks that assess orientation to time and place (20, 26). The administration of MoCA takes ten minutes to complete (20).

In screenings for dementia, the MoCA seems to achieve high sensitivity (94 per cent, 97 per cent) and modest specificity (50 per cent, 60 per cent), at a threshold of 26 (and above it) out of 30 (39, 40). But when the cut-off point is lowered to 23, that increases the test specificity to 88 per cent for dementia screening, while reducing the sensitivity to 83 per cent (41). The MoCA demonstrated predictive validity in a six-month follow-up, where it detected mild dementia in people with MCI with 94 per cent sensitivity and 50 per cent specificity (39). The MoCA is reported to have adequate test–retest reliability (20).

The MoCA has been translated into more than sixty languages (42). Moreover, normative data have been established in English in a large population (43), and also other languages (44–53). It is worth mentioning that the cut-off point varies greatly between different ethnic groups (54).

Rowland Universal Dementia Assessment Scale

The Rowland Universal Dementia Assessment Scale (RUDAS) is a brief cognitive screening tool that is suitable for use in culturally and linguistically diverse populations with
a potentially low level of education. The RUDAS measures memory, gnosis, praxis,
visuospatial skills, judgement, and language (55, 56). Its administration takes approximately ten minutes and requires minimal training (55). It has high inter-rater (0.99) and
test–retest (0.98) reliability (55).

The RUDAS was validated in community-dwelling persons in Australia who had
been recruited from clinics and healthcare programs. It showed a score of 88 per cent
sensitivity and 90 per cent specificity at a cut-off of 23/30 (57).

The RUDAS has been validated in more than thirteen languages apart from English
(58–66).

Mini-Cog

The Mini-Cog is a dementia screening tool that combines three-item word memory and
clock drawing. It was developed in a community sample that over-represented people
with dementia, low education, non-white ethnicity, and non-English speakers (67).

In mild dementia, the Mini-Cog has lower sensitivity (76 per cent vs 79 per cent) and
specificity (89 per cent vs 88 per cent) than the MMSE, at a cut-off point of 25 (68). The
Mini-Cog may not be appropriate for use with individuals who have severe visual
impairments or have difficulty holding a writing implement. It has no value in either
monitoring disease progression or rating severity (26). It has an inter-rater reliability
between 0.93 and 0.95 (69).

The Mini-Cog takes approximately three minutes to complete. It may be used
appropriately by relatively untrained raters as a first-stage dementia screen.

Frontal Assessment Battery

Given the lack of sensitivity of the tools available at the time to detect frontotemporal
dementia, Dubois and colleagues (22) developed the frontal assessment battery (FAB) as
a brief and simple tool that can assess executive functions. This instrument requires
approximately ten minutes to administer. The FAB was designed with a focus on the
assessment of six core neurocognitive domains that are strongly related to the prefrontal
region of the brain. Moreover, the FAB seems to be able to profile the extent of any
possible executive function impairment and the regions implicated in it.

The analysis of the FAB's psychometric properties has shown that it can discriminate
between patients with the prefrontal disease and healthy participants with a sensitivity of
77 per cent and a specificity of 87 per cent, at a cut-off point of 11/12.

The FAB has been translated into Italian (70) and Spanish (71). It has age- and
education-related normative data published in the Italian version (70).

Depression Scales

Despite its higher prevalence among hospitalised elderly patients and its negative impact,
depression continues to remain underdetected and undertreated (72).

There are various screening instruments in everyday use in general hospitals – for
example the Geriatric Depression Scale (GDS) (73). These scales have usually been

developed in community and primary care settings, but there is some doubt regarding their reliability and validity in an acute hospital setting.

Dennis and colleagues (74) reviewed thirteen different depression screening instruments. The most commonly cited depression screening tool was the GDS (73), which has multiple versions with different numbers of items. Other instruments examined were the Brief Assessment Schedule Depression Cards (BASDEC) score (75, 76) and the Hospital Anxiety and Depression Scale (HADS) (77). In the National Institute for Health and Care Excellence (NICE) guidance on depression in adults with a chronic physical health problem, the authors suggested the use of different versions of Patient Health Questionnaire (PHQ). We will provide an overview of all four.

The Geriatric Depression Scale

The original GDS was developed using one hundred questions related to depression in older people, then selecting the thirty that correlated best with the total score. Each question has a yes/no answer, the scoring being dependent on the answer given.

When comparison was made with the Zung and Hamilton Depression Scales, it was found that the GDS had a higher internal consistency. Its test–retest reliability was 0.83. The GDS has 84 per cent sensitivity and 95 per cent specificity rates at a cut-off of 10, whereas at a cut-off of 14 the sensitivity rate was mildly reduced, namely to 80 per cent, but the specificity rate increased to 100 per cent (78).

In hospital-based patients, the GDS-30 best performance was achieved with a cut-off of either 10 or 11, at a sensitivity rate of 85 per cent and a specificity rate of 82 per cent.

A shorter 15-item version of the GDS was developed by Shiekh and Yesavage (79). At a cut-off point of 3/4, the sensitivity and specificity of the GDS-15 were 88 respectively per cent and 76 per cent.

In hospital settings, Cullum and colleagues (80) found that the optimum cut-off point for diagnosing depression in older people in the general hospital was 6/7, which gave a sensitivity of 74 per cent and a specificity of 81 per cent.

The GDS does not appear to be a valid tool for assessing depression in patients who live with dementia (81).

Brief Assessment Schedule Depression Cards

Adshead and colleagues (75) developed the BASDEC using the Brief Assessment Schedule (82). Because of the risk of question items being overheard on inpatient units, the patients themselves would choose from a deck of cards the answers to particular questions. The BASDEC has nineteen cards with enlarged black print on a white background. The cards are presented one at a time. 'True' responses gain one point, except for 'I have given up hope' and 'I seriously considered suicide' responses. Those receive a score of two points for each. The 'Don't know' answers are scored as half a point. The maximum score available is twenty-one points. The BASDEC has a sensitivity of 71 per cent and a specificity of 78 per cent at a cut-off of 6/7 (82). BASDEC takes approximately three minutes, ranging between two and eight minutes (83).

In general hospital settings, BASDEC had a sensitivity of 80 per cent and a specificity 86 per cent, at a cut-off point of 6/7 (75, 76).

Hospital Anxiety and Depression Scale

The HADS was originally developed by Zigmond and Snaith, (77) to determine the levels of anxiety and depression in hospital settings or in patients with physical illnesses. The HADS is a fourteen-item scale. Seven of the items relate to anxiety and seven relate to depression. The scale avoids enquiring about depression and anxiety symptoms such as easy fatiguability and sleep problems, which might be common in physical illness. The HADS takes two to five minutes to complete (84).

The HADS appears to have very good reliability, as indicated by Cronbach's alpha of 0.83 for HADS-A and 0.82 for HADS-D. Its split half between the HADS-Anxiety (HADS-A) and HADS-Depression (HADS-D) is approximately 0.56. An optimal cut-off point of 8/9 for both HADS-A and HADS-D has sensitivity and specificity of approximately 80 per cent (85). Although not devised initially to assess depression or anxiety in older adults, the HADS seems to be valid among a community-dwelling population aged 65–80 years (86). In hospital settings, it seems that HADS-D continued to be a valid tool for measuring depressive symptoms in elderly patients, but the same is not true when it comes to anxiety symptoms as measured on the HADS-A subscale (87). In patients living with dementia, HADS may not be a good tool for measuring anxiety and depression symptoms (88).

Patient Health Questionnaire

The Patient Health Questionnaire (PHQ-9) is a self-administered nine-question instrument used in the primary care setting and designed to screen for the presence and severity of depression. The PHQ-9 may be used to diagnose depression according to DSM4 criteria and to assess its severity. The PHQ-9 takes less than three minutes to complete (89).

The two-item PHQ (PHQ-2) is an ultra-short screening instrument that uses the first two questions from the PHQ-9. Those two questions assess the presence of a depressed mood and a loss of interest or pleasure in routine activities. This ultra-short version of the PHQ has been shown to have good diagnostic sensitivity but poor specificity (90). NICE has advocated screening of those who suffer from chronic physical conditions (83). NICE suggested the use of two simple screening questions: the Whooley questions from PHQ-2. Those questions are: 'During the past month, have you often been bothered by feeling down, depressed or hopeless?' and 'During the last month, have you been bothered by having little interest or pleasure in doing things?' (90). In their review, Dennis and colleagues (74) found no evaluation of the PHQ-2 in older people in the acute general hospital setting. Moreover, the same NICE guidance indicated a lack of data on PHQ-9, PHQ-2, and Whooley questions in older adults in general hospital settings.

Assessment of Activities of Daily Living

The primary aim of using activities of daily living (ADL) scales with the elderly is to assess the degree of impairment secondary to cognitive decline. Activities of daily living can be categorised into two types: basic physical activities such as eating, toileting, washing, walking, and dressing (sometimes referred to as physical self-maintenance) and instrumental activities, which are more complex tasks that include shopping, using the telephone, cooking, housekeeping, self-medicating, and using transport.

There are three modes of obtaining information for measuring ADL:

1. self-reporting,
2. proxy response or informant-based response, and
3. performance measures.

Self-reporting measures are problematic in patients with dementia because of concerns over whether such patients can respond competently.

For the proposes of this section, we will only discuss the most commonly used informant-based scales, that assess both basic and instrumental ADL.

The Bayer Activities of Daily Living Scale

The Bayer-ADL Scale (Bayer-ADLS) has a total of twenty-five questions. The two introductory questions evaluate everyday activities, questions 3–20 assess direct problems concerning specific tasks of everyday living, and the final five items relate to cognitive functions. The scoring is done on a ten-point scale by asking the caregiver to draw a line through one of the appropriate circles marked '110'. The administration of this test takes approximately twenty minutes (83).

The Bristol Activities of Daily Living Scale

The Bristol-ADL Scale (Bristol-ADLS) was designed specifically for use with patients with dementia and consists of twenty daily living abilities. Each item is scored from 0 (totally independent) to 3 (totally dependent). The total score is calculated by summing the scores of all questions. The Bristol-ADLS has a minimum possible score of 0 (indicating total independence) and a maximum score of 60 (indicating total dependence) (91). The administration of this test takes approximately fifteen minutes (83). The Bristol-ADLS has good test–retest reliability as measured by Cohen's kappa, and it correlates well with the MMSE (91).

The Cleveland Scale for Activities of Daily Living

The Cleveland Scale for Activities of Daily Living (CSADL) was designed specifically to reflect changes in the nature and extent of the broad spectrum of functional difficulties seen in individuals with dementia. The scale focuses on aspects of behaviour that are affected by cognitive and physical impairments (92). The scale consists of forty-eight main items, broken down into sixteen domains that cover most of required daily activities. The CSADL takes approximately twenty-five minutes to administer (83).

The Dependence Scale

The Dependence Scale (DS) was developed by Stern and colleagues (93) to assess the amount of assistance needed by patients with Alzheimer's disease and the impact on patients and their caregivers. The DS can be used to assess the degree of functional impairment from mild to the most advanced stages of the disease (94).

The DS consists of thirteen items that represent a range of severity from mild (e.g. 'Does the patient need frequent help finding misplaced objects?') to moderate (e.g. 'Does the patient need to be watched when awake?') to severe (e.g. 'Does the patient have to be fed?') levels of dependency. The dependence level is calculated using a separate scale, which converts the scores of the thirteen items into a score ranging from 0 to 5, where higher scores indicate greater dependency. The application of the scale takes five minutes (83).

The Disability Assessment for Dementia

The Disability Assessment for Dementia (DAD) scale was developed and validated by Gélinas and colleagues (95), as a measure of functional ability in community-dwelling individuals with dementia. It is rated by a trained observer and takes twenty minutes to be administered. The DAD is a functional scale specifically developed for persons with Alzheimer's disease. It has forty items, which cover six different domains with a high degree of internal consistency and excellent inter-rater and test–retest reliability. (96).

Assessment of the Behavioural and Psychological Symptoms of Dementia

Behavioural and psychological symptoms of dementia (BPSD), also known as neuropsychiatric symptoms, are a heterogeneous group of non-cognitive and behavioural symptoms that occur in patients with dementia. They are highly correlated with the degree of functional and cognitive impairment and caregiver stress (97). A comprehensive review of BPSD can be found in Chapter 10.

We will discuss the three most commonly cited BPSD assessments (98).

The Neuropsychiatric Inventory

Cummings and colleagues originally developed and validated the Neuropsychiatric Inventory (NPI) in order to assess psychopathology in patients with dementia in inpatient settings (99). The NPI is based on a structured interview with a health worker or caregiver who has direct knowledge of the person's behaviour in the recent past. There is a nursing home version, the NPI-NH, and a shortened version, the NPI-Q.

The NPI assesses twelve different behavioural domains. The presence of challenging behaviours in each domain is assessed by asking the caregiver a screening question followed by a series of yes/no questions. The caregiver is then asked to rate the frequency of occurrence of that domain of behaviours. An NPI total score is obtained by summing all the individual domain total scores (144 points maximum). A measure of the level of caregiver distress is also given, but is not included in the NPI-Carer version (NPI-C) total score. The NPI has shown good content validity, concurrent validity, inter-rater reliability (93.6 per cent to 100 per cent for different behaviours) and three-week test–retest reliability (correlation = 0.79 for frequency and 0.86 for severity ratings) (99, 100). Currently the NPI is regarded as the gold standard in the measurement of BPSD and is widely used in clinical trials, community investigations, and large-scale population studies (98).

Behavioural Pathology in Alzheimer's Disease Rating Scale

The Behavioural Pathology in Alzheimer's Disease Rating Scale (BEHAVE-AD) is a clinician-rated scale developed to measure psychopathology in patients with Alzheimer's disease over the previous two weeks on the basis of an informant interview (101). It comprises twenty-five symptoms grouped into seven categories: paranoid and delusional ideation, hallucinations, activity disturbance, aggressiveness, diurnal rhythm disturbances, affective disturbances, and anxieties and phobias.

The scale has been validated in community-dwelling individuals with dementia and in nursing home residents with dementia (102, 103). It has also been validated for administration by telephone (104).

The BEHAVE-AD may not adequately measure apathy, disinhibition, and emotional inappropriateness, which are seen more in frontotemporal dementia (105).

The Consortium to Establish a Registry for Alzheimer's Disease Behaviour-Rating Scale for Dementia

The Consortium to Establish a Registry for Alzheimer's Disease Behaviour-Rating Scale for Dementia (CERAD-BRSD) is a standardized instrument to measure BPSD in people with dementia or cognitive impairment (106). It has forty-six items grouped into the following six domains: depressive features, inertia, psychotic features, vegetative features, irritability/aggression, and behavioural dysregulation.

The CERAD-BRSD was developed for use in both clinical and research settings (107, 108) and it measures comorbidity psychiatric comorbidities in individuals with Alzheimer's disease (109–111). The CERAD-BRSD has good test–retest reliability. Over one month it has correlation coefficients between 0.7 and 0.89 for patients with Alzheimer's disease (106).

Conclusion

In conclusion, there are a plethora of validated instruments for measuring how the elderly function in the following domains: cognition; depression; ADLs; and BPSD.

Each of these instruments has its pros and cons. If you want to be able to make a decision as to which instrument to use, we advise you to check the instrument's psychometric properties. We recommend following the American Psychological Association's guidance on psychological testing of the elderly for practical guide to delivering assessment instruments.

References

1. Fitzpatrick, R., Davey, C., Buxton, M.J., and Jones, D.R. Evaluating patient-based outcome measures for use in clinical trials: A review. *Health Technol Assess (Rockv)* 1998, 2(14): i–iv, 1–74. https://doi.org/10.3310/hta2140.

2. Munro, L., and Rodwell, J. Validation of an Australian sign language instrument of outcome measurement for adults in mental health settings. *Aust N Z J Psychiatry* 2009, 43(4): 332–9. https://doi.org/10.1080/00048670902721111.

3. Erickson, P., Taeuber, R.C., and Scott, J. Operational aspects of Quality-of-Life Assessment. Choosing the right instrument. *Pharmacoeconomics* 1995, 7 (1): 39–48. https://doi.org/10.2165/00019053-199507010-00005.

4. Testa, M.A., and Simonson, D.C. Assessment of quality-of-life outcomes. *N Engl J Med* 1996, 334(13): 835–40. https://doi.org/10.1056/nejm199603283341306.

5. Jaeschke, R., Singer, J., and Guyatt, G.H. Measurement of health status. Ascertaining the minimal clinically important difference. *Control Clin Trials* 1989, 10(4): 407–15. https://doi.org/10.1016/0197-2456(89)90005-6.

6. Streiner, D.L., Norman, G.R., and Cairney, J. *Health Measurement Scales:*

A Practical Guide to Their Development and Use (5th ed.). Oxford: Oxford University Press. 2015.

7. Fleiss, J.L. Measuring nominal scale agreement among many raters. Psychol Bull 1971, 76(5): 378–82. https://doi.org/10.1037/h0031619.

8. Regier, D.A., Narrow, W.E., Clarke, D.E., Kraemer, H.C., Kuramoto, S.J., Kuhl, E.A. et al. DSM-5 field trials in the United States and Canada, Part II: Test–retest reliability of selected categorical diagnoses. Am J Psychiatry 2013, 170(1): 59–70. https://doi.org/10.1176/appi.ajp.2012.12070999.

9. Calamia, M., Markon, K., and Tranel, D. Scoring higher the second time around: Meta-analyses of practice effects in neuropsychological assessment. Clin Neuropsychol 2012, 26(4): 543–70. https://doi.org/10.1080/13854046.2012.680913.

10. Gessmann H.-W., and Sheronov, E.A. Psychological test validity. J Mod Foreign Psychol 2013, 2(4): 20–31.

11. Cronbach, L.J., and meehl, P.E. Construct validity in psychological tests. Psychol Bull 1955, 52(4): 281–302. https://doi.org/10.1037/h0040957.

12. Kazis, L.E., Anderson, J.J., and Meenan, R.F. Effect sizes for interpreting changes in health status. Med Care 1989, 27(3 Suppl.): S178–89. https://doi.org/10.1097/00005650-198903001-00015.

13. Šimundić, A.-M. Measures of diagnostic accuracy: Basic definitions. EJIFCC 2009, 19(4): 203–11.

14. American Psychological Association. Guidelines for psychological practice with older adults. Am Psychol 2014, 69(1): 34–65. https://doi.org/10.1037/a0035063.

15. Tsoi, K.K.F., Chan, J.Y.C., Hirai, H.W., Wong, S.Y.S., and Kwok, T.C.Y. Cognitive tests to detect dementia: A systematic review and meta-analysis. JAMA Intern Med 2015, 175(9): 1450–8. https://doi.org/10.1001/jamainternmed.2015.2152.

16. Roebuck-Spencer, T.M., Glen, T., Puente, A.E., Denney, R.L., Ruff, R.M., Hostetter,

G. et al. Cognitive screening tests versus comprehensive neuropsychological test batteries: A national academy of neuropsychology education paper†. Arch Clin Neuropsychol 2017, 32(4): 491–8. https://doi.org/10.1093/arclin/acx021.

17. Carnero-Pardo, C. Should the Mini-Mental State Examination be retired? Neurol [English Ed 2014, 29(8): 473–81. https://doi.org/10.1016/j.nrl.2013.07.003.

18. Hsieh, S., Schubert, S., Hoon, C., Mioshi, E., and Hodges, J.R. Validation of the Addenbrooke's Cognitive Examination III in frontotemporal dementia and Alzheimer's disease. Dement Geriatr Cogn Disord 2013, 36(3–4): 242–50. https://doi.org/10.1159/000351671.

19. Hsieh, S., McGrory, S., Leslie, F., Dawson, K., Ahmed, S., Butler, C.R. et al. The Mini-Addenbrooke's Cognitive Examination: A new assessment tool for dementia. Dement Geriatr Cogn Disord 2015, 39(1–2): 1–11. https://doi.org/10.1159/000366040.

20. Nasreddine, Z.S., Phillips, N.A., Bédirian, V., Charbonneau, S., Whitehead, V., Collin, I. et al. The Montreal Cognitive Assessment, MoCA: A brief screening tool for mild cognitive impairment. J Am Geriatr Soc 2005, 53(4): 695–9. https://doi.org/10.1111/j.1532-5415.2005.53221.x.

21. Rowland, J.T., Basic, D., Storey, J.E., and Conforti, D.A. The Rowland Universal Dementia Assessment Scale (RUDAS) and the Folstein MMSE in a multicultural cohort of elderly persons. Int psychogeriatrics 2006, 18(1): 111–20. https://doi.org/10.1017/s1041610205003133.

22. Dubois, B., Slachevsky, A., Litvan, I., and Pillon, B. The FAB: A frontal assessment battery at bedside. Neurology 2000, 55 (11): 1621–6. https://doi.org/10.1212/wnl.55.11.1621.

23. Nilsson, F.M. Mini mental state examination (MMSE): Probably one of the most cited papers in health science. Acta Psychiatr Scand 2007, 116 (2): 156–7. https://doi.org/10.1111/j.1600-0447.2007.01037.x.

24. Folstein, M.F., Folstein, S.E., and McHugh, P.R. 'Mini-mental state': A practical method for grading the cognitive state of patients for the clinician. *J Psychiatr Res* 1975, 12(3): 189–98. https://doi.org/10.1016/0022-3956(75)90026-6.

25. Tombaugh, T.N., McIntyre, N.J. The Mini-Mental State Examination: A comprehensive review. *J Am Geriatr Soc* 1992, 40(9): 922–35. https://doi.org/10.1111/j.1532-5415.1992.tb01992.x.

26. Velayudhan, L., Ryu, S.H., Raczek, M., Philpot, M., Lindesay, J., Critchfield, M. et al. Review of brief cognitive tests for patients with suspected dementia. *Int Psychogeriatrics* 2014, 26(8): 1247–62. https://doi.org/10.1017/s1041610214000416.

27. Mathuranath, P.S., Nestor, P.J., Berrios, G.E., Rakowicz, W., and Hodges, J.R. A brief cognitive test battery to differentiate Alzheimer's disease and frontotemporal dementia. *Neurology* 2000, 55(11): 1613–20. https://doi.org/10.1212/01.wnl.0000434309.85312.19.

28. Qassem, T., Khater, M.S., Emara, T., Rasheedy, D., Tawfik, H.M., Mohammedin, A.S. et al. Normative data for healthy adult performance on the Egyptian–Arabic Addenbrooke's Cognitive Examination III. *Middle East Curr Psychiatry* 2015, 22(1): 27–36. http://dx.doi.org/10.1097/01.XME.0000457267.05731.0f.

29. Qassem, T., Khater, M.S., Emara, T., Rasheedy, D., Tawfik, H.M., Mohammedin, A.S. et al. Validation of the Egyptian–Arabic version of the Addenbrooke's Cognitive Examination III (ACE-III) in diagnosing dementia. *Dement Geriatr Cogn Disord* 2020, 49(2): 179–84. https://doi.org/10.1159/000507758.

30. Wang, B.R., Ou, Z., Gu, X.H., Wei, C.S., Xu, J., and Shi, J.Q. Validation of the Chinese version of Addenbrooke's Cognitive Examination III for diagnosing dementia. *Int J Geriatr Psychiatry* 2017, 32(12):e173–9. https://doi.org/10.1002/gps.4680.

31. Mekala, S., Paplikar, A., Mioshi, E., Kaul, S., Divyaraj, G., Coughlan, G. et al. Dementia diagnosis in seven languages: The Addenbrooke's Cognitive Examination-III in India. *Arch Clin Neuropsychol* 2020, 35(5): 528–38. https://doi.org/10.1093/arclin/acaa013.

32. Pigliautile, M., Chiesi, F., Stablum, F., Rossetti, S., Primi, C., Chiloiro, D. et al. Italian version and normative data of Addenbrooke's Cognitive Examination III. *Int Psychogeriatrics* 2019, 31(2): 241–9. https://doi.org/10.1017/s104161021800073x.

33. Takenoshita, S., Terada, S., Yoshida, H., Yamaguchi, M., Yabe, M., Imai, N. et al. Validation of Addenbrooke's cognitive examination III for detecting mild cognitive impairment and dementia in Japan. *BMC Geriatr* 2019, 19(1): 1–8. https://doi.org/10.1186/s12877-019-1120-4.

34. Peixoto, B., Machado, M., Rocha, P., Macedo, C., Machado, A., Baeta, É. et al. Validation of the Portuguese version of Addenbrooke's Cognitive Examination III in mild cognitive impairment and dementia. *Adv Clin Exp Med* 2018, 27(6): 781–6. https://doi.org/10.17219/acem/68975.

35. Matías-Guiu, J.A., Fernández-Bobadilla, R., Fernández-Oliveira, A., Valles-Salgado, M., Rognoni, T., Cortés-Martínez, A. et al. Normative data for the Spanish version of the Addenbrooke's Cognitive Examination III. *Dement Geriatr Cogn Disord* 2016, 41(5–6): 243–50. https://doi.org/10.1159/000445799.

36. Charernboon, T., Jaisin, K., and Lerthattasilp, T. The Thai version of the Addenbrooke's Cognitive Examination III. *Psychiatry Investig* 2016, 13(5): 571–3. https://dx.doi.org/10.4306%2Fpi.2016.13.5.571.

37. Waheed, W., Mirza, N., Waheed, M.W., Malik, A., and Panagioti, M. Developing and implementing guidelines on culturally adapting the Addenbrooke's cognitive examination version III (ACE-III): A qualitative illustration. *BMC*

Psychiatry 2020, 20(1): 1–13. https://doi
.org/10.1186/s12888-020-02893-6.

38. Beishon, L.C., Batterham, A.P., Quinn, T.J., Nelson, C.P., Panerai, R.B., Robinson, T. et al. Addenbrooke's Cognitive Examination III (ACE-III) and mini-ACE for the detection of dementia and mild cognitive impairment. *Cochrane Database Syst Rev* 2019, 12(12): CD013282. https://doi.org/10.1002/14651858.cd013282.pub2.

39. Smith, T., Gildeh, N., and Holmes, C. The Montreal Cognitive Assessment: Validity and utility in a memory clinic setting. *Can J psychiatry* 2007, 52(5): 329–32. https://doi.org/10.1177/070674370705200508.

40. Larner, A.J. Screening utility of the Montreal Cognitive Assessment (MoCA): In place of – or as well as – the MMSE? *Int Psychogeriatrics* 2012, 24(3): 391–6. https://doi.org/10.1017/s1041610211001839.

41. Carson, N., Leach, L., and Murphy, K.J. A re-examination of Montreal Cognitive Assessment (MoCA) cutoff scores. *Int J Geriatr Psychiatry* 2018, 33(2): 379–88. https://doi.org/10.1002/gps.4756.

42. Xu, Y., Mirelman, A., Saunders-Pullman, R., Mejia-Santana, H., Caccappolo, E., Raymond, D. et al. Differences in performance on English and Hebrew versions of the MoCA in Parkinson's patients. *Clin Park Relat Disord* 2020, 3: 100042. https://doi.org/10.1016/j.prdoa.2020.10.004.

43. Nasreddine, Z.S., Rossetti, H., Phillips, N., Chertkow, H., Lacritz, L., Cullum, M. et al. Normative data for the Montreal Cognitive Assessment (MoCA) in a population-based sampleAuthor Response. *Neurology* 2012, 78(10): 765–6. https://doi.org/10.1212/01.wnl.0000413072.54070.a3.

44. Hayek, M., Tarabey, L., Abou-Mrad, T., Fadel, P., and Abou-Mrad, F. Normative Data for the Montreal Cognitive Assessment in a Lebanese Older Adult Population. *J Clin Neurosci* 2020, 74: 81–6. https://doi.org/10.1016/j.jocn.2020.01.050.

45. Kopecek, M., Stepankova, H., Lukavsky, J., Ripova, D., Nikolai, T., and Bezdicek, O. Montreal cognitive assessment (MoCA): Normative data for old and very old Czech adults. *Appl Neuropsychol Adult* 2017, 24(1): 23–9. https://doi.org/10.1080/23279095.2015.1065261.

46. Larouche, E., Tremblay, M.P., Potvin, O., Laforest, S., Bergeron, D., Laforce, R. et al. Normative data for the Montreal Cognitive Assessment in middle-aged and elderly French-Quebec people. *Arch Clin Neuropsychol* 2016, 31(7): 819–26. https://doi.org/10.1093/arclin/acw076.

47. Thomann, A.E., Goettel, N., Monsch, R.J., Berres, M., Jahn, T., Steiner, L.A. et al. The Montreal Cognitive Assessment: Normative data from a German-speaking cohort and comparison with international normative samples. *J Alzheimer's Dis* 2018, 64(2): 643–55. https://doi.org/10.3233/jad-180080.

48. Konstantopoulos, K., Vogazianos, P., and Doskas, T. Normative Data of the Montreal Cognitive Assessment in the GreekpPopulation and Parkinsonian dementia. *Arch Clin Neuropsychol* 2016, 31(3): 246–53. https://doi.org/10.1093/arclin/acw002.

49. Conti, S., Bonazzi, S., Laiacona, M., Masina, M., and Coralli, M.V. Montreal Cognitive Assessment (MoCA)-Italian version: Regression based norms and equivalent scores. *Neurol Sci* 2015, 36(2): 209–14. https://doi.org/10.1007/s10072-014-1921-3.

50. Santangelo, G., Siciliano, M., Pedone, R., Vitale, C., Falco, F., Bisogno, R. et al. Normative data for the Montreal Cognitive Assessment in an Italian population sample. *Neurol Sci* 2015, 36 (4): 585–91. https://doi.org/10.1007/s10072-014-1995-y.

51. Narazaki, K., Nofuji, Y., Honda, T., Matsuo, E., Yonemoto, K., Kumagai, S. Normative data for the Montreal Cognitive Assessment in a Japanese community-dwelling older population. *Neuroepidemiology* 2013, 40(1): 23–9. https://doi.org/10.1159/000339753.

52. Freitas, S., Simões, M.R., Alves, L., and Santana, I. Montreal Cognitive Assessment (MoCA): Normative study for the Portuguese population. *J Clin Exp Neuropsychol* 2011, 33(9): 989–96. https://doi.org/10.1080/13803395.2011.589374.

53. Borland, E., Nägga, K., Nilsson, P.M., Minthon, L., Nilsson, E.D., and Palmqvist, S. The Montreal Cognitive Assessment: Normative data from a large Swedish population-based cohort. *J Alzheimer's Dis* 2017, 59(3): 893–901. https://dx.doi.org/10.3233%2FJAD-170203.

54. Milani, S.A., Marsiske, M., Cottler, L.B., Chen, X., and Striley, C.W. Optimal cutoffs for the Montreal Cognitive Assessment vary by race and ethnicity. *Alzheimer's Dement (Amsterdam, Netherlands)* 2018, 10: 773–81. https://doi.org/10.1016/j.dadm.2018.09.003.

55. Storey, J.E., Rowland, J.T.J., Conforti, D.A., Dickson, H.G. The Rowland Universal Dementia Assessment Scale (RUDAS): A multicultural cognitive assessment scale. *Int Psychogeriatrics* 2004, 16(1): 13–31. https://doi.org/10.1017/s1041610204000043.

56. Goudsmit, M., Van Campen, J., Schilt, T., Hinnen, C., Franzen, S., and Schmand, B. One size does not fit all: Comparative diagnostic accuracy of the Rowland Universal Dementia Assessment Scale and the mini mental state examination in a memory clinic population with very low education. *Dement Geriatr Cogn Dis Extra* 2018, 8(2): 290–305. https://doi.org/10.1159/000490174.

57. Basic, D., Rowland, J.T., Conforti, D.A., Vrantsidis, F., Hill, K., LoGiudice, D. et al. The validity of the Rowland Universal Dementia Assessment Scale (RUDAS) in a multicultural cohort of community-dwelling older persons with early dementia. *Alzheimer Dis Assoc Disord* 2009, 23(2): 124–9. 10.1097/wad.0b013e31818ecc98.

58. Chaaya, M., Phung, T.K.T., El Asmar, K., Atweh, S., Ghusn, H., Khoury, R.M. et al. Validation of the Arabic Rowland Universal Dementia Assessment Scale (A-RUDAS) in elderly with mild and moderate dementia. *Aging Ment Health* 2016, 20(8): 880–7. https://doi.org/10.1080/13607863.2015.1043620.

59. Chen, C.W., Chu, H., Tsai, C.F., Yang, H.L., Tsai, J.C., Chung, M.H. et al. The reliability, validity, sensitivity, specificity and predictive values of the Chinese version of the Rowland Universal Dementia Assessment Scale. *J Clin Nurs* 2015, 24(21–22): 3118–28. https://doi.org/10.1111/jocn.12941

60. Nielsen, T.R., Andersen, B.B., Gottrup, H., Lützhøft, J.H., Høgh, P., and Waldemar, G. Validation of the Rowland Universal Dementia Assessment Scale for multicultural screening in Danish memory clinics. *Dement Geriatr Cogn Disord* 2013, 36(5–6): 354–62. https://doi.org/10.1159/000354375.

61. Iype, T., Ajitha, B.K., Antony, P., Ajeeth, N.B., Job, S., and Shaji, K.S. Usefulness of the Rowland Universal Dementia Assessment scale in South India. *J Neurol Neurosurg Psychiatry* 2006, 77(4): 513–4. https://doi.org/10.1136/jnnp.2005.069005.

62. Nepal, G.M., Shrestha, A., and Acharya, R. Translation and cross-cultural adaptation of the Nepali version of the Rowland universal dementia assessment scale (RUDAS). *J Patient-Reported Outcomes* 2019, 3(1): 1–7. https://doi.org/10.1186/s41687-019-0132-3.

63. De Araujo, N.B., Nielsen, T.R., Engedal, K., Barca, M.L., Coutinho, E.S., and Laks, J. Diagnosing dementia in lower educated older persons: Validation of a Brazilian Portuguese version of the Rowland Universal Dementia Assessment Scale (RUDAS). *Brazilian J Psychiatry* 2018, 40(3): 264–9. https://doi.org/10.1590/1516-4446-2017-2284.

64. Custodio, N., Montesinos, R., Lira, D., Herrera-Perez, E., and Chavez, K., Reynoso-Guzman, W. et al. Validation of the RUDAS for the identification of dementia in illiterate and low-educated older adults in Lima, Peru. *Front Neurol* 2020, 11: 374. https://dx.doi.org/10.3389%2Ffneur.2020.00374.

65. Ayan, G., Afacan, C., Poyraz, B.C., Bilgic, O., Avci, S., Yavuzer, H. et al. Reliability and validity of Rowland Universal Dementia Assessment Scale in Turkish population. *Am J Alzheimers Dis Other Demen* 2019, 34(1): 34–40. https://doi.org/10.1177/1533317518802449.

66. Nielsen, T.R., Segers, K., Vanderaspoilden, V., Bekkhus-Wetterberg, P., Bjørkløf, G.H., Beinhoff, U. et al. Validation of the Rowland Universal Dementia Assessment Scale (RUDAS) in a multicultural sample across five Western European countries: Diagnostic accuracy and normative data. *Int Psychogeriatrics* 2019, 31(2): 287–96. https://doi.org/10.1017/s1041610218000832.

67. Borson, S., Scanlan, J., Brush, M., Vitaliano, P., and Dokmak, A. The Mini-Cog: A cognitive 'vital signs' measure for dementia screening in multi-lingual elderly. *Int J Geriatr Psychiatry* 2000, 15(11): 1021–7. https://doi.org/10.1002/1099-1166(200011)15:11%3C1021::AID-GPS234%3E3.0.CO;2-6.

68. Borson, S., Scanlan, J.M., Chen, P., and Ganguli, M. The Mini-Cog as a screen for dementia: Validation in a population-based sample. *J Am Geriatr Soc* 2003, 51(10): 1451–4. https://doi.org/10.1046/j.1532-5415.2003.51465.x.

69. Scanlan, J., Borson, S. The Mini-Cog: Receiver operating characteristics with expert and naïve raters. *Int J Geriatr Psychiatry* 2001, 16(2): 216–22. https://doi.org/10.1002/1099-1166(200102)16:2%3C216::AID-GPS316%3E3.0.CO;2-B.

70. Appollonio, I., Leone, M., Isella, V., Piamarta, F., Consoli, T., Villa, M.L. et al. The Frontal Assessment Battery (FAB): Normative values in an Italian population sample. *Neurol Sci* 2005, 26(2): 108–16. https://doi.org/10.1007/s10072-005-0443-4.

71. Hurtado-Pomares, M., Valera-Gran, D., Sánchez-Pérez, A., Peral-Gómez, P., Navarrete-Muñoz, E.M., and Terol-Cantero, M.C. Adaptation of the Spanish version of the Frontal Assessment Battery for detection of executive dysfunction.

Med Clin (Barc) 2021, 156(5): 229–32. https://doi.org/10.1016/j.medcli.2020.04.028.

72. Rentsch, D., Dumont, P., Borgacci, S., Carballeira, Y., DeTonnac, N., Archinard, M. et al. Prevalence and treatment of depression in a hospital department of internal medicine. *Gen Hosp Psychiatry* 2007, 29(1): 25–31. https://doi.org/10.1016/j.genhosppsych.2006.08.008.

73. Yesavage, J.A., Brink, T.L., Rose, T.L., Lum, O., Huang, V., Adey, M. et al. Development and validation of a geriatric depression screening scale: A preliminary report. *J Psychiatr Res* 1983, 17(1): 37–49. https://doi.org/10.1016/0022-3956(82)90033-4.

74. Dennis, M., Kadri, A., and Coffey, J. Depression in older people in the general hospital: A systematic review of screening instruments. *Age and Ageing* 2012, 41(2): 148–54. https://doi.org/10.1093/ageing/afr169.

75. Adshead, F., Cody, D.D., and Pitt, B. BASDEC: A novel screening instrument for depression in elderly medical inpatients. *BMJ* 1992, 305(6850): 397. https://doi.org/10.1136/bmj.305.6850.397.

76. Loke, B., Nicklason, F., and Burvill, P. Screening for depression: Clinical validation of geriatricians' diagnosis, the Brief Assessment Schedule Depression Cards and the 5-item version of the Symptom Check List among non-demented geriatric inpatients. *Int J Geriatr Psychiatry* 1996, 11(5): 461–5. https://doi.org/10.1002/(SICI)1099-1166(199605)11:5%3C461::AID-GPS336%3E3.0.CO;2-F.

77. Zigmond, A.S., and Snaith, R.P. The hospital anxiety and depression scale. *Acta Psychiatr Scand* 1983, 67(6): 361–70. https://doi.org/10.1111/j.1600-0447.1983.tb09716.x.

78. Brink, T.L., Yesavage, J.A., Lum, O., Heersema, P.H., Adey, M., and Rose, T.L. Screening tests for geriatric depression. *Clin Gerontol* 1982, 1(1): 37–43. https://doi.org/10.1300/J018v01n01_06.

79. Sheikh, J.I., Yesavage, J.A. Geriatric Depression Scale (GDS): Recent evidence and development of a shorter version. *Clin Gerontol* 1986, 5(1–2): 165–73. https://doi.org/10.1300/J018v05n01_09.

80. Cullum, S., Tucker, S., Todd, C., and Brayne, C. Screening for depression in older medical inpatients. *Int J Geriatr Psychiatry* 2006, 21(5): 469–76. https://doi.org/10.1002/gps.1497.

81. Burke, W.J., Houston, M.J., Boust, S.J., and Roccaforte, W.H. Use of the Geriatric Depression Scale in dementia of the Alzheimer type. *J Am Geriatr Soc* 1989, 37 (9): 856–60. https://doi.org/10.1111/j.1532-5415.1989.tb02266.x.

82. Macdonald, A.J.D., Mann, A.H., Jenkins, R., Richard, L., Godlove, C., and Rodwell, G. An attempt to determine the impact of four types of care upon the elderly in London by the study of matched groups. *Psychol Med* 1982, 12(1): 193–200. https://doi.org/10.1017/s0033291700043452.

83. Burns, A., Lawlor, B., and Craig, S. *Assessment Scales in Old Age Psychiatry* (2nd ed.). London: CRC Press, 2004.

84. Snaith, R.P. The Hospital Anxiety and Depression Scale. *Health Qual Life Outcomes* 2003, 1: 29. https://doi.org/10.1186/1477-7525-1-29.

85. Bjelland, I., Dahl, A.A., Haug, T.T., and Neckelmann, D. The validity of the Hospital Anxiety and Depression Scale: An updated literature review. *J Psychosom Res* 2002, 52(2): 69–77. https://doi.org/10.1016/S0022-3999(01)00296-3.

86. Djukanovic, I., Carlsson, J., and Årestedt, K. Is the Hospital Anxiety and Depression Scale (HADS) a valid measure in a general population 65–80 years old? A psychometric evaluation study. *Health Qual Life Outcomes* 2017, 15(1): 193. https://doi.org/10.1186/s12955-017-0759-9.

87. Kenn, C., Wood, H., Kucyj, M., Wattis, J., and Cunane, J. Validation of the hospital anxiety and depression rating scale (HADS) in an elderly psychiatric population. *Int J Geriatr Psychiatry* 1987,

2(3): 189–93. https://doi.org/10.1002/gps.930020309.

88. Stott, J., Spector, A., Orrell, M., Scior, K., Sweeney, J., and Charlesworth, G. Limited validity of the Hospital Anxiety and Depression Scale (HADS) in dementia: Evidence from a confirmatory factor analysis. *Int J Geriatr Psychiatry* 2017, 32 (7): 805–13. https://doi.org/10.1002/gps.4530.

89. Kroenke, K., Spitzer, R.L., and Williams, J.B.W. The PHQ-9: Validity of a brief depression severity measure. *J Gen Intern Med* 2001, 16(9): 606–13. https://doi.org/10.1046/j.1525-1497.2001.016009606.x.

90. Whooley, M.A., Avins, A.L., Miranda, J., and Browner, W.S. Case-finding instruments for depression: Two questions are as good as many. *J Gen Intern Med* 1997, 12(7): 439–45. https://doi.org/10.1046/j.1525-1497.1997.00076.x.

91. Bucks, R.S., Ashworth, D.L., Wilcock, G.K., and Siegfried, K. Assessment of activities of daily living in dementia: Development of the Bristol Activities of Daily Living Scale. *Age and Ageing* 1996, 25(2): 113–20. https://doi.org/10.1093/ageing/25.2.113.

92. Patterson, M.B., Mack, J.L., Neundorfer, M.M., Martin, R.J., Smyth, K.A., and Whitehouse, P.J. Assessment of functional ability in Alzheimer disease: A review and a preliminary report on the Cleveland Scale for Activities of Daily Living. *Alzheimer Dis Assoc Disord* 1992, 6(3): 145–63. https://doi.org/10.1097/00002093-199206030-00003.

93. Stern, Y., Albert, S.M., Sano, M., Richards, M., Miller, L., Folstein, M. et al. Assessing patient dependence in Alzheimer's disease. *Journals Gerontol* 1994, 49(5): M216–M222. https://doi.org/10.1093/geronj/49.5.M216.

94. Bavazzano, A., Magnolfi, S.U., Calvani, D., Valente, C., Boni, F., Baldini, A. et al. Functional evaluation of Alzheimer patients during clinical trials: A review. *Arch Gerontol Geriatr* 1998, 26(SUPPL.1):

27–32. https://doi.org/10.1016/S0167-4943(98)80005-8.

95. Gélinas, I., Gauthier, L., McIntyre, M., and Gauthier, S. Development of a functional measure for persons with Alzheimer's disease: the disability assessment for dementia. *Am J Occup Ther* 1999, 53(5): 471–81. https://doi.org/10.5014/ajot.53.5.471.

96. Desai, A.K., Grossberg, G.T., and Sheth, D.N. Activities of daily living in patients with dementia: Clinical relevance, methods of assessment and effects of treatment. *CNS Drugs* 2004, 18(13): 853–75. https://doi.org/10.2165/00023210-200418130-00003.

97. Kales, H.C., Gitlin, L.N., and Lyketsos, C.G. Assessment and management of behavioral and psychological symptoms of dementia. *BMJ* 2015, 350: h369. https://doi.org/10.1136/bmj.h369.

98. Jeon, Y.H., Sansoni, J., Low, L.F., Chenoweth, L., Zapart, S., and Marosszeky, N. Recommended measures for the assessment of behavioral disturbances associated with dementia. *Am J Geriatr Psychiatry* 2011, 19(5): 403–15. https://doi.org/10.1097/jgp.0b013e3181ef7a0d.

99. Cummings, J.L., Mega, M., Gray, K., Rosenberg-Thompson, S., Carusi, D.A., and Gornbein, J. The Neuropsychiatric Inventory: Comprehensive assessment of psychopathology in dementia. *Neurology* 1994, 44(12): 2308. https://doi.org/10.1212/WNL.44.12.2308.

100. Connor, D.J., Sabbagh, M.N., and Cummings, J.L. Comment on administration and scoring of the Neuropsychiatric Inventory (NPI) in clinical trials. *Alzheimer's Dement* 2008, 4(6): 390–4. https://dx.doi.org/10.1016%2Fj.jalz.2008.09.002

101. Reisberg, B., Borenstein, J., Salob, S.P., Ferris, S.H., and Franssen, E.H., Georgotas, A. Behavioral symptoms in Alzheimer's disease: Phenomenology and treatment. *J Clin Psychiatry* 1987, 48(5, Suppl): 9–15.

102. Brodaty, H., Draper, B., Saab, D., Low, L.F., Richards, V., Paton, H. et al. Psychosis, depression and behavioural disturbances in Sydney nursing home residents: Prevalence and predictors. *Int J Geriatr Psychiatry* 2001, 16(5): 504–12. https://doi.org/10.1002/gps.382.

103. De Deyn, P.P., Katz, I.R., Brodaty, H., Lyons, B., Greenspan, A., and Burns, A. Management of agitation, aggression, and psychosis associated with dementia: a pooled analysis including three randomized, placebo-controlled double-blind trials in nursing home residents treated with risperidone. *Clin Neurol Neurosurg* 2005, 107(6): 497–508. https://doi.org/10.1016/j.clineuro.2005.03.013.

104. Monteiro, I.M., Boksay, I., Auer, S.R., Torossian, C., Sinaiko, E., and Reisberg, B. Reliability of routine clinical instruments for the assessment of Alzheimer's disease administered by telephone. *J Geriatr Psychiatry Neurol* [Internet] 1998, 11(1): 18–24. https://doi.org/10.1177/089198879801100105.

105. Chiu, M.J., Chen, T.F., Yip, P.K., Hua, M.S., and Tang, L.Y. Behavioral and psychologic symptoms in different types of dementia. *J Formos Med Assoc* 2006, 105(7): 556–62. https://doi.org/10.1016/s0929-6646(09)60150-9.

106. Patterson, M.B., Mack, J.L., Mackell, J.A., Thomas, R., Tariot, P., and Weiner, M. et al. A longitudinal study of behavioral pathology across five levels of dementia severity in Alzheimer's disease. *Alzheimer Dis Assoc Disord* 1997, 11(Suppl2): 40–4. https://doi.org/10.1097/00002093-199700112-00006.

107. Teri, L., Logsdon, R.G., Peskind, E., Raskind, M., Weiner, M.F., Tractenberg, R.E. et al. Treatment of agitation in AD: A randomized, placebo-controlled clinical trial. *Neurology* 2000, 55(9): 1271–8. https://doi.org/10.1212/wnl.55.9.1271.

108. Higgins, M., Koch, K., Hynan, L.S., Carr, S., Byrnes, K., and Weiner, M.F. Impact of an activities-based adult dementia care program. *Neuropsychiatr Dis Treat* 2005, 1(2): 165–9. https://dx.doi.org/10.2147%2Fnedt.1.2.165.61050.

109. Tractenberg, R.E., Weiner, M.F., Patterson, M.B., Teri, L., and Thal, L.J. Comorbidity of psychopathological domains in community-dwelling persons with Alzheimer's disease. *J Geriatr Psychiatry Neurol* 2003, 16(2): 94–9. https://doi.org/10.1177/0891988703016002006.

110. Wilkosz, P.A., Miyahara, S., Lopez, O.L., DeKosky, S.T., and Sweet, R.A. Prediction of psychosis onset in Alzheimer disease: The role of cognitive impairment, depressive symptoms, and further evidence for psychosis subtypes. *Am*

J Geriatr Psychiatry 2006, 14(4): 352–60. https://doi.org/10.1097/01.jgp.0000192500.25940.1b.

111. Neundorfer, M.M., McClendon, M.J., Smyth, K.A., Stuckey, J.C., Strauss, M.E., and Patterson, M.B. A longitudinal study of the relationship between levels of depression among persons with Alzheimer's disease and levels of depression among their family caregivers. *J Gerontol B Psychol Sci Soc Sci* 2001, 56 (5): 301–13. https://doi.org/10.1093/geronb/56.5.p301.

Index

Numbers: **bold**=table, *italics*=figure.

Printed in the United States
by Baker & Taylor Publisher Services